Handbook of ICU Therapy
Second Edition

This new, expanded and thoroughly updated edition of *Handbook of ICU Therapy* builds on the success of the first edition and continues to provide concise information on a broad spectrum of issues relating to care of the critically ill patient. There are also several new, topical chapters. As with the first edition, it is equally applicable to anaesthetists, intensivists, operating department practitioners and anaesthetic/theatre/recovery nurses, and the heart of the book focuses on providing practical information in a readable and easily accessible format. All of the authors are directly involved in intensive care unit (ICU) practice and/or research and are familiar with the most recent developments in this fast-moving area of medicine.

Ian McConachie has been a consultant in anaesthesia and intensive care for over 15 years. Prior to this, he lectured extensively in anaesthesia and he is now a primary examiner for the Royal College of Anaesthetists.

Handbook of ICU Therapy

Second Edition

Edited by

Dr Ian McConachie
Consultant in Anaesthesia & Intensive Care
Blackpool Victoria Hospital

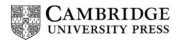

CAMBRIDGE UNIVERSITY PRESS
Cambridge, New York, Melbourne, Madrid, Cape Town, Singapore, São Paulo

CAMBRIDGE UNIVERSITY PRESS
The Edinburgh Building, Cambridge CB2 2RU, UK

Published in the United States of America by Cambridge University Press, New York

www.cambridge.org
Information on this title: www.cambridge.org/9780521

First published 1998
Second edition 2006

Printed in the United Kingdom at the University Press, Cambridge

A record for this publication is available from the British library

Library of congress in Publication data

ISBN-13 978-0-521-68247-3
ISBN-10 0-521-68247-9

Contents

List of contributors

Editor

Dr I. McConachie, FRCA
Consultant in Anaesthesia and Intensive Care, Blackpool Victoria Hospital

Contributors

Anaesthesia and Intensive Care
Dr R. Brits, FRCA
Dr C. Clarke, FRCA
Dr J. Cupitt, FRCA
Dr V. Godbole, FRCA
Dr C. Harle, FRCA
Dr D. Kelly, FRCA
Dr R. Markham, FRCA
Dr R. Morgan, FRCA
Dr T. Owen, FRCA
Dr N. Randall, FRCA
Dr N. Sharma, FRCA
Dr S. Vaughan, MRCP FRCA
Dr S. Wiggans, FRCA

Intensive Care and Surgery
Dr J. Naisbitt, MB ChB

Intensive Care and A + E
J. Costello, MRCPI

Cardiology
Dr R. Beynon, MRCP
Dr D. Hesketh Roberts, FRCP

Cardiothoracic Surgery
Mr J. Dunning, MRCS

Blackpool Victoria Hospital
Whinney Heys Road
Blackpool FY3 8NR

Special Contributions from

Dr R. Kishen, FRCA, Intensive Care Unit, Hope Hospital, Salford
Dr G. Brear, FRCP, Intensive Care Unit, Wythenshawe Hospital, Manchester
Dr J. Barker, FRCA, Intensive Care Unit, Wythenshawe Hospital, Manchester
Dr P. Nightingale, FRCP, FRCA, Intensive Care Unit, Wythenshawe Hospital,
    Manchester

Preface

This text:

- Is aimed primarily at trainees working in intensive care. Hopefully will appeal to multidisciplinary trainees being exposed to ICU for the first time under joint college guidelines for ICU training. May also be of interest to ICU nurses looking for information on modern medical (in the strictest sense) approaches to ICU therapy. A basic knowledge of physiology and pharmacology is assumed as well as either a medical background or advanced nursing experience in intensive care.
- May also be a useful "aide memoire" for ICU examinations especially for the FRCA and diplomas in intensive care.
- The First Edition arose out of a series of ICU study days organised by the editor in the North West region since 1992. Many of the authors have been lecturers on these courses.
- The authors are all either experienced ICU practitioners or invited experts on specialist issues. Being involved in ICU research was not a prerequisite although many of the authors have been or are involved in ICU research – a clinical commitment at the bedside was thought to be more important for this text.
- Aims to provide practical information on the management of common and/or important problems in the critically ill patient as well as sufficient background information to enable understanding of the principles and rationale behind their therapy. We hope it will prove useful at the bedside but we would like to emphasise that this, or any other book, is no substitute for experienced supervision, support and training.
- Throughout, the importance of cardiac function is emphasised.
- Does not aim to cover all of ICU practice and is not a substitute to the major ICU reference textbooks. For example, practical aspects of monitoring techniques are not covered (best learnt at the bedside) but, however, the philosophy of

monitoring is covered where necessary to illustrate important management points. Similarly, pathophysiology is included to help understand management principles.

- The Second Edition contains several new chapters on topical aspects of ICU therapy as well as revisions of older chapters – many have been completely rewritten.
- The format is designed to provide easy access to information presented in a concise manner. We have tried to eliminate all superfluous material. Selected important or controversial references are presented as well as suggestions for further reading.

Part I

Basic principles

Cardiac function, monitoring, oxygen transport

I. McConachie

Stroke volume and cardiac output

Cardiac output (CO) is the volume of blood pumped by the ventricle per minute. It ranges from 4–7 l/min in a normal adult at rest and can increase up to 17 l/min during exercise. CO is normally indexed to body surface area (BSA) to allow comparisons of "normal" CO between patients of different height and weight – Cardiac index (CI):

$$CO = \text{Heart rate (HR)} \times \text{Stroke volume (SV)}$$

Factors governing SV include preload, afterload and the contractility of the cardiac muscle.

HR and rhythm

- Therefore bradycardia will impair CO. Conversely, increases in HR, although arithmetically increasing CO, may impair overall cardiac function by increasing myocardial oxygen demand, causing ischaemia and reducing time for diastolic filling. Some units therefore use the response of SV to therapy as being more appropriate for overall cardiac function.
- An arrhythmia may also be detrimental to cardiac function, for example, in atrial fibrillation (AF) the loss of the atrial contribution to ventricular filling may be significant. SV is the volume of blood ejected by the ventricle per heartbeat. It is the end-diastolic volume minus the end-systolic volume. Normally 70–80 mls for a 70 kg man at rest.

Preload

- The force of ventricular contraction is related to the myocardial fibre length (Frank Starling relationship).
- Myocardial fibre length is related to end-diastolic ventricular volume (EDV). This is commonly referred to as "preload". The heart beats efficiently with adequate preload and thus fluid therapy may increase cardiac function.
  Note: The active force needed for ejection of blood from the ventricle is greater for a large ventricle than a small one. This is explained by the Law of Laplace which states for a sphere $P = 2T/R$. Thus ventricular cardiac muscle must generate a greater tension when the heart is dilated compared to a normal sized heart to produce the same intraventricular pressure.
- EDV is difficult to quantify though an assessment can be made by echocardiography.
- Vascular pressures can be measured more easily and both central venous pressure (CVP) and pulmonary artery occlusion or capillary "wedge" pressure (PAOP or PCWP) are used clinically to reflect the end-diastolic pressure (EDP) and thus the EDV.
- Graphs can be constructed of CO against filling pressure. Filling pressure can then be increased until there are no further increases in CO. Preload can then be considered to be optimal.
- One problem is that with decreased compliance (increased stiffness) of the ventricle wall, for example, following myocardial infarction (MI) the pressure may be increased relative to the volume. Therefore, the EDP may overestimate true preload.

Note: Preload gives information about the filling pressure of the heart. It does not give any information about the blood volume.

Afterload

This is the force that opposes ventricular muscle contraction, that is, the ventricular wall tension that must develop in order to eject blood from the ventricle.
   Afterload is increased by:

- Anatomical obstruction, for example, aortic stenosis.
- Peripheral resistance in the circulatory system. Clinically this is reflected by systemic vascular resistance (SVR).

$$SVR = \frac{\text{Mean arterial pressure (MAP)} - CVP}{CO}$$

The SVR accounts for approximately 95% of the resistance to ejection and is used clinically to estimate afterload.

- Decreased distensibility of the vascular system. Blood pressure (BP) although convenient to measure is a poor reflection of afterload and gives no information about volume and flow to organs.
- Enlarged ventricle (Laplace).
- Increased blood viscosity, which is largely dependent on haematocrit. The greater the viscosity, the greater the resistance to flow.
- Decreased intrathoracic pressure, see Chapter 9.

Increased afterload will increase the workload of the heart and oxygen consumption and reduce SV.

Afterload is reduced by:

- Reduced SVR.
- Vasodilator drugs, the peripheral vasodilator drugs, can improve the SV of failing hearts by reducing afterload and ventricular work; vasodilators also reduce preload via venous dilatation.
- Anaemia.
- Increased intrathoracic pressure.

Contractility

This is the effective pumping ability of the heart muscle. The force and velocity of cardiac contraction is one definition of contractility although this is very difficult to measure in practice as most clinical measurements, for example, CO, ejection fraction, etc. are influenced by preload and afterload.

Contractility is increased by the following:

- increased sympathetic activity,
- positive inotropes,
- increased preload.

Contractility is reduced by the following:

- decreased filling,
- hypoxia and hypercapnia (although both will cause sympathetic stimulation),
- acidosis and alkalosis,
- electrolyte disturbances,
- negative inotropes.

The ejection fraction is often used as an indirect index of contractility:

$$\text{Ejection fraction} = \frac{\text{end-diastolic volume} - \text{end-systolic volume}}{\text{end-diastolic volume}}.$$

The normal value is greater than 60%.

The CO, SV, left ventricular stroke work and ejection fraction are best thought of as measures of overall cardiac performance, probably clinically more useful.

Ventricular interdependence

Both ventricles share a common septum. Studies have shown that about 20–40% of the pulmonary systolic pressure and volume outflow result from left ventricular contraction [1]:

- If right ventricular end-diastolic volume increases this shifts the septum towards the left ventricle (LV) decreasing left ventricular diastolic compliance.
- Right ventricular volumes can increase with pulmonary hypertension.

Heart/lung interactions

In the past, medicine encouraged a systems approach to disease. Thus diseases of the heart would be taught in one unit and then diseases of the lungs would be taught in another. Although not without merit this approach has limitations. It is increasingly recognised that the organ systems work in series rather than in parallel, that is, disease or therapy of one directly influences one or more other organs. Nowhere is this more apparent than with the heart and lung which after all are connected by their vasculature and share the thoracic cavity. Indeed, the lungs are the only organ which receives the whole CO. Forces acting on the lungs also act on the heart. Pinsky has done much to investigate these issues and popularised the fact that the heart is a "pressure chamber within a pressure chamber" (see Further reading). This emphasises that pressure applied to the lungs is automatically applied to and affects the heart. This has several implications:

- It is intuitively obvious that respiratory function and ventilation must have an effect on cardiac function. This has especial relevance to intermittent positive pressure ventilation (IPPV) and is discussed in Chapter 9.
- As airway pressure increases, this pressure is transmitted to the right atrium and acts as a backpressure opposing venous return, that is, venous return and CO decreases. During normal quiet respiration this effect is minimal but is

measurable. The effects are of course magnified with IPPV when high pressures are applied to the lungs (see Chapter 9).

- The other main effect of respiration on cardiac function is by changes in tidal volume. Again during quiet respiration these effects are minimal but with disease and IPPV effects can be clinically significant.

If one takes the linkage of the heart and lungs to its logical conclusion and considers the overall cardiopulmonary unit, the main function of which is to deliver oxygen to the cells, then one must also take factors such as haemoglobin (Hb) and blood viscosity into account when assessing the patient. The increase in CO and minute volume with anaemia is a perfect example of the linkage of different organ systems to act as an overall cardiopulmonary unit.

Respiratory failure and the heart

Shallow breathing in respiratory failure can increase pulmonary vascular resistance (PVR), partly by collapsing alveoli causing a fall in diameter of extra alveolar pulmonary blood vessels, and partly by development of hypoxic pulmonary vasoconstriction. The worsening PVR exacerbates the development of hypoxia and acidosis which further worsens PVR! Thus, heart/lung interactions in respiratory failure can result in a progressive, downward spiral of the patient's condition.

Increased work of breathing and the heart

Any condition increasing work of breathing requires oxygen and energy. This requires increased blood flow and, in essence, the heart has to work harder. Thus it is perhaps not surprising that respiratory failure causes a strain on cardiac function. The potential for myocardial ischaemia is also present especially when there is associated tachycardia and hypoxaemia.

Shock and respiratory failure

In severe shock, the reduced blood flow to the diaphragm coupled with the increased minute volume and respiratory energy expenditure causes respiratory failure, even in normal lungs. This is convincingly demonstrated in animal studies for example, much of the lactic acid accumulating in shock comes from the respiratory muscles [2]. IPPV, by reducing the work of breathing, lessens the blood lactate levels compared with spontaneous breathing. In cardiogenic shock the mode of death is often from respiratory arrest secondary to diaphragmatic fatigue, again due to the increased work of breathing.

Changes in CO and oxygenation

A pitfall is to wrongly ascribe a measured hypoxaemia to a respiratory illness when the true cause is cardiovascular in origin.

Falls in CO lead to a compensatory increase in oxygen extraction by the tissues. This results in a decrease in mixed venous Hb saturation (SvO_2). This directly results in a decrease in *arterial* saturation, especially in the absence of supplemental inspired oxygen. This, in itself, is one rationale for the administration of oxygen following MI.

An exception to this effect is in the presence of physiological shunting through the lungs. Here a decrease in CO causes a decrease in the fraction of output shunting through the lungs and *no* change in PO_2.

Monitoring

Monitoring may be described as the intermittent or continuous observation of a patient using clinical examination and appropriate equipment to assess progress of the condition:

- The most useful and reproducible monitor remains the thorough and repeated clinical examination by the doctor.
- Not all critical care environments are the same, and all models of monitoring equipment are slightly different. The clinician must take time to become familiar with the equipment in his or her own hospital.

Invasive monitoring

By definition a urinary catheter or a nasogastric tube is a form of invasive monitoring. However, by common convention, invasive monitoring is usually taken to refer to vascular cannulation. Mainly it is vascular pressures which are measured using pressure transducers although use of the pulmonary artery catheter permits many other measurements, calculations and sampling of blood. Before instituting invasive monitoring one must always ask "What are we monitoring and why?" The answer should be that we monitor something to do with one or more of the following:

- intervene therapeutically in emergency situations,
- guide and plan future therapy,

- establish diagnoses,
- establish prognosis.

Monitoring is not a therapy in itself which explains the argument that invasive monitoring does not in itself improve survival. Of course, survival will not be improved by any monitoring and measurements. Survival will only be improved if appropriate therapeutic measures are taken on the basis of the measurements taken. It should also be self evident that the right measurements must be made and the information acted upon in the right manner. Much of the current debate regarding the usefulness of the pulmonary artery or Swan–Ganz catheter revolves around lack of knowledge on the part of the physician inserting the catheter and inappropriate therapeutic interventions based on the data obtained (see later).

Invasive monitoring is not without complications although these can be reduced by careful technique and practice. Therefore, one should always monitor non-invasively if possible. For example:

- The use of pulse oximetry has reduced (but not eliminated) the need for regular blood gas analysis.
- Automatic non-invasive BP measurement negates the need for direct arterial pressure measurements in many patients.
- Non-invasive CO measurements are reducing the frequency of insertion of pulmonary artery flotation catheters (PAFCs).

However, in the critically ill patient non-invasive monitoring may not suffice as discussed below.

Direct arterial BP measurement

- The insertion of a small (common sizes are 20 or 22 gauge) teflon coated catheter into an artery (usually the radial, ulnar, brachial, dorsalis pedis or femoral are used) allows direct beat to beat assessment of the systemic BP.
- The presence of an arterial line also provides access for the measurement of arterial blood gas samples.
- When BP is low the "true" arterial pressure may be underestimated by non-invasive measurements. A common pitfall is to prefer the non-invasive reading as more accurate – presumably due to the reassurance of a better reading!
- The decision to use invasive BP monitoring is based on the clinical indication, together with an assessment of the ease with which it can be safely undertaken and the ability of the staff in the critical care area to look after the set up.

- It is probably inappropriate to run infusions of inotropic and vasoactive drugs without direct BP measurement. It is also strongly advised that any ventilated patient have arterial access both for BP measurement and blood gas analysis.
- Common complications include local bleeding and infection. Serious complications include embolisation and thrombosis and development of arterio-venous (AV) fistulae. Fortunately, serious complications are rare and can be minimised by choosing Teflon, small bore catheters inserted percutaneously.
- Intra arterial pressure measurements are not always accurate, usually due to failure of calibration or wrong height of transducer. In general, the Mean pressure is less prone to error, variation and excessive damping than the Systolic and Diastolic.

The pros and cons of this monitoring modality can be assessed by comparison with the non-invasive cuff pressure alternative.

Invasive Arterial BP	Non-Invasive BP
Beat-to-beat control	"Stat" mode cycles c. 20–30 s.
Unaffected by rhythm	Difficulty reading BP in AF
Automatic pulse measurement	Not always available
Almost always possible	Difficult in obese patients
Accuracy unaffected by patient	Inaccurate in obese patients
Movement artefact clearly visible	Unable to read if moving
Allows blood sampling	Not applicable
Susceptible to over and under damping	Not applicable
Requires training and practice	Easy to use
Potential ischaemic damage	Cuff compression injury rare
Danger of accidental injection	Not applicable
Massive blood loss if disconnection	Not applicable

Echocardiography

Echocardiography, especially by the transoesophageal route, is a useful, comparatively non-invasive, means of assessing cardiac function. Advantages include:

- Dynamic as opposed to static assessment, for example, one can see how the heart functions globally and see regional wall motion abnormalities.
- Easy assessment of cardiac, valvular and major vessel structures.
- Helps to provide the "missing link" between pressure and volume within the cardiac chambers.

Intermittent assessment of cardiac function on intensive care unit (ICU) is becoming increasingly common technique for ICU specialists.

Indices of tissue perfusion and oxygenation

Measurement of pHi (gastric mucosal pH) may be an indicator of splanchnic perfusion and may predict outcome [3]. Both pHi and blood lactate may be superior to oxygen transport variables in predicting outcome [4].

CVP monitoring

The central (or great) veins within the neck and mediastinum may be thought of as a manometer tube with four accessible branches: the right and left internal jugular veins, and the right and left subclavian veins.

Factors involved in the choice of site of CVP monitoring are discussed in Chapter 4.

The pressure measured within this "venous manometer" is the filling pressure responsible for ventricular filling during diastole. The CVP may be judged clinically as the jugular venous pressure (JVP). This is very difficult to quantify and trends or sudden changes in the filling pressures are easier to assess directly.

Many critical care conditions cause the CVP to rise and fall. The usefulness of this monitoring system may be assessed from the following list.

Conditions causing increase in CVP:

- *Cardiac failure*: If the right ventricle is unable to efficiently eject a SV there will be increased back pressure in the systemic venous system.
- *Cardiac tamponade*: Again if the right ventricle is compressed by fluid in the pericardial sac back pressure in the great veins will cause the CVP to rise.
- *Positive pressure ventilation*: Increased intrathoracic pressure produced during inspiration and the application of positive end expiratory pressure (PEEP) both result in elevation of the CVP.
- *Fluid resuscitation*: This is one of the commonest causes for CVP monitoring. To assess response to fluid resuscitation.
- *Superior vena cava (SVC) obstruction*: This is caused due to tumour or trauma to the root of the neck.

Conditions causing decrease in CVP:

- *Hypovolaemia*. Any condition resulting in reduced venous return to the heart, for example, exsanguination, sepsis, gastrointestinal (GI) tract losses, sweating.

- *Fall in intrathoracic pressure.* At the end of a period of positive pressure ventilation and during spontaneous inspiration.

CVP monitoring should be considered in all critically ill patients in whom knowledge of the filling pressures of the right heart will assist in the resuscitation and maintenance of an adequate circulating volume to ensure optimal oxygen delivery.

CVP lines allow for the infusion of vasoactive drugs that would cause constriction of small peripheral veins. They may also be used for the infusion of irritant substances, for example, parenteral nutrition and potassium.

After insertion of CVP lines via the above routes, a chest X-ray (CXR) must be obtained reasonably promptly both to rule out pneumothorax and also to check catheter tip position (within the SVC is ideal). If during and after CVP line insertion there is clinical deterioration of the patient the possibility of a Pneumothorax *must* be entertained.

Long catheters can be threaded into the thorax via the basilic and cephalic veins in the antecubital fossae. The advantages are the little risk of bleeding and zero risk of pneumothorax. However, the complication rate is *higher* than that of other routes of central venous access; that is, high infection rate and a high rate of thrombosis. The success rate is also low, 60% in some series.

Limitations of CVP monitoring or why we need the Pulmonary artery catheter

CVP reflects right atrial pressure (RAP) which is usually taken to reflect RV end diastolic pressure (RVEDP). CVP provides useful information regarding the status of the right side of the heart. This is valuable in cases of RV failure or in assessing the RV response to pulmonary hypertension:

- It does *not* necessarily reflect LV preload and also poorly correlates with blood volume. CVP is often used as a guide to LV function and, indeed, directional changes in CVP may reflect alterations in LV performance. However, if either ventricle becomes selectively depressed, or in the presence of severe pulmonary disease, changes in CVP will *not* reflect changes in LV function.
- CVP is "several steps" away from LV end-diastolic ventricular volume (LVEDV) or true preload and each approximation is influenced by pathological conditions, for example, LV compliance, mitral valve disease, intrathoracic pressures, tricuspid regurgitation.
- There are many studies showing a poor relationship between CVP and PCWP derived from a Pulmonary Artery Catheter in various disease states.

Pulmonary artery flotation catheter

In 1970 Swan, Ganz and colleagues described a balloon tipped catheter which could be inserted through the great veins via the heart to the pulmonary circulation. By means of the balloon the tip of the catheter could be isolated from the pressure generated by the right ventricle. Various additions and modifications including further infusion ports, CVP monitoring port, thermistor connection, heating coil, continuous venous oximetry cable and pacing facilities.

The information gained from the PAFC is of three types:

(1) Pressures derived from catheter placement.
(2) Measurement of CO.
(3) Mathematically derived data.

Pressures derived from catheter placement

During the insertion of the PAFC the pressures produced from the transduced catheter tip as it "floats" (balloon inflated during insertion) through the right heart are as follows:

- CVP;
- right atrial (RA) pressure;
- right ventricular (RV) pressure;
- pulmonary artery pressure;
- PCWP.

The PCWP is the pressure measured by the tip of the catheter when the forward pressure from the right ventricle is obstructed by the balloon (this pressure should be measured for no longer than 30 s at a time as the pulmonary blood flow is ceased down stream of the inflated balloon making pulmonary infarction a possibility). The PCWP is also known as the Pulmonary artery occlusion pressure (PAOP).

Provided the tip of the catheter is contained within a continuous column of blood between it and the LV, then at the end of diastole with the mitral valve open, the PCWP measures the LV end-diastolic pressure (LVEDP). From Starling's law, the force of contraction of the LV is dependent on the degree of muscle fibre stretch during diastolic filling. Thus provided the ventricle wall is of normal compliance the pressure developed within the ventricle at end diastole is directly proportional to the LVEDV and hence to preload. Under these conditions PCWP directly reflects LVEDV.

Clearly there are situations in which the above relationship does not hold:

- In patients undergoing positive pressure mechanical ventilation with high airway pressures the alveolar pressure may exceed the pulmonary venule pressure. In this state the continuous column of blood is "broken" and the wedged PAFC is measuring the alveolar pressure.
- Mitral valve disease affects PCWP. Mitral stenosis causes a large-back pressure ("a" wave) on the PCWP trace as the atrium contracts against the stenotic valve. Mitral regurgitation causes a large "v" wave as the ventricular outflow passes back up the pulmonary venous system.
- The compliance of the ventricle wall is altered in states of cardiac and systemic disease. MI, cardiac tamponade, aortic valve disease, the cardiomyopathies and systemic sepsis all cause the PCWP not to reflect LVEDV. This observation may be used clinically to assess the severity of the causative condition.

Pitfalls in the PCWP

- Upper limit of "normal" is 12 mmHg. The optimal PCWP is the PCWP which provides the best CO without increases in lung water or pulmonary oedema. The optimal PCWP is rarely above 18 mmHg.
- It is only a guide to the LA pressure. Pulmonary artery (PA) diastolic pressure usually approximates to PCWP and may sometimes be used if there is difficulty getting the catheter to "wedge".
- If compliance is increased, for example after previous MI, it is accepted that PCWP will usually have to be greater than "normal" for optimal SV.
- It can reflect transmitted intrathoracic pressure, especially in the presence of PEEP. To minimise the effect of intrathoracic pressure on PCWP the catheter tip should be positioned in the lower third of the lung (if higher, alveolar pressure may exceed pulmonary artery pressure). All PCWP measurements should be made at end of expiration (EE):

    During spontaneous respiration, EE = *highest* part of waveform.
    During IPPV, EE = *lowest* part of pressure waveform.
- The PCWP is *not* a measurement of blood volume although changes in PCWP correlate with changes in blood volume.

Thermodilution CO

Thermodilution PAFC measures temperature in the pulmonary artery (a useful source of an accurate core temperature). 10 ml of cold fluid is injected through the proximal port of the catheter. Blood flow is calculated from the temperature drop sensed by the Thermistor at the tip of the catheter in the Pulmonary artery after mixing has occurred. Modern catheters can measure CO continuously by the same principle but in reverse, that is, heated filament to produce small increases in blood temperature:

- The CO measured in this way is still currently viewed as the "Gold Standard" method of this measurement in the critically ill patient. A full discussion of non-invasive methods of measuring CO is beyond the scope of this text (see Further reading).
- Due to the differences in CO with changes in Intrathoracic Pressure during IPPV, some recommend timing the measurement at EE. However, this begs the question: Which is the "correct" CO; the one during inspiration or the one during expiration? It seems sensible to make the measurements randomly and obtain an "average" CO. Continuous methods do the "averaging" for us.
- CO varies with height and weight. To enable one patient to be compared with another the CO is usually indexed to BSA, that is the CI. In theory every patient has the same "normal" CI.

Mathematically derived haemodynamic data

From the measured data produced by the PAFC together with knowledge of the systemic mean BP (from the arterial line) and the central venous pressure (from the CVP line) a further set of derived data may be produced:

- SVR and PVR
- LV and RV stroke work
- LV and RV stroke volume
- RV ejection fraction and RV end-diastolic ventricular volume (RVEDV) (rapid response thermistor catheters only).

Although mathematical formulae for each of the above figures exists (see below), modern monitoring systems calculate them automatically.

- *Stroke work index (SWI)*: It is the work generated by each ventricle during one cardiac cycle. It is a function of the pressure generated in systole and the SV ejected. Increases in SWI may be beneficial but also increases myocardial oxygen demand.
- *Vascular Resistance, Systemic or Pulmonary*: Resistance is determined by dividing the pressure drop across the system by flow. There is controversy as to

whether SVR and PVR should be indexed to BSA. The main use of the SVR is to help sort out the specific problem in cases of hypotension, especially in septic shock but one should treat the BP rather than the SVR. SVR may be increased by vasoconstriction or hypertension. Reductions occur in sepsis, cirrhosis and AV fistulae. Changes in calculated SVR may be seen with changes in CVP without any change in vascular tone.

Normal values

$$\text{LVSWI} = (\text{MAP} - \text{PCWP}) \times \text{SVI} \times 0.0136 \quad 44\text{–}56 \, \text{gm.m/m}^2$$

$$\text{RVSWI} = (\text{PAP} - \text{CVP}) \times \text{SVI} \times 0.0136 \quad 7\text{–}10 \, \text{gm.m/m}^2$$

$$\text{SVR} = \frac{\text{MAP} - \text{CVP}}{\text{CO}} \times 80 \qquad 900\text{–}1200 \, \text{dynes.s/cm}^5$$

$$\text{PVR} = \frac{\text{MPAP} - \text{PCWP}}{\text{CO}} \times 80 \qquad 100\text{–}200 \, \text{dynes.s/cm}^5$$

MPAP = mean pulmonary artery pressure.

Indications for the PAFC

- Monitor preload.
- Optimise preload prior to the use of inotropes.
- Pulmonary oedema not responsive to simple measures or where therapy produces hypotension.
- Shock.
- Complicated MI.
- To enable manipulation of oxygen transport variables.
- Differentiate cardiogenic and non-cardiogenic pulmonary oedema.
- More rarely, after acute MI, to differentiate between acute ventricular septal defect (VSD) and mitral regurgitation.
- May be inserted prophylactically for high-risk surgery especially cardiac surgery.

Complications associated with the PAFC

During insertion:

- See Chapter 4.

  During passage of the catheter:

- Arrhythmias
- Intracardiac knotting
- Cardiac or PA perforation.

Catheter in situ:

• Pulmonary embolism (PE) and infarction
• Valve damage
• Thrombocytopenia (not such a problem with modern catheters)
• Endocarditis
• PA rupture, increased risk with pulmonary hypertension.

Inaccurate measurements and false interpretations.

Hints on safe use of PAFC

• Balance risk versus benefit.
• Slowly inflate balloon while watching waveform.
• On wedging trace stop further inflation of balloon.
• If catheter overwedges, immediately deflate balloon and withdraw catheter 1–2 cm.
• Minimise duration of balloon inflation.
• If balloon inflates with less than 1.5 ml of air, withdraw 1 cm.
• Continuously monitor PA trace for spontaneous migration and wedging.
• Minimise number of wedgings in patients with pulmonary hypertension.

Newer techniques of preload assessment

The aim of preload assessment, in general, is to predict and quantify the improvement in SV in response to a fluid challenge. Neither the CVP or the PCWP are thought to reliably *predict* an improvement in cardiac function following administration of fluid.

The role of the RV end diastolic volume index (RVEDVI) as measured by a rapid thermistor PAFC in assessing preload has received much attention. The results from different studies are conflicting:

• The RVEDVI may be a better predictor of preload than the PCWP in trauma patients during large-volume shock resuscitation. When the RVEDVI is 130 ml/m^2 or less, volume administration will likely increase the CI [5].
• The RVEDVI may not be a reliable predictor of the response to fluid. As a predictor of fluid responsiveness, PCWP was superior to RVEDVI [6].
• RVEDV from the rapid response PAFC may overestimate left ventricular preload. If RVEDV is used as an absolute value for determining preload,

patients may be under-resuscitated. Transesophageal echocardiography may assist in determining preload and cardiac performance in critically ill patients [7].

- CI correlates significantly better with RVEDVI than PCWP at all levels of PEEP up to 50 cmH$_2$O. RVEDVI is a more reliable predictor of volume depletion and preload especially in patients receiving higher levels of PEEP where PCWP is difficult to interpret [8].

Another simpler method of preload assessment looks promising:

- Recent studies suggest that the presence of arterial pulse pressure variation (PPV) during the respiratory cycle indicates a relative hypovolaemia [9] and, indeed, predicts an increase in CO with fluid. Most monitors can "freeze" the arterial trace and quantify this PPV or one can simply view the "swing" on the arterial trace.
- Additionally and importantly, it is suggested that if there is *no* PPV there will be no increase in CO no matter how much fluid is given [10]. This technique only seems to apply in the patient undergoing IPPV.

The PAFC controversy

Detractors of the PAFC, state that their benefit in terms of increased survival is unproven. Of course, survival will not be improved by any monitoring or measurements. (It would be ludicrous to blame thermometers for the high-death rate from septic shock.) Survival will only be improved if appropriate therapeutic measures are taken on the basis of the measurements taken. The use of a PA catheter is only of value if used as part of an overall management plan.

- An important paper by Connors was published in 1996 and caused considerable discussion (including the front page of the *New York Times*). The paper claimed to show an increased mortality associated from the use of the PAFC [11]. Direct complications, for example, arrhythmias, pulmonary infarction were not thought to be responsible as these are, in general, low in experienced hands. The increased mortality was thought to arise from inappropriate use of the information obtained especially inappropriate use of "supranormal goals" of oxygen transport as discussed below. Although there is disagreement with the methodology of this study (e.g. it was retrospective) there arose calls for formal controlled studies of the use of the PAFC in critically ill patients (which might previously have been considered unethical).

- In addition, inappropriate use of the information obtained from the PAFC may be compounded by the ignorance of doctors inadequately trained in their use [12].
- A large-retrospective study from the UK failed to find an association between the use of the PAFC and mortality [13].
- Meta-analysis of 12 randomised trials found a statistically significant reduction in morbidity using PA catheter-guided strategies [14].
- A French study [15] is the first to show that patients in whom the PAFC is used are sicker and, therefore, have a higher mortality than other patients. This study did not get as much publicity as the Connors study!
- A randomised trial of 200 catheters from the UK has also shown no evidence of increased mortality in those patients receiving a PAFC [16].
- In the most recent published large study, the use of PAFCs inserted preoperatively and used to guide the achievement of high oxygen delivery (see below) failed to show an improved outcome compared with "conventional" therapy [17].
- The UK PACMAN study is as yet unpublished but early presentations at scientific meetings suggests that there is no benefit (and no harm either) from the use of PAFCs in ICU patients. This is the first adequately powered trial (approximately 1000 patients prior to the trail being stopped) to address this issue and broadly supports the other trials in this area.

However, there is no doubt that the PAFC gives us invaluable information, not readily obtained elsewhere. For example:

- In one study [18] physicians were only able to correctly predict values for PCWP, CI and PA pressure about 50% of the time. Treatment was changed in 48.4% of patients after catheterisation. This is not meant to suggest that all critically ill patients should have a PAFC since the most important role of the experienced physician is in deciding who should be catheterised, and when.
- A French study found correctly predicted haemodynamic profiles in only 56% of patients prior to catheterisation. Changes of treatment were prompted in 63% of patients who were unresponsive to standard therapy. The mortality rate was significantly less when the assessment of haemodynamic data led to a change in therapy despite identical precatheterisation characteristics [19].

Some final points:

- Many physicians continue to use the PAFC despite the conflicting evidence and believe it benefits their patients.

- Even if the PAFC were to be withdrawn from use there are other methods now widely available to measure CO.
- The PACMAN trial examines the use of PAFCs as part of their units' current practice. Should we not now be looking at what constitutes best practice? Should we throw away the PAFC or learn to use it better? Are the documented changes in practice after insertion of the PAFC useless? Surely no information cannot be better than some information?

Further studies may help define the best therapies in differing circumstances and define the overall value of the PAFC in terms of survival.

Oxygen transport

Oxygen delivery or DO_2 is the oxygen content of the arterial blood (CaO_2) multiplied by the blood flow or CO. Thus

$$DO_2 = CO \times CaO_2$$

The normal CaO_2 of 20 ml is the Hb concentration multiplied by 1.34 (the constant for the amount of O_2 each gram of Hb can combine with) and the % oxy-Hb saturation (SaO_2). Dissolved O_2 is usually considered to be negligible. This is the CaO_2 per decilitre which must, therefore, be multiplied by 10 to unify the units because CO is measured in l/min. That is,

$$DO_2 = CO \times Hb \times SaO_2 \times 1.34 \times 10$$

Normal DO_2 therefore

$$5 \times 15 \times 100\% \times 1.34 \times 10 \cong 1000\,ml/min$$

If CI is used the resultant DO_2 is also indexed to BSA. That is,

$$DO_2 \cong 600\,ml/min\,m^2.$$

Adequate DO_2 is achieved by attention to cardiac function, Hb and oxygenation. Note that the PaO_2 contributes little to oxygen content and DO_2. (The PaO_2 is not an important measure of arterial oxygenation. The SaO_2 is more significant in assessing oxygenation of arterial blood while the PaO_2 is important in evaluating gas exchange in the lungs.)

Oxygen release from Hb at the tissues is increased by factors shifting the oxy-Hb dissociation curve to the right, for example, acidosis, fever, increased 2,3-diphosphoglyceraldehyde (2,3-DPG) while factors which shift the curve to the left, for example, alkalosis, hypothermia, reduced 2,3-DPG (stored blood) impair oxygen release at the tissues.

In patients who are fully oxygenated and have an adequate Hb the only logical way to increase DO_2 is to increase CI. This has practical implications for therapy.

Normal mixed venous SvO_2 is 75% (68–77%) and therefore venous oxygen content (CvO_2) is 15 ml. Thus the oxygen extraction ratio (OER) is 25%. Oxygen consumption (VO_2) of the whole body (indexed) is therefore:

$$VO_2 = CI \times (CaO_2 - CvO_2) \times 10$$

$$\cong 150\,ml/min\,m^2$$

VO_2 reflects metabolic rate and as such is increased in thyrotoxicosis, fever, physiological stress response, feeding and by a direct calorigenic effect of inotropes [20]. Anaesthesia, cyanide and carbon monoxide poisoning, and hypothermia reduce VO_2. Sedation of ventilated patients reduces VO_2 partly by direct sedative effect and partly by reducing the work of breathing.

Supply dependency

- The normal response to a fall in DO_2 (low CI, anaemia, hypoxaemia) is to maintain VO_2 by increases in OER and decreases in SvO_2. Thus, normally, VO_2 is "supply independent".
- VO_2 is "supply dependent" when extraction does not change in response to alterations in delivery; that is, further increases in DO_2 result in increases in VO_2, revealing potential tissue hypoxia. Supply dependency was widely identified in early studies where DO_2 and VO_2 were calculated using the shared variables of CI and CaO_2. This leads to a potential error due to "mathematical coupling". This finding led to many studies of increasing DO_2 to "supranormal" levels which is generally no longer recommended [21]. More recent studies, using truly independent methods of measuring DO_2 and VO_2, have mainly failed to substantiate the claims for widespread existence of supply dependency [22].
- In addition, if dobutamine has a direct calorigenic effect to raise VO_2 [20], then this response need not reflect tissue hypoxia.
- There are frequent "spontaneous" changes in DO_2 and VO_2 in ventilated patients [23]. This limits the value of studies showing that VO_2 is dependent on DO_2.
- There are still areas of controversy, for example, if the studies showing supply dependency were due to mathematical coupling why did studies of some groups of patients show this (e.g. septic and acute respiratory distress syndrome (ARDS) patients) while other groups (e.g. heart failure) did not?

At the other end of the scale, with decreases of DO_2:

- Where DO_2 is low and lactic acidosis present, increasing DO_2 will lead to increases in VO_2 [24], that is supply dependency. In haemorrhagic or cardiogenic shock, VO_2 is maintained by increases in OER down to a critical level of DO_2 (below which further decreases in DO_2 lead to the rapid demise of the patient) at the expense of low levels of SvO_2.
- This mechanism of increased extraction is only a short-term answer and the O_2 debt has to be repaid. Studies have shown that the magnitude of O_2 debt and its clearance is linked to ultimate survival [25].

Supranormal goals

- The team led by W.C. Shoemaker identified values of CI, DO_2 and VO_2 and blood volume retrospectively associated with increased survival of trauma and high-risk surgical patients [26]. The "goals" were:
  - $CI > 4.5 \, l/min \, m^2$
  - $DO_2 > 600 \, ml/min \, m^2$
  - $VO_2 > 170 \, ml/min \, m^2$
  - Normal BP
  - Blood volume 500 ml > normal unless PCWP > 20 mmHg
- They then attempted to achieve these goals prospectively in an attempt to improve survival in a similar group of patients with considerable success [27].
- Others attempted to apply these goals in other groups of patients with lesser success.
- Indeed, it now seems that this approach may be detrimental in some groups of patients e.g. the elderly in whom attempts to aggressively raise CI may promote myocardial ischaemia [28].
- Thus it has been concluded that this approach cannot be universally recommended [21] but there may be benefits in specific groups of patients especially trauma patients and high-risk surgical patients when applied preoperatively. This will be explored later in this text.
- A key issue may be timing: early correction of oxygen debt may be helpful but late intervention will not be. Shoemaker has suggested that "no amount of extra oxygen can restore irreversible oxygen debt, failed debt or dead cells" [29]. His recent meta-analysis [29] suggested that there can be significant reductions in mortality in critical illness when patients are treated early to achieve optimal goals before the development of organ failure, when there were control group mortalities of >20% (otherwise the patients are not sick

enough) and when therapy produced differences in oxygen delivery between the control and protocol groups.

Monitoring of venous oxygenation

Mixed venous oxygen saturation: SvO_2

This may be measured from a fibreoptic PAFC or by taking a sample from a PAFC and running it through a blood gas co-oximeter.

- In general if the peripheral tissues are unable to utilise oxygen (e.g. sepsis, hypothermia) the SvO_2 will rise. If the heart is unable to deliver oxygen the tissues will extract as much as possible from what is available and the SvO_2 will fall.
- If the critically ill patient is to survive DO_2 must be restored to such a level that VO_2 can be maintained without critically low levels of SvO_2. SvO_2 levels $<60\%$ are dangerous and levels of $<40\%$ are incompatible with long-term survival.
- SvO_2 is therefore obviously related to the balance of DO_2 and VO_2 or more accurately to the balance between the *ability* to extract oxygen and DO_2.
- SvO_2 does not necessarily vary with CO. Not all patients can increase their OER if DO_2 falls, for example, septic patients with loss of vasoregulation and maldistribution of flow.
- Thus the value of mixed venous oxygenation measurements is that it reflects the balance between CO and OER. As CO is the most important index of DO_2 in most patients, many physicians monitor oxygen transport by measuring CO and assessing its adequacy to metabolic needs with measurements of venous oxygenation [30].
- The main flaw in this approach is that global measurements take little notice of regional disturbances.
- Most recently the monitoring of venous saturation from the central veins via a modified CVP catheter has been shown to be of value in guiding early goal-directed therapy in severe sepsis [31]. The use of such measurements is the subject of much research and seems to offer a relatively less invasive (and quick) guide to the balance of overall oxygen transport.

FURTHER READING

Kuper M, Soni N. Non invasive cardiac output monitors. *CPD Anaesth* 2003; 5: 17–25.

Pinsky MR. The hemodynamic consequences of ventilation: an evolving story. *Intens Care Med* 1997; 23: 493–503.

Shephard JN, Brecker SJ, Evans TW. Bedside assessment of myocardial performance in the
critically ill. *Intens Care Med* 1994; 20: 513–21.

Soni N, Fawcett WJ, Halliday FC. Beyond the lung: oxygen delivery and tissue oxygenation.
Anaesthesia 1993; 48: 704–11.

Tobin M. Principles and Practice of Intensive Care Monitoring. McGraw Hill, 1998.

REFERENCES

1. Santamore WP, Dell'talia LJ. Ventricular interdependence: significant left ventricular contributions to right ventricular systolic function. *Prog Cardiovas Dis* 1998; 40: 289–308.

2. Aubier M, Vines N, Syllie G, Mozes R, Roussos C. Respiratory muscle contribution to
lactic acidosis in low cardiac output. *Am Rev Resp Dis* 1982; 126: 648–52.

3. Doglio GR, Pusajo JF, Egurrola MA, Bonfigli GC, Parra C. Gastric mucosal pH as a prognostic index of mortality in critically ill patients. *Crit Care Med* 1991; 19: 1037–40.

4. Friedman G, Berlot G, Kahn RJ, Vincent JL. Combined measurements of blood lactate
concentrations and gastric intramucosal pH in patients with severe sepsis. *Crit Care
Med* 1995; 23: 1184–93.

5. Chang MC, Blinman TA, Rutherford EJ, Nelson LD et al. Preload assessment in trauma
patients during large-volume shock resuscitation. *Arch Surg* 1996; 131: 728–31.

6. Wagner JG, Leatherman JW. Right ventricular end-diastolic volume as a predictor of
the hemodynamic response to a fluid challenge. *Chest* 1998; 113: 1048–54.

7. Kraut EJ, Owings JT, Anderson JT, Hanowell L et al. Right ventricular volumes overestimate left ventricular preload in critically ill patients. *J Trauma* 1997; 42: 839–45.

8. Cheatham ML, Nelson LD, Chang MC, Safcsak K. Right ventricular end-diastolic volume index as a predictor of preload status in patients on positive end-expiratory pressure. *Crit Care Med* 1998; 26: 1801–6.

9. Tavernier B, Makhotine O, Lebuffe G, Dupont J et al. Systolic pressure variation as a
guide to fluid therapy in patients with sepsis-induced hypotension. *Anesthesiology*
1998; 89: 1313–21.

10. Michard F, Teboul JL. Predicting fluid responsiveness in ICU patients: a critical analysis
of the evidence. *Chest* 2002; 121: 2000–8.

11. Connors A, Speroff T, Dawson N, Thomas C, Harrell Jr FE, Wagner D et al. The effectiveness of right heart catheterisation in the initial care of critically ill patients. *J Am Med
Assoc* 1996; 276: 889–97.

12. Gnaegi A, Feihl F, Perret C. Intensive care physicians' insufficient knowledge of right
heart catheterisation at the bedside: Time to act? *Crit Care Med* 1997; 25: 213–20.

13. Murdoch SD, Cohen AT, Bellamy MC. Pulmonary artery catheterization and mortality
in critically ill patients. *Br J Anaesth* 2000; 85: 611–5.

14. Ivanov R, Allen J, Calvin JE. The incidence of major morbidity in critically ill patients managed with pulmonary artery catheters: a meta-analysis. *Crit Care Med* 2000; 28: 615–9.

15. Viellard-Baron A, Girou E, Valente E et al. Predictors of mortality in acute respiratory distress syndrome: Focus on the role of right heart catheterisation. *Am J Resp Crit Care Med* 2000; 161: 1597–1601.

16. Rhodes A, Cusack RJ, Newman PJ, Grounds RM et al. A randomised, controlled trial of the pulmonary artery catheter in critically ill patients. *Intensive Care Med* 2002; 28: 256–64.

17. Sandham JD, Hull RD, Grant RF et al. A randomised, controlled trial of the use of pulmonary artery catheters in high risk surgical patients. *New Eng J Med* 2003; 348: 5–14.

18. Connors AF, McCaffree DR, Gray BA. Evaluation of right heart catheterisation in the critically ill patient without myocardial infarction. *New Eng J Med* 1983; 308: 263–7.

19. Mimoz O, Rauss A, Rekik N, Brun-Buisson C, Lemaire F, Brochard L. Pulmonary artery catheterization in critically ill patients: a prospective analysis of outcome changes associated with catheter-prompted changes in therapy. *Crit Care Med* 1994; 22: 573–9.

20. Bhatt SB, Hutchinson RC, Tomlinson B, Oh TE, Mak M. Effect of dobutamine on oxygen supply and uptake in healthy volunteers. *Br J Anaesth* 1992; 69: 298–303.

21. Heyland DK, Cook DJ, King D, Kernerman P, Brun-Buisson C. Maximizing oxygen delivery in critically ill patients: a methodologic appraisal of the evidence. *Crit Care Med* 1996; 24: 517–24.

22. Hanique G, Dugernier T, Laterre PF, Dougnac A, Roeseler J et al. Significance of pathologic oxygen supply dependency in critically ill patients: comparison between measured and calculated methods. *Inten Care Med* 1994; 20: 12–8.

23. Villar J, Slutsky AS, Hew E, Aberman A. Oxygen transport and oxygen consumption in critically ill patients. *Chest* 1990; 98: 687–92.

24. Vincent JL, Roman A, De Backer D, Kahn RJ. Oxygen uptake/supply dependency. Effects of short-term dobutamine infusion. *Am Rev Respir Dis* 1990; 142: 2–7.

25. Shoemaker WC, Appel PL, Kram HB. Role of oxygen debt in the development of organ failure sepsis, and death in high-risk surgical patients. *Chest* 1992; 102: 208–15.

26. Shoemaker WC. Relation of oxygen transport patterns to the pathophysiology and therapy of shock states. *Inten Care Med* 1987; 13: 230–43.

27. Shoemaker WC, Appel PL, Kram HB, Waxman K, Lee TS. Prospective trial of supranormal values of survivors as therapeutic goals in high-risk surgical patients. *Chest* 1988; 94: 1176–86.

28. Hayes MA, Timmins AC, Yau EH, Palazzo M, Hinds CJ et al. Elevation of systemic oxygen delivery in the treatment of critically ill patients. *New Engl J Med* 1994; 330: 1717–22.

29. Kern JW, Shoemaker WC. Meta-analysis of hemodynamic optimization in high-risk patients. *Crit Care Med* 2002; 30: 1686–92.

30. Vincent JL. The relationship between oxygen demand, oxygen uptake, and oxygen supply. *Inten Care Med* 1990; 16(Suppl 2): S145–8.

31. Rivers E, Nguyen B, Havstad S et al. Early goal-directed therapy in the treatment of severe sepsis and septic shock. *New Engl J Med* 2001; 345: 1368–77.

2

Shock

I. McConachie

Shock is a very imprecise term for a common, life-threatening condition.

A modern, acceptable definition of shock might be "a clinical syndrome resulting from tissue dysfunction secondary to inadequate perfusion and oxygenation" (i.e. inadequate DO_2 and VO_2). Note that hypotension is not part of this definition; shock and hypotension are commonly linked but not synonymous. One can be hypotensive without being shocked and one can be shocked without being hypotensive. Some authorities would insist that unless lactic acidosis is present (indicating tissue hypoxia) one cannot be said to be "shocked".

Signs of shock include:

Clinical   Low blood pressure (BP) (e.g. <90 mmHg or 60 mmHg below a previous basal level)
             Oliguria <½ml/kg/h
             Pale, sweaty skin, cool peripheries
             Rapid, thready pulse
             Reduced conscious level
O_2 transport DO_2 and VO_2 reduced
             SVO_2 <50%
             Lactic acidosis

Studies have shown that VO_2 decreases before any changes in BP, urine output, etc. Four main types of shock have classically been described:

(1) Hypovolaemic: Often haemorrhagic in nature
(2) Cardiogenic
(3) Septic

All will be discussed in the appropriate section of this volume.

Less commonly

(4) Anaphylactic: See below

In addition some recognise:

- Traumatic: Effect of tissue injury in addition to haemorrhage.
- Obstructive: A special form of cardiogenic shock due to failure of left ventricular (LV) filling due to cardiac tamponade, pneumothorax or venocaval obstruction. Massive pulmonary embolus leads to a form of obstructive shock.
- Spinal: Not described in this text but the haemodynamic picture is mainly one of vasodilatation.

Massive pulmonary embolism

Acute circulatory failure is the commonest cause of death from pulmonary embolism (PE). This is believed to follow acute right ventricular (RV) failure secondary to the acute increase in RV afterload (acute cor pulmonale). Other factors include the development of RV ischaemia, decreased LV filling because of ventricular interdependence, hypoxaemia and vasoactive mediator release. Fluid therapy in acute PE is controversial. On the one hand, the further increase in right atrial pressure (RAP) should partially restore venous return and improve cardiac output (CO). However, further increases in right atrial (RA) and RV volumes may further impede LV filling. Inotropes may be useful by increasing ventricular contractility and vasopressors may improve right coronary perfusion. However, these interventions only serve to buy time for definitive intervention (e.g. thrombolysis).

Pathophysiology

Although it is common and in many ways appropriate to think of shock in haemodynamic terms (see below) shock is simultaneously a systemic and a cellular disease leading ultimately to:

- decreased adenosine triphosphate (ATP) production,
- membrane dysfunction,
- cellular swelling,
- cell death.

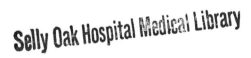

Once cellular swelling occurs, restoration of local tissue perfusion may not be possible leading to continuing secondary ischaemia. Damage to other organs such as the lungs results from leucocyte sequestration and deposition in the pulmonary capillaries leading to increased pulmonary shunting and increased capillary permeability from release of inflammatory mediators. The reticulo endothelial system function is depressed which decreases clearance of toxic materials (e.g. endotoxin, foreign proteins, immune complexes and platelet aggregates).

   Tissue trauma from trauma and surgery has additional effects:

- complement activation,
- coagulation cascade activation,
- cytokine release,
- granulocyte activation leading to the production of oxygen free radicals and endothelium dysfunction.

During recovery from shock after successful resuscitation there will be an oxygen debt to be repaid. Studies have shown that failure to repay this debt is associated with ongoing tissue hypoxia and organ failure [1].

Therapeutic approach to the shocked patient

Unfortunately, our knowledge of the pathophysiological cellular events in shock outweigh our ability to modify these events. Therapy is still largely "macroscopic" (i.e. restoration of tissue perfusion not "microscopic").

(1) *Airway, oxygenation and ventilation.* The threshold for intubation and ventilation of shocked patients should be low:
   - Patients are unlikely to be able to guard their own airway. Frank vomiting is uncommon but silent aspiration common.
   - IPPV will reduce the work and oxygen consumption associated with breathing and hopefully ensure oxygenation.
   - Severe shock will cause hypoxia in the absence of respiratory disease due to a reduction in pulmonary blood flow and low SVO_2.
(2) *Circulatory support* including attention to:
   - heart rate and rhythm,
   - preload,
   - contractility,
   - afterload,

- coronary perfusion and cerebral perfusion pressures,
- haematocrit.

Simple haemodynamic patterns may help in diagnosis of the cause of shock and guide cardiovascular management although mixed pathology may coexist. For example:

hypovolaemic shock: low pulmonary capillary wedge pressure (PCWP), low cardiac index (CI), high systemic vascular resistance (SVR); *cardiogenic shock*: high PCWP, low CI, high SVR; *septic shock*: low PCWP, high CI, low SVR.

A fluid challenge is appropriate in virtually all patients unless obviously suffering from gross congestive cardiac failure.

(3) *Specific therapy* according to cause.

Progressive or refractory shock

Even in young patients it has been shown that myocardial failure contributes to the shocked state if the shock is maintained; that is eventually all shock states will have a degree of cardiogenic aetiology. This is due to a combination of poor coronary perfusion, acidosis or possibly a depressant factor released from ischaemic tissue. This will proceed to the so-called refractory shock where loss of capillary vasomotor control leads to reduced tissue blood flow, sludging in the microcirculation and cellular hypoxia, and death. It has also been suggested that refractory shock may partly have a septic component from bacterial or endo-toxin translocation across the gut wall.

The golden hour

- The original concept of a "golden hour" or a critical therapeutic "window" of opportunity was applied to shock following traumatic injury but probably applies to outcome following shock due to any cause. Although generally accepted as a principle, it was originally based solely on animal studies backed up later by circumstantial patient evidence.
- In general, if the duration of shock exceeds an hour, mortality increases pro-gressively due to development of refractory shock or from the insidious devel-opment of organ failure. If shock is prolonged the patient is likely to die at a

later stage from organ failures, even if the original "shock" is subsequently reversed.

- Thus, speed is of extreme importance in resuscitating shocked patients.
- Therefore, it is common to initiate treatment empirically while the specific cause is being identified although common sense should tell one that the young man presenting with a large gastrointestinal (GI) bleed is suffering from haemorrhagic shock! The urgency of the situation may warrant the use of vasopressors to maintain coronary perfusion pressure while other therapies and diagnostic procedures are being instituted.

Anaphylactic shock

In anaphylactic shock the trigger stimulus causes release of histamine, serotonin, slow release substance, kinins and other vasoactive materials mainly from mast cells. These substances act primarily on smooth muscle leading to peripheral and airway oedema (stridor may not appear until 80% of the airway is obstructed), bronchospasm and vasodilatation, and capillary leakage. Some of the mediators may also act directly on the myocardium.

The two major causes of death are "shock" including cardiac depression and laryngeal oedema.

Management includes:

- Withdrawing the trigger stimulus, basic life support and cardiopulmonary resuscitation (CPR).
- Laryngeal oedema may require intubation or cricothyrotomy or may settle with nebulised adrenaline in less severe reactions.
- IV fluids especially colloids should be administered to restore plasma volume.

    A 1 mm layer of subcutaneous fluid over the whole body is equivalent to a loss of approximately 1.5 l of extracellular fluid.

- The agent of choice in severe reactions is adrenaline by incremental dosage as required. Infusions may be required after the initial treatment especially following reactions to agents with a long plasma half-life such as artificial colloids. In addition to its beneficial cardiac effects it is a specific antidote as it blocks mediator release from mast cells. If the intravenous route is not immediately available, adrenaline may be administered down the tracheal tube.
- Steroids are usually administered but take several hours to have an effect.

- Salbutamol may help for persistent bronchospasm but aminophylline should probably be avoided as there is an increased risk of serious arrhythmias when given in the presence of increased adrenaline blood levels.
- Antihistamines such as piriton are of little value in acute anaphylaxis as they do not reverse the effect of histamine already released and have no effect on the actions of mediators other than histamine. Logically, many authors contend that if antihistamines are desired to be given, both H1 and H2 receptors must be blocked for maximum therapeutic effect.

FURTHER READING

Fisher M. Treatment of acute anaphylaxis. *Br Med J* 1995; 311: 731–3.

REFERENCE

1. Shoemaker WC, Appel PL, Kram HB. Role of oxygen debt in the development of organ failure sepsis, and death in high-risk surgical patients. *Chest* 1992; 102: 208–15.

3

Oxygen therapy

D. Kelly

Gas flow into the lung varies sinusoidally. The flow rate at its peak can vary enormously and reach values over $100 \, l/min$. However values of around $50–60 \, l/min$ are more common. The flow rate depends on several factors such as:

- patient size,
- muscle power and endurance,
- disease state,
- presence or absence of airflow obstruction,
- compliance of lung.

Intratracheal oxygen concentrations will only stay constant if the total gas flow is high enough to meet the demands of the patient at all points of the inspiratory cycle. Environmental air will be entrained to make up the shortfall if the delivery system fails to deliver a high enough flow.

Very few oxygen delivery systems meet these requirements and consequently intratracheal oxygen concentrations can vary enormously:

- both between patients using the same device,
- within the same patient using the same device but under different circumstances.

As the delivered flow rate is not high enough at some point during inspiration, air is entrained which dilutes the actual FiO_2 as Table 3.1 illustrates.

Delivery devices

Nasal catheters

Can be single or double pronged. The single catheters are more recent and are better tolerated due to a foam collar around their distal end. Nasal catheters are

Table 3.1. O_2 concentrations prescribed compared with O_2 concentrations delivered to trachea

| Apparatus | % O_2 delivered | % in trachea | | |
		Quiet breathing	Normal breathing	Hyperventilation
Face mask with	44	39.5	32.7	26
nebuliser at 10 l/min	60	53.4	50.3	41
	100	62.7	52	42
Face mask with	44	41.1	34.2	29.1
nebuliser at 15 l/min	60	52.5	46.1	40.1
	100	68.1	54	50.2
Venturi mask	24	23.1	22	21
at 4 l/min	28	24.2	23	21.4
Venturi mask	35	32.3	30	26.2
at 8 l/min	40	36.4	33.1	29.4

Adapted with permission from Gibson RL, Comer PB, Beckham RW, Mcgraw CP. Actual tracheal oxygen concentrations with commonly used oxygen equipment. *Anesthesiology* 1976; 44: 73.

better tolerated by patients and are more likely to be kept on. However, as can be seen from Table 3.1, the intratracheal FiO_2 varies with gas flow rate and patients' inspiratory flows.

Low-flow masks

Masks such as the Hudson rely on the entrainment of air around the mask and through holes in the mask to meet the patients demand for gas and as explained earlier this can vary enormously. The higher the inspiratory flow rate, the more air is entrained and the lower the inspired FiO_2.

Low-flow masks with reservoirs

Adding a reservoir for oxygen to these masks diminishes the amount of air that needs to be entrained to match the inspired flow rates and consequently the FiO_2 is higher. Oxygen has to be supplied at a high enough rate to keep the reservoir bag inflated. If this is achieved then the FiO_2 can be as high as 85%.

High-flow masks

These masks entrain air using the oxygen supply as a jet stream. The fast moving gas imparts energy to the static gas, that is air and some of this gas is dragged along with the faster stream. These masks were traditionally known as venturi masks although it is not strictly a venturi effect which entrains the air [1]. The oxygen concentration is preset if the oxygen flows to the mask are set correctly. These masks are more likely to provide a more reliable intratracheal oxygen concentration. However if the inspiratory flow rates are high even these delivery systems will not meet the needs of the patient and the intratracheal FiO_2 will be lower than prescribed.

T-pieces

These are connected to endotracheal or tracheostomy tubes and are supplied with humidified air and oxygen from a variable entrainment device. At the higher oxygen concentrations the total gas flow is much less and dilution of the inspired FiO_2 from the open end of the T-piece can be considerable. This can be reduced by adding a length of tubing to this open end which will then act as a reservoir of oxygen enriched air.

Constant positive airway pressure

This refers to CPAP. These systems aim to maintain the airway pressure positive relative to atmospheric pressure at all phases of the respiratory cycle. They do this by utilising expiratory valves which raise the pressure and either high-flow rates or a mixture of high-flow rates and a pressurised reservoir to minimise the fluctuations in pressure during the respiratory cycle. The work of breathing is minimised by keeping the degree of pressure fluctuation to a minimum. In order to maintain the system pressure it is important to minimise leakage. Tight fitting face masks are mandatory and avoiding pressure effects from these can be difficult. Owing to the closed nature of these systems and high gas flows utilised the FiO_2 is a much more reliable predictor of intratracheal oxygen concentrations.

Benefits of CPAP

- A predictable FiO_2.
- An increase in FRC.

- A reduction in the work of breathing because the increase in lung volume moves the lung to a more favourable part of its pressure volume curve.
- A reduction in pulmonary vascular resistance secondary to the improvement in lung volume and relief of hypoxaemia.

Disadvantages of CPAP

- It increases mean intrathoracic pressure which reduces venous return to the heart.
- It requires a certain amount of technical expertise to assemble the circuit correctly.
- The high-gas flows are difficult to humidify.
- The tight fitting face masks are sometimes poorly tolerated and cause pressure effects.

Hypoxic drive

During an exacerbation of chronic obstructive pulmonary disease (COPD) ventilatory drive can be four times normal [2]. Administering oxygen will reduce the drive but it does not return to normal and remains elevated [3]. The reduction in drive however will lead to a rise in the $PaCO_2$. If this is clinically significant then consideration should be given to some form of ventilatory support. A saturation of 90% should be aimed for. This will avoid most of the consequences of hypoxaemia without reducing the respiratory drive unduly. However, some patients with COPD will develop CO_2 narcosis when given oxygen therapy, even at low concentrations. This may sometimes be managed by reducing the concentration of inspired oxygen. Otherwise, Doxapram may produce a slight and temporary improvement in blood gases in some patients. Ventilation, by invasive and non-invasive means, is the only other reasonable alternative at present.

It should be borne in mind that a hypoxaemic arrest is much more damaging than a hypercapnic respiratory arrest.

Oxygen toxicity

Oxygen toxicity in critically ill patients is perhaps controversial but there is *no* doubt that in certain situations an excess of oxygen is toxic (before discussing oxygen toxicity one must not forget other hazards of high concentrations of oxygen, e.g. fire hazard).

In general, clinical evidence for oxygen toxicity revolves around three situations:

(1) *Oxygen convulsions (the Paul Bert effect)*
    Exposure to oxygen at greater than 2 atmospheres of pressure may cause convulsions. The mechanisms are unclear.
(2) *Retrolental fibroplasia (RLF)*
    The observation that hyperoxia is the major aetiological factor in the above condition has led to tight control of oxygen therapy in neonates. In rare cases a similar pathology can occur in adults.
(3) *Pulmonary oxygen toxicity of major relevance to intensive care unit (ICU) therapy*
    There are considerable problems in investigating pulmonary oxygen toxicity, not least in distinguishing between the effects of hyperoxia and of the pulmonary pathology requiring ventilation. Many of the studies demonstrating oxygen toxicity were done on animals or human volunteers.

Certainly breathing 100% oxygen produces:

- slight respiratory depression;
- painful tracheitis;
- mild depression of both heart rate and cardiac output;
- constriction of blood vessels;
- with prolonged inhalation, depression of red blood cells (RBC) formation;
- reduced secretion of surfactant;
- capillary endothelium permeability may also be increased leading to interstitial oedema;
- absorption atelectasis due to loss of nitrogen "splinting" small airways blocked by secretions.

In the 1940s it became accepted that the threshold for safety was an exposure to an inspired concentration of 60% oxygen. However, there is evidence that pulmonary toxicity may be related to high PaO_2 rather than inspired oxygen. During manned spaceflight, exposure to 100% oxygen at 0.3 atmospheres of pressure produces no great problems.

Thus it is suggested that, at least in part, the mechanism of pulmonary damage in patients requiring high inspired concentrations of oxygen may be the associated ventilatory manoeuvres required for patients with significant pulmonary pathology, that is the high pressures, shearing forces and high lung volumes generated.

In addition, some of the postulated harmful effects may be due to toxic oxygen free radicals. It has been suggested that a stepwise increase in FiO_2 (as is normally seen in the face of deteriorating gas exchange) results in the stimulation of protective enzymes, for example superoxide dismutase which "mop up" the free radicals, thus preventing many of the harmful effects [4]. Certainly there must be some protective mechanism at work or no patient ventilated with 100% oxygen should recover (and some eventually do).

Another problem is that there are some drugs whose ability to cause alveolitis is enhanced by a high oxygen environment. Bleomycin is the best known but there are a number of reports implicating amiodarone in acute pulmonary toxicity when the lung is exposed to an increased FiO_2 [5]. In these circumstances the inspired oxygen should be kept as low as possible.

Conclusion

- Hyperoxia may produce harmful pulmonary effects, but it is very difficult to separate these effects from the effects of the pathology which necessitates the high FiO_2 in the first place or the associated mechanical ventilation.
- It is obviously sensible to limit the FiO_2 where possible (oxygen should be treated as any other drug with the correct dose being administered and unnecessary overdose avoided) to that producing the minimal acceptable PO_2.
- However, there is no excuse for allowing a patient to become hypoxic for fear of the risk of oxygen toxicity.

FURTHER READING

Murphy R, Mackway-Jones K, Sammy I, Driscoll P, Gray A et al. Emergency oxygen therapy for the breathless patient. Guidelines prepared by North West Oxygen Group. *Emerg Med J* 2001; 18: 421–3.

Powell JF, Menon DK, Jones JG. The effects of hypoxaemia and recommendations for postoperative oxygen therapy. *Anaesthesia* 1996; 51: 769–72.

REFERENCES

1. Scacci R. Air entrainment masks: jet mixing is how they work; the Bernoulli and venturi principles are how they don't. *Respir Care* 1979; 24: 928.
2. Aubier M, Murciano D, Fournier M, Milil-Emili J, Pariente R, Derenne J. Central respiratory drive in acute respiratory failure of patients with chronic obstructive pulmonary disease. *Am Rev Respir Dis* 1980; 122: 191–9.

3. Schmidt G, Hall J. Assessment and management of patients with COPD in the emergent setting. *J Am Med Assoc* 1989; 261: 3444–53.

4. Crapo JD, Barry BE, Foscue HA. Structural and biochemical changes in rat lungs occurring during exposures to lethal and adaptive doses of oxygen. *Am Rev Respir Dis* 1980; 112: 123–8.

5. Donica SK, Paulsen AW, Simpson BR et al. Danger of amiodarone therapy and elevated oxygen concentrations in mice. *Am J Cardiol* 1996; 77: 109–10.

4

Central venous access

T. Owen

Over 200,000 Central venous catheters (CVC's) are inserted in the UK each year [1] and many of these are either inserted in, or cared for in the intensive care setting. Therefore a comprehensive knowledge of any complications and methods of minimising these complications are essential for the intensive care physician.

Indications

The indications are as follows:

- haemodynamic monitoring,
- intravenous infusion of fluids,
- intravenous infusion of drugs (e.g. inotropes, antibiotics),
- total parenteral nutrition (TPN),
- renal replacement therapy,
- intravenous access in patients with poor peripheral access (e.g. IV drug abusers).

Sites used for insertion

Sites used for central venous cannulation include:

- internal jugular vein (IJV),
- subclavian vein (SV),
- femoral vein (FV),
- external jugular vein,

- axillary vein,
- peripherally-inserted central catheter (PICC).

The first three of the above are the most commonly used, and this chapter will concentrate mainly on these. The fact that there is such a choice of sites suggests that there is not one site that is significantly better for CVC insertion than any other. Indeed each one has its own advantages and disadvantages, and choosing which site to use is also discussed in this chapter.

Insertion technique: landmark or ultrasound?

The standard technique for CVC placement is using the "landmark" method – the relationship of the chosen vein to known anatomical landmarks is used to guide the needle in the right direction. However this is now changing with the increasing use of ultrasound guidance to aid insertion. The recent National Institute for Clinical Excellence (NICE) guidelines on use of ultrasound guidance for CVC placement [1] have caused considerable controversy amongst both anaesthetists and intensivists [2–4].

The NICE recommendations are as follows:

- 2-D imaging ultrasound guidance is the preferred method for CVC insertion in the IJV in elective situations.
- 2-D imaging ultrasound guidance should be considered in most clinical circumstances, elective or emergency.
- Those using 2-D imaging ultrasound guidance should be appropriately trained to achieve competence.
- Audio-guided Doppler ultrasound guidance not recommended.

The potential advantages of the use of ultrasound-guided cannulation include:

- *Identification of anatomical variations in vein position and vein thrombosis*: studies have shown that the IJV does not follow the traditional landmarks, with abnormal anatomy or thrombosis seen in up to 10–20% of patients [5–7], even more commonly in some subgroups [8, 9].
- *Fewer failed catheter placements*: this can lead to potentially critical delays in instigation of treatment.
- *Fewer attempts to pass catheter*: it has been shown that the risk of complications increases with the number of attempts required to pass the CVC [10].

- *Avoidance of arterial puncture and other immediate complications.*
- *Less time taken*: as fewer failed placements and fewer attempts required.
- *Cost-effective*: due to less time and avoiding the economic impact of treating complications.

NICE commissioned a meta-analysis by Hind et al [11] to "assess the evidence for the clinical effectiveness of US-guided central venous cannulation" which looked at five outcomes: failed catheter placement, complications from placement, failed first attempt at placement, number of attempts required and time to successful cannulation.

The results showed that US-guided cannulation was more effective than the landmark method in all five outcomes for IJV cannulation. Risk of failed catheter placement for subclavian and femoral approaches was also shown to be less with ultrasound guidance but from more limited evidence, so no recommendations were made for these approaches.

The cost-effectiveness of ultrasound guidance was assessed by use of an economic model that look into account initial outlay, maintenance, training and the cost savings of fewer complications. This suggested a saving of £2 per patient when ultrasound guidance was used.

Although the Royal College of Anaesthetists (RCA) were consulted at the draft stage of the report, many anaesthetists and intensivists remained critical of a number of areas of the guidelines:

- The meta-analysis included some unblinded and some under-powered trials.
- The quoted frequency of carotid puncture was considered not wholly accurate.
- Potential for de-skilling of trainees in the landmark approach.
- The potential medico-legal implications of not using ultrasound if one was available.
- The initial outlay required, and the validity of the analytical model used to show cost-effectiveness.

Many of these concerns were covered in an RCA statement [12] and a *British Journal of Anaesthesia* editorial [2], but the concerns still remain and ultrasound-guided cannulation is not yet the standard technique the Department of Health (DoH) would like it to be.

Further studies have been undertaken since the meta-analysis by Hind et al, with conflicting results. A prospective randomised trial compared IJV cannulation using anatomical landmarks or prepuncture ultrasound [13]. Pre-puncture ultrasound only improved complication and success rate in patients where respiratory jugular venodilation could not be identified. A prospective analysis by Martin et al [14] also goes against the use of ultrasound, showing no improvement in CVC placement by junior residents (whatever their year of training).

Two prospective analyses [15, 16] with 29 and 493 patients, respectively did however support the use of ultrasound, one claiming a change in management rate of 14% when ultrasound was used, and the other, using a two person technique showing a significant decrease in complication and failure rate when the "sonographer" was familiar with the method.

The axillary vein is also becoming more popular, being easier to visualise with ultrasound and having a lower complication rate than the subclavian approach [17].

It is clear then that the controversies surrounding the use of ultrasound guidance are set to continue. A recent postal survey of Scottish and Merseyside ICU's [18], with a 73% and 100% response respectively, showed that 65% of Scottish and all Merseyside ICU's used ultrasound only in difficult situations, most thought it took longer and about half were concerned about de-skilling of staff. Very little formal training was given in either region. However, the majority were planning to implement the NICE guidelines despite their reservations.

Complications of CVCs

Insertion of a CVC is not a benign procedure and is associated with complications that can cause considerable morbidity. Death due to a pneumothorax caused during CVC insertion has been reported. The following is one of numerous ways of classifying the complications associated with insertion and use of CVCs.

(1) Mechanical complications (6–19% of patients):
    (a) arterial puncture,
    (b) haematoma formation,
    (c) pneumothorax,
    (d) haemothorax,
    (e) nerve injury,
    (f) arrhythmias,
    (g) cardiac tamponade,
    (h) arterio-venous fistula,
    (i) air embolism,
(2) Failure of cannulation (1–35%);
(3) Malposition of CVC (5–37%);
(4) Thrombosis (2–40%);

Table 4.1. Frequency of mechanical complications at different insertion sites
From McGee et al [19]

Complication	Frequency		
	IJV	SV	FV
Arterial puncture	6.3–9.4	3.1–4.9	9.0–15.0
Haematoma	0.1–2.2	1.2–2.1	3.8–4.4
Haemothorax	0	0.4–0.6	0
Pneumothorax	0.1–0.2	1.5–3.1	0
Total	6.3–11.8	6.2–10.7	12.8–19.4

(5) Infective complications (5–26%):
   (a) local infection,
   (b) catheter colonisation,
   (c) catheter-related blood stream infection (CR-BSI).

Mechanical complications

Table 4.1 summarises the frequency of the main mechanical complications at the three main insertion sites. As can be seen, the risk of complications is similar with SV and IJV and higher with the FV approach. The SV has the lowest risk of arterial puncture but the greatest risk of pneumo/haemothorax, whilst the IJV has a lower rate of pneumo/haemothorax, but a higher risk of arterial puncture. The FV has no risk of pneumo/haemothorax but the highest risk of arterial puncture or haematoma.

The consequence of each complication is also different at each site. For example, arterial puncture can cause uncontrolled, concealed haemorrhage if occurring via the SV approach as the subclavian artery is relatively incompressible and may track into the pleural space. The same complication with the IJV approach can lead to cerebrovascular accidents (CVA) if there is severe carotid artery disease or even airway obstruction if a large haematoma were to form but it is however more compressible therefore much easier to control any bleeding.

Failure of cannulation

Failed cannulation, as well as being a blow to personal pride, can lead to considerable time consumption and potentially fatal delays in instigation in treatment of the patients underlying problems. More attempts at cannulation also increase the risks of mechanical complications [10]. There is also an economic cost.

Methods to minimise this risk include appropriate training in insertion techniques, correct choice of insertion site, correct positioning of patient and use of ultrasound-guided cannulation.

Malposition of CVC

CVC's are ideally positioned either in the superior vena cava (SV/IJV approaches) or thoracic inferior vena cava (FV approach). Insertion into the right atrium risks arrhythmias and erosion through the atrial wall leading to cardiac tamponade, whereas if it is not far enough in the risk of thrombosis is increased [20]. When checking the position on a chest X-ray, the tip should be level with the carina, which has been shown to be a consistent anatomical landmark in relation to the pericardial sac [21].

Placement of CVC's in the opposite subclavian or neck vein, axillary or even internal mammary vein is possible and this may require resiting of the CVC. It may also mean incorrect central venous pressure (CVP) measurements, delivery of irritant drugs to the peripheral circulation and subsequent inflammation or thrombosis.

According to one meta-analysis, malposition is significantly less common with the IJV approach than the SV approach [22] (5.3% versus 9.3%) though other studies could detect no difference or found the opposite [10, 22–24]. The FV approach appears to have the highest malposition rate, one study showing 17% of CVC's in the right atrium, and only 63% in the thoracic inferior vena cava [26].

Thrombosis

Thrombosis of CVC's is a frequent (<10–66%) complication, but is asymptomatic in two-thirds of cases. Although most studies in this area looked at long-term catheters in cancer patients, thrombosis occurred within the first 8 days in around 64–98% of those in whom thrombosis developed [27]. The main sequelae of catheter thrombosis are:

- *Catheter-related sepsis*: the risk of catheter-related sepsis is 2.6 times greater in those catheters with thrombosis than those without [28].
- *Pulmonary embolism*: seen in 7–31% of patients, of which half are asymptomatic. They are not usually fatal [27, 28].
- *Postphlebitic syndrome*: seen in 15–35%, though the long-term consequence of this is not known [27].

Prevention of thrombosis can be achieved in the following ways:

- *Choice of insertion site*: the SV has the lowest frequency of thrombosis (1.9–10%), with IJV and SV catheter thrombosis much higher (20–40%) [22, 26–28].
- *Position of tip*: thrombosis is less common when the CVC tip is placed in the distal superior vena cava rather than proximal [20, 27].
- *Anticoagulation*: the use of low molecular weight heparin (LMWH) or low dose warfarin has been shown to decrease the incidence of catheter-related thrombosis [27].

Infective complications

Catheter-related sepsis is a major cause of morbidity and mortality in ICU patients, and is the most common cause of hospital-acquired bacteraemia. As stated earlier catheter-related infection is generally divided as follows:

- *Local infection*: presents as local inflammation or pus formation around the site of insertion.
- *Catheter colonisation*: can be defined as greater than 15 colony-forming units (CFU's) from culture of either the catheter tip or subcutaneous portion of the catheter.
- *CR-BSI*: culture of the same organism from the catheter and from blood taken from a peripheral site.

Pathogenesis of CR-BSI

Infections can develop in one of three ways:

- *Migration from insertion site*: spread from the insertion site along the catheter track is responsible for most cases of early (<10 days) CR-BSI.
- *Contamination of catheter hubs*: this generally causes CR-BSI in catheters that have been inserted for longer periods.
- *Seeding of catheter from distant location*: a focus of infection elsewhere in the body can occasionally cause CR-BSI.

The organisms responsible include:

- coagulase-negative staphylococci (32–41%),
- *Staphylococcus aureus* (18–31%),

- Gram-negative bacilli (10–18%),
- yeasts (9–11%),
- pseudomonas (4–6%),
- Entero/Streptococci (3–14%).

Prevention of CR-BSI

The most recent guidelines for prevention of catheter-related infections are from the DoH in 2001 [30] and US equivalent in 2002 [31]. There is however continued research into new methods of prevention published on a regular basis. A brief summary of the recommendations from these guidelines, together with more recent research, is summarised as follows:

- *Education*: Ensuring that all staff are aware and are trained in procedures to decrease the risk of catheter-related infection is well proven, as are the use of infection-control teams [31].
- *Site of insertion*: Despite a lack of randomised studies, the SV approach is generally excepted as at lowest risk of developing catheter-related infection, while the FV is the site most likely [29–31]. Use of peripheral venous catheters or PICC's will result in a much lower risk of infection.
- *Aseptic technique*: Use of maximal barrier precautions during insertion (cap, mask, sterile gown, sterile gloves and large sterile drape) decreases the risk of infection [30, 31].
- *Skin antisepsis*: 2% chlorhexidine gluconate has been shown to be more effective at preventing catheter colonisation than both povidine-iodine and 70% alcohol [31].
- *Catheter site dressings*: No difference has been shown between transparent and gauze dressings [31]. A logical approach would be to use gauze dressings if there was any ooze or bleeding after initial insertion and then replace with a transparent dressing so that the site could be observed for signs of infection without further disturbance. One study has shown a decrease in CR-BSI with the use of chlorhexidine-impregnated sponge dressing [32].
- *Antimicrobial/antiseptic impregnated catheters*: CVC's coated externally with chlorhexidine and silver sulfadiazine decrease risk of CR-BSI in short-term catheters [33], but are ineffective in the longer term as would be expected according to the pathogenesis described previously. Minocycline/rifampin impregnated CVC's are coated both internally and externally, and are effective

in preventing CR-BSI for up to 30 days and appear cost-effective [33]. An as yet unproven concern is that of potential antimicrobial resistance.

- *Single-lumen versus multi-lumen catheters*: The requirement for multi-lumen catheters on intensive therapy/treatment unit (ITU) far outweigh the few studies that suggest an increased risk of infection.
- *Antibiotic prophylaxis*: No convincing evidence for this has been found [31].
- *Anticoagulant prophylaxis*: As discussed earlier, thrombosis has been shown to increase risk of infection. Most ITU patients have indications for LMWH and there is enough evidence to suggest it may well decrease the risk of catheter-related infection [33].
- *Routine replacement of CVC*: There is no evidence that routine replacement of CVC's either at a new site or by guide-wire exchange reduces the risk of catheter-related infection [30, 31].
- *Silver iontophoretic device*: May be effective but not proven [33].
- *Iodinated alcohol-containing catheter hub*: Evidence not convincing, though a povidine-iodine impregnated sponge over the hub may be effective [33].
- *Antimicrobial locks*: Vancomycin has been used in long-term catheters with some success, but routine use on ITU inadvisable due to risk of developing Vancomycin resistant Enterococci [33].
- *Silver impregnated subcutaneous cuff*: May prevent CR-BSI for first 10 days [33].

Management of suspected CR-BSI

Diagnosis

Infection in an ITU patient can be from many sources, of which a CVC must always be considered, however well the above recommendations have been adhered to. There is unfortunately no quick and easy way to identify whether a CVC is the source of infection or not. An ideal approach would let the diagnosis or exclusion of a CR-BSI be achieved without the need for removal of the catheter thereby reducing risks of new catheter placement.

At present, the most common method of diagnosing a CR-BSI is by culture of the catheter tip (or subcutaneous portion of the CVC) along with a blood culture from a peripheral site; CR-BSI being assumed if the same organism is grown from both. This results however in many catheters being removed unnecessarily.

The simplest approach that would avoid CVC removal involves simultaneous blood cultures from the CVC and a peripheral site. If the time difference to a positive culture between the two is <2 h this would suggest the CVC as the source of infection and has specificity and sensitivity >90% [34].

Treatment

If a CVC is thought to be infected and diagnosis is uncertain (a not uncommon problem), various different methods of treatment have been suggested:

- *Removal +/- resiting of CVC*: This is the treatment of choice if there is obvious exit site infection, if it is no longer required or if there is severe sepsis with no obvious cause. If there are only mild signs of sepsis however, this method is not the only option.
- *Rewiring of CVC*: The DoH guidelines recommend this if there are no signs of local infection or proven CR-BSI. The CVC should be removed if subsequent microbiology proves positive for CR-BSI. A systematic review did show a (non-significant) trend towards increased risk of catheter-related infection with this technique [35].
- *Antibiotics without CVC removal*: one study has suggested that CR-BSI caused by coagulase-negative *staphylococcus* can be treated without removal of CVC [36], though other organisms will persist if the CVC is not removed.

The antibiotic of choice depends partly on local policy and partly on the clinical status of the patient. First-line treatment is generally flucloxacillin or a first-generation cephalosporin unless they are high-risk for methicillin resistant *Staphylococcus aureus* (MRSA) or are penicillin allergic in which case a glycopeptide would be appropriate.

Which insertion site to use?

As stated previously the three most common sites used for insertion are the FV, SV, IJV. When deciding which site to use the following questions need to be considered:

- *How good is the access to the site?*
  Obese patients may well have difficult access to the IJV due to obscuring of landmarks, whilst their groin regions may often be infected, excluding femoral catheterisation. Patients may have deformity due to trauma, previous surgery or congenital disease that will make a particular site less favourable.
- *What is the frequency of complications at that site?*
  As described earlier in the chapter, there is an important variation in frequency of different complications at different sites.
- *Which complications do you most want to avoid?*
  Even if a complication is less common at one site, the potential for harm if it does occur could be much greater than at other sites. Therefore patient factors

that may make a particular complication much more serious should have taken into consideration. Examples include pneumothorax in a patient with severe respiratory failure, subclavian artery puncture in the coagulopathic patient, carotid artery puncture in a patient with severe carotid atherosclerosis and infection in a neutropenic patient.

- *Why is a CVC required?*
  If central venous access is required solely for TPN, a PICC may be more appropriate to minimise the risk of infection. If required for haemodialysis the SV can sometimes be problematic as kinking under the clavicle may prevent adequate flow rates.
- *How experienced are you in insertion at different sites?*
  If not trained or experienced in a particular approach, then this approach should be avoided, although Lefrant et al did not identify operator's training as predictive of immediate complications or failure [9].

It is clear from these points that choice of site must be made on a case-by-case basis, taking into account both technical and patient factors.

A good general approach for the "typical" ICU patient, in whom central venous access is likely to be required for a considerable time, could be as follows:

- If appropriately experienced, and there are no patient contra-indications (coagulopathy, respiratory compromise etc.), then the subclavian approach should be the first choice as this has the lowest risk of infection. Use of the lateral approach may well help in visualisation of the vein with ultrasound [17].
- If the SV approach fails or is thought inappropriate then the IJV would be preferable, but the FV could be used if risks of the IJV were considered unacceptable (unable to lie flat, severe carotid disease, respiratory compromise etc.).
- Consider alternative sites such as axillary, external jugular and PICC's.

FURTHER READING

Cicalini S, Palmieri F, Petrosillo N. Clinical review: new technologies for prevention of intravascular catheter-related infections. *Crit Care* 2004; 8: 157–62.

Managing bloodstream infections associated with intravascular catheters. *Drug Therap Bull* 2001; 39(10): 75–80.

National Institute for Clinical Excellence. *Guidance on the Use of Ultrasound Guiding Devices for Placing Central Venous Catheters.* Technology Appraisal Guidance No. 49, September 2002.

Timsit JF. What is the best site for central venous catheter insertion in critically ill patients? *Crit Care* 2003; 7: 397–9.

REFERENCES

1. National Institute for Clinical Excellence. *Guidance on the Use of Ultrasound Guiding Devices For Placing Central Venous Catheters.* Technology Appraisal Guidance No. 49, September 2002.

2. Scott DHT. "It's NICE to see in the dark". *Br J Anaesth* 2003; 90(3): 269–72.

3. Scott DHT. "The king of the blind extends his frontiers". *Br J Anaesth* 2004; 93(2): 175–7.

4. White SM. Correspondence. *Anaesthesia* 2003; 58: 295–6.

5. Denys BG, Uretsky BF. Anatomical variations of internal jugular vein location: impact on central venous access. *Crit Care Med* 1991; 19(12): 1516–9.

6. Gordon AC, Saliken JC, Johns D, Owen R et al. US-guided puncture of the internal jugular vein: complications and anatomic considerations. *J Vasc Interv Radiol* 1998; 9(2): 333–8.

7. Caridi JG, Hawkins Jr IF, Wiechmann BN, Pevarski DJ et al. Sonographic guidance when using the right internal jugular vein for central vein access. *Am J Roentgenol* 1998; 171(5): 1259–63.

8. Lin BS, Kong CW, Tarng DC, Huang TP et al. Anatomical variation of the internal jugular vein and its impact on temporary haemodialysis vascular access: an ultrasonic survey in uraemic patients. *Nephrol Dial Transplant* 1998; 13: 134–8.

9. Benter T, Teichgraber UK, Kluhs L, Papadopoulos S et al. Anatomical variations in the internal jugular veins of cancer patients affecting central venous access. Anatomical variation of the internal jugular vein. *Ultraschall Med* 2001; 22(1): 23–6.

10. Lefrant JY, Muller L, De La Coussaye JE, Prudhomme M et al. Risk factors of failure and immediate complication of subclavian vein catheterisation in critically ill patients. *Intens Care Med* 2002; 28: 1036–41.

11. Hind D, Calvert N, McWilliams R, Davidson A et al. Ultrasonic locating devices for central venous cannulation: meta-analysis. *Br Med J* 2003; 327: 361.

12. NICE Technology Appraisal. Guidance No. 49 on the use of ultrasound locating devices for placing central venous catheters. Comment from the Royal College of Anaesthetists. http://www.rcoa.ac.uk

13. Hayashi H, Amano M. Does ultrasound imaging before puncture facilitate internal jugular vein cannulation? Prospective randomised trial comparison with landmark-guided puncture in ventilated patients. *J Cardiothoracic Vasc Anaesth* 2002; 16(5): 572–5.

14. Martin MJ, Husain FA, Piesman M, Mullenix PS et al. Is routine ultrasound guidance for central line placement beneficial? A prospective analysis. *Curr Surg* 2004; 61(1): 71–4.

15. Gann M, Sardi A. Improved results using ultrasound guidance for central venous access. *Am Surg* 2003; 69(12): 1104–7.

16. Mey U, Glasmacher A, Hahn C, Gorschluter M et al. Evaluation of an US-guided technique for central venous access via the internal jugular vein in 493 patients. *Support Care Cancer* 2004; 11(3): 148–55.

17. Sharma A, Bodenham AR, Mallick A. Ultrasound-guided infraclavicular axillary vein cannulation for central venous access. *Br J Anaesth* 2004; 93(2): 188–92.

18. Sundaram R, Smyth CCA, Noble JS. Ultrasound guidance for central venous access – impact of NICE guidance on current practice. *J Int Care Soc* 2004; 5(2): 62–3.

19. McGee DC, Gould MK. Preventing complications of central venous catheterisation. *N Engl J Med* 2003; 348: 1123–33.

20. Cadman A, Lawrance JA, Fitzsimmons L, Spencer-Shaw A et al. To clot or not to clot? That is the question in central venous catheters. *Clin Radiol* 2004; 59(4): 349–55.

21. Albrecht K, Nave H, Breitmeier D, Panning B et al. Applied anatomy of the superior vena cava – the carina as a guide to central venous catheter placement. *Br J Anaesth* 2004; 92: 75–77.

22. Ruesch S, Walder B, Tramer MR. Complications of central venous catheters: internal jugular versus subclavian access – a systematic review. *Crit Care Med* 2002; 30: 454–60.

23. Mansfield PF, Hohn DC, Fornage BD, Gregurich MA et al. Complications and failures of subclavian vein catheterization. *N Eng J Med* 1994; 331: 1735–8.

24. Iovino F, Pittiruti M, Buononato M, Lo Schiavo F. Central venous catheterization: complications of different placements. *Ann Chir* 2001; 126: 1001–6.

25. Gladwin MT, Slonim A, Landucci DL, Gutierrez DC et al. Cannulation of the IJV: is post-procedural chest radiography always necessary? *Crit Care Med* 1999; 27: 700–7.

26. Durbec O, Viviand X, Potie F, Vialet R et al. A prospective evaluation of the use of femoral venous catheters in critically ill adults. *Crit Care Med* 1997; 25: 1986–9.

27. Kuter DJ. Thrombotic complications of central venous catheters in cancer patients. *The Oncologist* 2004; 9(2): 207–16.

28. Timsit JF, Farkas JC, Boyer JM, Martin JB et al. Central vein catheter – related thrombosis in intensive care patients. *Chest* 1998; 114: 207–13.

29. Merrer J, De Jonge B, Golliot et al. Complications of femoral and subclavian catheterization in critically ill patients: a randomized controlled trial. *JAMA* 2001; 286:700–7

30. Pratt RJ et al. Guidelines for preventing infections associated with the insertion and maintenance of central venous catheters. *J Hosp Inf* 2001; 47(Suppl): S47–67.

31. Centres for Disease Control and Infection. *Guidelines for the Prevention of Intravascular Catheter-Related Infections.* MMWR August 9, 2002; 51(RR-10): 1–29.

32. Garland JS, Alex CP, Mueller CD et al. A randomised control trial comparing povidine–iodine to a chlorhexidine gluconate impregnated dressing for prevention of central venous catheter infections in neonates. *Paediatrics* 2001; 107: 1431–7.

33. Cicalini S, Palmieri F, Petrosillo N. Clinical review: new technologies for prevention of intravascular catheter-related infections. *Crit Care* 2004; 8: 157–62.

34. Blot F et al. Diagnosis of catheter-related bacteraemia: a prospective comparison of the time to positivity of hub-blood to peripheral-blood cultures. *Lancet* 1999; 354: 1071–7.

35. Cook D et al. Central venous catheter replacement strategies: a systematic review of the literature. *Crit Care Med* 1997; 25: 1417–24.

36. Raad I et al. Impact of central venous catheter removal on the recurrence of catheter-related coagulase-negative staphylococcal bacteraemia. *Infect Control Hosp Epid* 1992; 13: 215–21.

5

Fluid therapy in ICU

I. McConachie

Fluid therapy in ICU

Maintenance of normal hydration and electrolyte composition is essential in intensive care unit (ICU) patients.

"Volume loading" is an important principle of cardiovascular management and is the cornerstone of management of surgical and trauma patients.

Conversely, overhydration may be a factor in poor outcome from ICU care.

Body fluid compartments

Water comprises approximately 60% of body weight. Approximately two-thirds of this is intracellular fluid and the remainder extracellular fluid. Extracellular fluid is mainly interstitial fluid with only 15–20% consisting of blood and plasma. In critically ill patients there are often considerable increases in extracellular fluid.

In order to understand the principles of fluid therapy one must be aware of which body fluid compartment one is wishing to maintain or resuscitate, for example:

- Intracellular space – deficits mainly H_2O.
- Interstitial space – deficits H_2O and electrolytes.
- Intravascular space – deficits of plasma volume and/or red blood cell (RBC).
- Surgical and trauma patients may suffer losses of so-called "third space" fluids (called because it represents a third extracellular space) due to tissue fluid sequestration of interstitial fluid (i.e. H_2O and electrolytes).

Fluid therapy involves the use of the following:

Crystalloids

- H_2O with electrolytes approximating the composition and osmolality of plasma.
- Crystalloids redistribute through the extracellular fluids and, therefore, only about 20% of the volume administered will remain in the intravascular space.
- Hartmann's solution (compound Ringer's lactate) is closest in electrolyte composition to that of plasma and interstitial fluid. It has a pH of 6.7. Osmolality slightly reduced compared to plasma. The administration of lactate containing fluids in shock was once considered controversial but does not seem to worsen acidosis.
- 0.9% Saline ("normal" saline) contains 150 mmol/l of both Na and Cl: that is, slightly increased Na but greatly increased Cl cf. plasma and interstitial fluid. Excess use can be associated with hyperchloraemic acidosis (see below) and hypernatraemia. It has a pH of 5.7.
- Dextrose 5%. No electrolytes, just dextrose and H_2O. Usually considered with the crystalloids but technically is not one because it contains no Na. It has a pH of 4.5. Its osmolality is lower than the other common crystalloids. May be useful in the Na overloaded patient to replace H_2O but otherwise plays little role in ICU therapy. Dextrose 5% is *not* a resuscitation fluid.
- Dextrose 4%/0.18% saline is commonly used as 2–3 l/day will approximate the body's requirement for H_2O and Na. This is superficially attractive as a maintenance fluid for the young and fit but probably not in critically ill patients. In addition, excessive use may place the elderly at risk of hyponatraemia due to its slightly reduced osmolality compared to plasma.

Saline-induced metabolic acidosis and choice of crystalloid

As little as 2 l saline per hour will produce acidosis in healthy young patients undergoing surgery [1]. The exact significance of this with regard to outcome is debatable.

- Compared with 0.9% saline, volume resuscitation with Hextend (starch with balanced electrolyte solution) was associated with less metabolic acidosis and longer survival in an experimental animal model of septic shock [2].
- In elderly surgical patients, the use of crystalloids and colloids containing balanced electrolyte solutions prevented the development of hyperchloremic metabolic acidosis and improved indices of gastric mucosal perfusion compared with saline-based crystalloid and colloid fluids [3].

Thus many would consider "balanced" Hartmann's solution to be superior to "unbalanced" saline for use as a routine fluid. However:

- The infusion of large volumes of Ringer's lactate solution during major surgery leads to postoperative mild hyponatraemia and respiratory acidosis [4].
- Large volumes of lactated Ringer's solution administered to volunteers produced small transient reductions in serum osmolality. Large volumes of sodium chloride did not change osmolality but resulted in lower pH [5].

In conclusion, excessive volumes of any one fluid may be associated with problems.

For a full account of the effects of electrolytes on acid–base balance (see Further reading).

Colloids

- H_2O, electrolytes and other particles (synthetic or natural) large enough to remain in the intravascular space for several hours.
- Albumin solutions are natural colloids and are discussed in detail below.
- Synthetic colloids are mainly starches or gelatin compounds.

Starches

- Molecular weight varies but most starches have a clinical effect within the intravascular space of about 6 h. Anaphylaxis is rare.
- The starch particles are taken up by the reticuloendothelial system but long-term effects of their retention in the body are not known. Itching is a problem with the long lasting starches [6].
- Opinions differ regarding effects on coagulation – main effect is probably to promote a dilutional coagulopathy if large volumes are administered. With large volumes there may also be a reduction in Factor VIII levels and a similar effect on platelet function to Von Willebrand's disease.
- Pentastarch 10% is a fluid with a lower molecular weight than Hydroxyethyl starch – more readily broken down by the kidney and excreted. There was some initial enthusiasm that smaller starches such as Pentastarch may "plug" the leaks in the capillaries in sepsis and other conditions with increases in endothelial permeability. However, convincing evidence is lacking.

Gelatins

- Relatively cheap and widely used. The clinical effect within the intravascular space lasts 3–4 h.
- Overuse should be limited by fear of excessive haemodilution which can reduce DO_2 after an initial rise [7].
- Coagulation effects are from haemodilution only. Haemaccel contains calcium and therefore citrated blood should not be mixed in the same IV giving set.
- Allergic reactions are rare and usually mild.
- Gelatin fluids are derived from bovine collagen but are considered free from risk of transmission of prions associated with Bovine Spongiform Encephalitis (BSE).

Dextrans

- Dextrans contain polysaccharides. Higher-molecular-weight dextrans (dextran 70–70,000 Daltons weight) are effective plasma volume expanders.
- Some practitioners make use of their antithromboembolic and antisludging properties in situations where peripheral perfusion is compromised.
- In general, they are not routinely used in ICU because they interfere with crossmatching and large volumes may cause a coagulopathy.

Small volume resuscitation

An initial bolus of 20 ml/kg is often recommended as the initial fluid volume in resuscitation. Small volume resuscitation aims to achieve the same initial haemodynamic response with 4 ml/kg of fluid with, of course, advantages in terms of time requirements for infusion and storage space required.

- Commonest fluid studied has been 7.5% saline – significantly hypertonic.
- Acts by many mechanisms including redistribution of interstitial fluid to the intravascular space and decreased cellular swelling, and tissue oedema.
- Increased blood pressure (BP), cardiac index (CI), renal blood flow.
- Short-lived effect unless combined with colloid. Ultimately the interstitial fluid will have to be replaced.
- Main role has been in field resuscitation to "buy time" [8].
- Excessive use will lead to hypernatraemia.
- Due to the reduced tissue oedema, may be useful in head injuries [9].

Crystalloid versus colloid debate

There has been controversy over the best type of fluid for resuscitation (i.e. crystalloids or colloids). Part of the problem is the lack of studies showing a sufficiently clear superiority of one fluid type over another, sufficient to convert its opponents and without reasonable criticisms of study methodology. There are several problems with most of the available studies for example, different species, fluids, injuries, illnesses, complications studied [10].

It is not widely appreciated that many of the original US studies of crystalloids versus colloids in trauma patients were flawed. This was because most patients in both groups were given blood transfusions. In the US, patients are commonly given *whole* blood (as opposed to packed red cells in the UK) that is, both groups received colloid from the whole blood (i.e. there was no such thing as a pure crystalloid group).

In most studies there is probably a skewed distribution of severity of sickness with a large group of patients who will do all right whichever fluid is given and a smaller group of patients who will die regardless of which fluid is given. These patients may mask (statistically speaking) a group of patients in whom choice of fluid may be critical. This possibility has been seized upon by the colloid enthusiasts!

There are certain statements regarding the colloid/crystalloid controversy which can be made which are reasonably accepted by both groups:

- Crystalloids replace interstitial losses. Colloids are superior at replacing plasma volume deficits – more quickly and lasting longer – giving greater increases in CI and DO_2. Crystalloid administration may also produce such increases but approximately three times as much will be needed with consequent delays in achieving goals of resuscitation.
- Crystalloids are cheap. Colloids are more expensive. Many centres in the US use crystalloids almost exclusively. However it has been pointed out that whole blood may be a significant source of colloid in studies purporting to use no colloid.
- In most situations: for example, routine surgery both potentially give excellent results if appropriate amounts are used.
- Many studies show similar effects on respiratory function. Overdose of either may produce respiratory failure.
- Colloids do have specific if uncommon side effects such as allergic reactions and impaired coagulation.

- Overdose of crystalloids certainly cause dramatic peripheral oedema. The importance of this with regard to outcome is disputed but some concerns are discussed below.
- In recent years concerns have been raised that the overuse of colloid fluids may be associated with a worsening of renal function. This has been termed "hyper-oncotic acute renal failure". The original reports concerned the use of Dextrans (and at that time it was thought that there was either direct toxicity or accumulation in the renal tubules) but may be seen with *excess* use of all colloids especially if the patient has other renal risk factors or is dehydrated. The problem may be worse with use of colloids in large volumes or high molecular weights. The theory proposed is that the resultant high plasma colloid osmotic pressure counteracts opposing hydrostatic filtration pressure in the glomerulus.
- Many believe in the "Golden Hour" for resuscitation and that, therefore, speed of resuscitation is crucial. Therefore, when restoration of blood volume, cardiac output (CO) and tissue perfusion is urgent colloids may be preferable to crystalloid.

Most reasonable people do not take extreme positions in the debate. In most situations close monitoring especially with regard to fluid overload is more important than absolute choice of fluid.

However, recent systematic reviews have failed to uncover any survival benefit from the use of colloids [11, 12]. Indeed, there seems to be a slight survival benefit associated with the use of crystalloids compared with colloids in trauma patients.

In the first edition of this text colloids, on balance, were favoured over crystalloids for many situations – especially in resuscitation. The author acknowledges that the pendulum seems to be swinging in favour of more routine use of crystalloids. However, the most important points to remember are that:

- Anaemia is better tolerated than hypovolaemia.
- There is no doubt that the best replacement for major blood loss is blood.

Fluid maintenance strategies

- Fluid intake comes from total parenteral nutrition (TPN), enteral nutrition, colloids, crystalloids and medications especially antibiotics. Thermodilution CO measurements at 10 ml of fluid per measurement must not be forgotten.
- Losses come from urine, faeces especially diarrhoea, skin and lung evaporation (increases in fever), haemorrhage, third space losses, N/G drainage and fistulae.

Vascular fluid may be lost to the circulation in ICU patients due to increased capillary endothelium permeability ("leaky capillaries"). Humidified gases reduce the insensible lung H_2O losses in ventilated patients. Abnormal surgical losses for example, from fistulae, diarrhoea should be replaced with crystalloids.
- Hormonal changes promote Na and H_2O retention following surgery.
- Less well appreciated is that some drugs promote fluid retention – notably steroids.

Volume-loading strategies

- Hypovolaemia must be treated promptly to restore organ perfusion.
- The consequences of hypovolaemia may be more difficult to treat and carry a higher mortality than the consequences of overhydration.
- In haemorrhage or hypovolaemia, 20 ml/kg fluid bolus should be administered rapidly.
- A volume challenge for example 5 ml/kg of colloid is probably indicated in all cases of acute haemodynamic compromise.
- Inotropes can have disastrous consequences in the presence of hypovolaemia. (see chapter on Inotropes and vasopressors)
- Fluid administration with for example, colloid is best guided by a response of increasing stroke volume (SV) as a result of increasing pulmonary capillary wedge pressure (PCWP); that is, stop administering colloid when there is no further increase in SV with more fluid.
- In the absence of a pulmonary artery flotation catheters (PAFC), central venous pressure (CVP) trends can be useful (the absolute CVP is not always that helpful in ventilated patients) for example:
  - No increase in CVP and BP with fluid   → Give more fluid
  - Increase in CVP and BP, and then decrease → Give more fluid
  - Increase in CVP but no increase in BP then → Give no more fluid
  - Increase in CVP but decrease in BP then   → Give no more fluid
- Overloaded, oedematous patients may still need colloid boluses to maintain CO and filling pressures (i.e. the intravascular volume may still be low). The use of vasopressors to maintain filling pressures in such patients is controversial as splanchnic vasoconstriction may occur.
- Although difficult to prove, many specialists believe that colloids are better than crystalloids in oedematous patients with "leaky capillaries" – if only

because less volume will probably need to be given and, therefore, be available to "leak out".

- Short, large bore cannula give best flows for rapid volume loading.
- Generous fluid loading in many patients may be appropriate. For example, Mythen and Webb showed in high-risk surgical patients that fluid loading after induction of anaesthesia to a maximum SV led to a reduction of the incidence of low pHi from 50% to 10% [13].
- Using Doppler ultrasonography to measure CO, Singer showed that intraoperative volume loading increased SV and CO, resulted in a more rapid postoperative recovery and a reduced hospital stay in a study group of fractured neck of femur patients [14].
- This approach must be tempered with caution in the elderly or patients with known heart failure due to the potential risk of fluid overload precipitating pulmonary oedema. In these patients perioperative invasive monitoring may be indicated.

The vexed question of albumin

Albumin is a natural colloid derived from pooled human plasma which has been heat treated to prevent human immunodeficiency virus (HIV) and other viral transmission. There remain concerns about the possible transmission of the BSE prion by albumin administration.

The use of albumin solutions in ICU is controversial, relates to both fluid therapy and nutritional support, and merits discussion in some detail.

Until relatively recently albumin solutions were the only readily available colloid solution available in the USA.

Albumin solutions are still relatively expensive and scarce in many areas. One American study had difficulty with patient inclusion due to an actual shortage of albumin.

In ICU patients, albumin synthesis is reasonably well maintained but the vascular permeability to albumin increases and the effective volume of distribution is dramatically increased. In addition, albumin metabolism is also increased. Thus, albumin blood levels fall rapidly in critical illness and reflect the severity of illness, and mortality rather than nutritional status [15]. Trends in albumin levels predict the difficulty of weaning from mechanical ventilation [16].

Albumin levels are relatively insensitive to nutritional support.

Albumin blood levels improve as the underlying condition resolves, often accompanied by a spontaneous diuresis.

Proponents of the use of albumin justify its use by citing:

- Increases in colloid oncotic pressure (COP).
- Free radical scavenging, binding of drugs and toxic substances [17].
- Increased incidence of diarrhoea in hypoalbuminaemia.
- Albumin is a "natural colloid".
- If it is appropriate to replace low levels of for example, haemoglobin (Hb), electrolytes etc., why not albumin?

However, the plasma/tissue COP gradient remains relatively well maintained and, thus, numerous studies have failed to find a relationship between low albumin levels and pulmonary oedema. Most studies, for example, by Rubin [18], have failed to find benefits from albumin supplementation in terms of length of stay, outcome etc. despite significant increases in albumin levels. The only significant increase in the albumin group in all studies has been in costs!

A controversial systematic review of the use of albumin concluded that "there is no evidence that albumin administration reduces mortality in critically ill patients with hypovolaemia, burns, or hypoalbuminaemia and a strong suggestion that it may increase mortality. These data suggest that use of human albumin in critically ill patients should be urgently reviewed and that it should not be used outside the context of rigorously conducted, randomised controlled trials" [19]. Many believed the conclusions to be unjustified and there are significant concerns that the analysis was based on studies of the use of albumin in ICU in two distinct circumstances:

- Use in nutritional support/to maintain serum albumin levels.
- Use as a resuscitation fluid.

A landmark study from Australia [20] challenges the conclusions of the above review. Almost 7000 patients were studied comparing 4% albumin with saline for intravascular resuscitation. There were no differences in outcome at 28 days. Thus the most recent (and arguably strongest) evidence suggests that albumin is, at the very least, safe to give for fluid resuscitation (at least as safe as saline).

Nevertheless, in many ICUs the use of albumin has declined to virtually zero.

Problems of fluid overload

During critical illness many patients' weight increases, probably reflecting increased endothelial permeability as well as excessive administration of fluids.

This is associated with a poor outcome [21]. Whether removing or preventing this extra fluid which has accumulated as oedema fluid can *improve* this reduced outcome back to "normal" is less certain. Certainly, the balance of opinion for ventilated patients with acute respiratory distress syndrome (ARDS) is shifting towards "keeping the patient dry" (as long as organ perfusion is well maintained) [22]. In addition, a pilot study has suggested that at least 1 day of negative fluid balance by the 3rd day of ICU admission predicts improved chances of survival in patients with septic shock [23]. A controlled trial of "normal" fluid administration versus fluid administration aiming to avoid increases in patient weight in colorectal surgery patients showed a dramatic increase in survival and less complications in patients treated with less intravenous fluids so as not to gain weight [24].

Harmful effects of the extra fluid may include:

- Increased lung H_2O, reduced pulmonary compliance and impaired gas exchange.
- Ileus may be promoted due to oedema of the gut. In one study of patients undergoing major bowel surgery, a positive balance sufficient to cause a 3 kg weight gain after surgery delayed return of gastrointestinal function and prolonged hospital stay [25].
- Tissue oxygenation [26] and, by association, wound healing may be impaired by the tissue oedema associated with excessive crystalloid administration.

Thus it is important to watch intake closely and match to output where possible. Useful points are:

- Weighing the patient daily is important.
- Minimise fluids required to administer medications.
- Once patient is established on nutritional support may not require "routine" maintenance crystalloids.
- Dramatic weight gain should be resisted if necessary by the judicious use of low-dose diuretics *if* haemodynamically tolerated.

FURTHER READING

Griffel MI, Kaufman BS. Pharmacology of colloids and crystalloids. *Crit Care Clin* 1992; 8: 235–53.

Holte K, Sharrock NE, Kehlet H. Pathophysiology and clinical implications of perioperative fluid excess. *Br J Anaesth* 2002; 89: 622–32.

Sirker AA, Rhodes A, Grounds RM, Bennett ED. Acid-base physiology: the "traditional" and the "modern" approaches. *Anaesthesia* 2002; 57: 348–56.

Wade CE, Kramer GC, Grady JJ, Fabian TC, Younes RN. Efficacy of hypertonic 7.5% saline
and 6% dextran-70 in treating trauma: a meta-analysis of controlled clinical studies.
Surgery 1997; 122: 609–16.

REFERENCES

1. Scheingraber S, Rehm M, Sehmisch C, Finsterer U. Rapid saline infusion produces
    hyperchloremic acidosis in patients undergoing gynecologic surgery. *Anesthesiology*
    1999; 90: 1265–70.
2. Kellum JA. Fluid resuscitation and hyperchloremic acidosis in experimental sepsis:
    improved short-term survival and acid-base balance with Hextend compared with
    saline. *Crit Care Med* 2002; 30: 300–5.
3. Wilkes NJ, Woolf R, Mutch M, Mallett SV et al. The effects of balanced versus saline-
    based hetastarch and crystalloid solutions on acid-base and electrolyte status and gas-
    tric mucosal perfusion in elderly surgical patients. *Anesth Analg* 2001; 93: 811–6.
4. Takil A, Eti Z, Irmak P, Yilmaz Gogus F. Early postoperative respiratory acidosis after
    large intravascular volume infusion of lactated ringer's solution during major spine
    surgery. *Anesth Analg* 2002; 95: 294–8.
5. Williams EL, Hildebrand KL, McCormick SA, Bedel MJ. The effect of intravenous lac-
    tated Ringer's solution versus 0.9% sodium chloride solution on serum osmolality in
    human volunteers. *Anesth Analg* 1999; 88: 999–1003.
6. Morgan PW, Berridge JC. Giving long-persistent starch as volume replacement can
    cause pruritus after cardiac surgery. *Br J Anaesth* 2000; 85: 696–9.
7. Beards SC, Watt T, Edwards JD, Nightingale P, Farragher EB. Comparison of the
    hemodynamic and oxygen transport responses to modified fluid gelatin and heta-
    starch in critically ill patients: a prospective, randomized trial. *Crit Care Med* 1994;
    22: 600–5.
8. Mattox KL, Maningas PA, Moore EE, Mateer JR, Marx JA et al. Prehospital hypertonic
    saline/dextran infusion for post-traumatic hypotension. The U.S.A. Multicenter Trial.
    Ann Surg 1991; 213: 482–91.
9. Vassar MJ, Perry CA, Gannaway WL, Holcroft JW. 7.5% sodium chloride/dextran for
    resuscitation of trauma patients undergoing helicopter transport. *Arch Surg* 1991; 126:
    1065–72.
10. Gammage G. Crystalloid versus colloid: is colloid worth the cost? *Int Anesthesiol Clin*
    1987; 25: 37–60.
11. Schierhout G, Roberts I. Fluid resuscitation with colloid or crystalloid solutions
    in critically ill patients: a systematic review of randomised trials. *Br Med J* 1998; 316:
    961–4.
12. Choi PT, Yip G, Quinonez LG, Cook DJ. Crystalloids vs. colloids in fluid resuscitation: a
    systematic review. *Crit Care Med* 1999; 27: 200–10.

13. Mythen MG, Webb AR. Perioperative plasma volume expansion reduces the incidence of gut mucosal hypoperfusion during cardiac surgery. *Arch Surg* 1995; 130: 423–9.

14. Sinclair S, James S, Singer M. Intraoperative intravascular volume optimisation and length of hospital stay after repair of proximal femoral fracture: randomised controlled trial. *Br Med J* 1997; 315: 909–12.

15. McCluskey A, Thomas AN, Bowles BJ, Kishen R. The prognostic value of serial measurements of serum albumin concentrations in patients admitted to an intensive care unit. *Anaesthesia* 1996; 51: 724–7.

16. Sapijaszko MJ, Brant R, Sandham D, Berthiaume Y. Nonrespiratory predictor of mechanical ventilation dependency in intensive care unit patients. *Crit Care Med* 1996; 24: 601–7.

17. Emerson Jr TE. Unique features of albumin: a brief review. *Crit Care Med* 1989; 17: 690–4.

18. Rubin H, Carlson S, DeMeo M, Ganger D, Craig RM. Randomized, double blind study of intravenous human albumin in hypoalbuminaemic patients receiving total parenteral nutrition. *Crit care Med* 1997; 25: 249–52.

19. Cochrane Injuries Group Albumin Reviewers. Human albumin administration in critically ill patients: systematic review of randomised controlled trials. *Br Med J* 1998; 317: 235–40.

20. Finfer S, Bellomo R, Boyce N, French J et al. A comparison of albumin and saline for fluid resuscitation in the intensive care unit. *N Engl J Med* 2004; 350: 2247–56.

21. Lowell JA, Schifferdecker C, Driscoll DF, Benotti PN, Bistrian BR. Postoperative fluid overload: not a benign problem. *Crit Care Med* 1990; 18: 728–33.

22. Schuster DP. Fluid management in ARDS: "keep them dry" or does it matter? *Intens Care Med* 1995; 21: 101–3.

23. Alsous F, Khamiees M, DeGirolamo A, Amoateng-Adjepong Y et al. Negative fluid balance predicts survival in patients with septic shock: a retrospective pilot study. *Chest* 2000; 117: 1749–54.

24. Brandstrup B, Tonnesen H, Beier-Holgersen R, Hjortso E et al. Effects of intravenous fluid restriction on postoperative complications: comparison of two perioperative fluid regimens: a randomized assessor-blinded multicenter trial. *Ann Surg* 2003; 238: 641–8.

25. Lobo DN, Bostock KA, Neal KR, Perkins AC et al. Effect of salt and water balance on recovery of gastrointestinal function after elective colonic resection: a randomised controlled trial. *Lancet* 2002; 359: 1812–8.

26. Lang K, Boldt J, Suttner S, Haisch G. Colloids versus crystalloids and tissue oxygen tension in patients undergoing major abdominal surgery. *Anesth Analg* 2001; 93: 405–9.

6

Anaemia and blood transfusion

I. McConachie

Anaemia is extremely common amongst critically ill patients, whether as a direct result of their admission diagnosis, as a complication of their stay in intensive care or, indeed, from iatrogenic causes:

- In the multicentre European ABC study (Anaemia and Blood transfusion in Critical care), 29% of patients were anaemic at some point in their stay (defined as an Hb (haemoglobin) concentration <10 g/dl [1]).
- In non-bleeding ICU patients the average fall in Hb concentration has been shown in one study [2] to be 0.52 g/dl/day. The decline was larger for the 1st 3 days than later days and was greater in septic patients.

Aetiology of anaemia on adult intensive care unit

Many factors are involved in the aetiology of anaemia in the critically ill:

- Surgical and traumatic blood loss.
- There is a blunted erythropoietin (EPO) response in critical illness [3]. EPO production will be further reduced if renal failure develops.
- Gastrointestinal blood loss; either as the admission diagnosis or occurring as a complication of critical illness. Even without overt melaena and despite the use of pharmacological prophylaxis a slow but continuous G-I mucosal blood loss may well be a major contributing factor to the anaemia seen on Intensive Care Unit (ICU). For example, an endoscopic study [4] performed at the time of ICU admission found that the frequency of acute gastric erosions was 21.7%. By the third day of admission the frequency had increased to 37.5% in patients receiving prophylaxis with Sucralfate and 88.9% in patients with no prophylaxis.

- With renal replacement therapy one can expect an increase in blood transfusion rate compared to patients not receiving renal support. This is correlated to the filter life span i.e. when the filter membranes become clotted red blood cells (RBCs) are lost [5]. The anticoagulation necessary for renal replacement therapy may also increase the risk of anaemia.
- Diagnostic blood sampling results in approximately 40 ml of blood loss per day [2]. This is reduced compared to previous studies suggesting that the now commonly used bedside micro-analyser systems may have an impact on the total blood loss during ICU stay.
- Spillage during vascular cannulation.
- Coagulopathy and haemolysis.
- Other factors (e.g. iron, B_{12} and folate availability).

Effects of anaemia

Chapter 1 has shown the role of Hb in overall oxygen delivery (DO_2). It can easily be seen that a fall in Hb may have a profound effect on global DO_2 unless compensatory mechanisms occur. It is on this premise that RBC are often transfused, that is, to augment DO_2. One must be careful to distinguish between the effects of anaemia and those of hypovolaemia – especially with acute blood loss. There is no doubt that hypovolaemia is much poor tolerated than anaemia. Thus, where hypovolaemia is present, restoration of blood volume and cardiac output is the first priority.

In the normovolaemic patient a rapid fall in Hb brings about certain compensatory changes:

- The decrease in plasma viscosity improves peripheral blood flow and thus enhances venous return to the right atrium. The reduced viscosity also reduces afterload, which may be an important mechanism in maintaining or increasing cardiac output.
- A rightward shift in the oxyhaemoglobin dissociation curve (ODC) is seen, which increases the O_2 unloading by Hb for a given blood PO_2. The primary reason for this is the increased red cell 2,3-diphosphoglycerate synthesis seen during anaemia.

Whether or not these compensatory mechanisms are as successful in maintaining oxygen consumption (VO_2) during critical illness as they are during other anaemic states is unknown.

There will be additional physiological responses if the anaemia results from acute haemorrhage leading to a fall in blood volume.

Role of anaemia in morbidity and mortality

Both critical illness and anaemia put stress on the myocardium to increase cardiac output and hence global DO_2. To do so myocardial DO_2 must increase to meet its own increased O_2 demand (MVO_2). As normal myocardial O_2 extraction runs at between 75% and 80% any increase in MVO_2 must be met primarily by an increase in coronary flow. In the presence of coronary artery disease fixed coronary stenoses may prevent any increase in myocardial flow, thus limiting myocardial DO_2. Thus, during anaemia the demands of an increased cardiac output may result in cardiac ischaemia with, at least the potential for increased morbidity and mortality:

- A retrospective analysis by Carson [6] involving Jehovah's Witnesses undergoing surgery demonstrated a significantly higher morbidity and mortality in patients with a preoperative Hb of <6 g/dl. This effect was substantially more significant in patients with pre-existing cardiac disease and in those who had a larger blood loss.
- A similar, more recent study [7] found that the risk of death was low in patients with postoperative Hb levels of 7.1–8.0 g/dl. As postoperative anaemia worsened, the risk of mortality rises and becomes extremely high below 5–6 g/dl.
- Elderly anaemic patients with myocardial infarction have a higher mortality rate [8] even when other factors have been taken into account.

Recent studies on the significance of anaemia in critically ill patients are difficult to separate from studies on the benefits or otherwise of transfusion and will be discussed below.

Management of anaemia in the critically ill

Prevention

A detailed account of perioperative methods of reducing surgical blood loss lies outside the scope of this text but these include:

- Hypotensive anaesthetic techniques.
- Improved surgical techniques including minimally invasive surgery.

- Appropriate attention to patient positioning and venous drainage.
- Use of tourniquets and infiltration of vasoconstrictors.
- Use of antibrinolytic and other drugs to reduce bleeding.
- Surgery under spinal or epidural anaesthesia as opposed to general anaesthesia.
- In addition, the loss of *RBCs* may be reduced by the use of haemodilution techniques and the use of cell-saver strategies.

In the critically ill patient, interest in prevention of anaemia has centred around:

- Improved membrane biocompatibility of extracorporeal technology such as for renal replacement therapy or cardiac bypass.
- Use of microanalyser systems for blood tests and other "point of care" laboratory systems.
- The routine use of pulse oximetry has reduced the need for arterial blood gas sampling.
- The potential for indwelling vascular oxygenation and pH sensors to reduce blood gas sampling.
- Preservation of gut mucosal integrity.
- EPO therapy. A study from Holland has shown that critically ill patients with low levels of endogenous EPO can respond to exogenous EPO by increasing reticulocytes [9]. Indeed, two randomised-controlled trials (RCTs) have shown that the prophylactic administration of EPO is potentially of value. The largest, over 1300 patients [10] showed that patients receiving weekly subcutaneous injections of 40,000 units of EPO were less likely to undergo transfusion, received less total number of units of blood over the 28-day study period and had an increased Hb from baseline to study end. EPO therapy is expensive and the benefits are, so far, controversial. However, if it reduces red cell transfusion requirements and avoids the harmful effects of transfusion it may well be a highly cost-effective therapy for the critically ill patient.

Transfusion in critically ill patients

Prevalence of transfusion in ICU

Transfusion of RBC is extremely common in ICU patients. In the ABC study mentioned earlier [1], 37% of ICU patients received one or more units during their

ICU stay. Older patients and those with a longer ICU stay received more transfusions.

Trauma patients, perhaps not surprisingly receive more units of blood [11].

Effect of transfusion on oxygen transport

It has been assumed that an increase in global DO_2 (e.g. by red cell transfusion) would result in an increase in VO_2 in critical illness:

- However, Dietrich [12] studied the increase of DO_2 by red cell transfusion in non-surgical intensive care patients. After volume resuscitation, patients were transfused if their Hb was <10 g/dl. He showed neither an increase in VO_2 nor a decrease in blood lactate levels in any patient and concluded that the shock state of this patient group was not improved by red cell transfusion.
- In postcardiac surgery patients, the oxygen transport responses to transfusion vary. Even in anaemic patients there is no consistent VO_2 response to transfusion [13].

Several studies have addressed this issue in patients with sepsis and septic shock:

- Conrad [14] studied augmentation of DO_2 by blood transfusion in septic patients. Transfusion resulted in a significant increase in Hb and DO_2. However, despite the increase in DO_2, there was no increase in VO_2 or decrease in lactate. Subset analysis showed that a pretransfusion oxygen extraction ratio (OER) under 24% *was* associated with an increase in VO_2, but the pretransfusion level of cardiac index, pulmonary capillary wedge pressure, lactate, or VO_2 was not. It was concluded that an isolated increase in arterial oxygen content as a means of increasing DO_2 does not improve VO_2 in septic shock following adequate fluid resuscitation. However, patients with a low OER represent a subset of patients which may improve consumption with transfusion, and may represent a different microcirculatory disturbance.
- Steffes [15] further studied the role of lactic acidosis (implying tissue hypoxia) as a predictor of response to augmenting DO_2 with transfusion. In patients with normal lactic acid both DO_2 and VO_2 increased. However, in patients with lactic acidosis VO_2 did not significantly change after transfusion despite increased DO_2. He concluded that lactic acidosis may predict patients who will not respond to transfusion. It was suggested that patients with lactic acidosis may have a peripheral oxygen utilisation defect that prevents improvement in VO_2 with increasing DO_2.

Thus, increasing DO_2 by red cell transfusion may not be of benefit and exposes the patient to the possible harmful effects of blood transfusion.

Harmful effects of blood transfusion

Problems such as hyperkalaemia, hypocalcaemia, metabolic acidosis, hypothermia, dilutional coagulopathy and citrate toxicity, although important, are related to massive blood transfusion only and will not be discussed further in this text.

Wrong blood

Sadly "wrong blood to patient" errors still occur – and are potentially lethal. Analysis of incident reports has revealed multiple errors of identification, often beginning when blood was collected from the blood bank [16]. The use of hospital protocols including systems for validation of patient identification by more than one person is vital.

Old blood

There may be several problems arising from the transfusion of old blood in critically ill patients though their exact clinical significance is still debated:

- Stored blood has reduced levels of 2,3-DPG levels causing a leftward shift in the ODC and a reduced unloading of O_2 from Hb.
- The reduced membrane deformability of red cells, brought about through their storage, is thought to impede their passage through the narrow confines of a capillary bed with potential implications for ischaemic organs and tissues. The high haematocrit of packed red cells will increase blood viscosity and further threaten perfusion of such areas.
- A small retrospective study of patients with severe sepsis found that the age of the stored transfused RBC was directly associated with mortality [17].
- Another retrospective study, this time of post coronary artery bypass grafting (CABG) patients, showed that the age of the stored blood was associated with the chance of developing pneumonia [18]. However, another study from the same group has found no evidence of increased morbidity in cardiac surgery patients when old blood is transfused [19].
- From a trauma unit database, multivariate analysis has identified that the mean age of blood transfused, number of units older than 14 days, and number of

units older than 21 days are independent risk factors for the development of organ failures [20]. They suggest that fresh blood may be more appropriate for the initial resuscitation of trauma patients requiring transfusion.

Haemolytic reactions

An estimated 1 in 250,000 transfusions result in an overt haemolytic reaction, most commonly secondary to minor RBC antigens. This is almost certainly an underestimate due to under reporting and failure to recognise such a reaction during either surgery or the course of a critical illness at a time when the signs (hypotension, tachycardia, disseminated intravascular coagulation (DIC), pyrexia) can be attributed to a more common pathology.

Transfusion related acute lung injury

Acute lung injury following blood transfusion is thought to result from the activation of recipient neutrophils by donor antibodies and donor RBC derived membrane lipids. Such neutrophil activation increases endothelial permeability with extravasation of inflammatory mediators and fluid. The resultant clinical picture is indistinguishable from acute respiratory distress syndrome (ARDS):

- In the perioperative or critically ill patient there are often other factors that could explain why a patient should develop ARDS and so the incidence of transfusion related acute lung injury (TRALI) is probably underestimated.
- It is possible that the use of leucodepleted blood may reduce the incidence of TRALI.

Increase in cytokines?

- Laboratory studies have shown that RBC transfusion activates neutrophils causing a release of inflammatory cytokines [21].
- Intraoperative transfusion in cardiac surgery patients increases the inflammatory response [22]. During storage the leucocytes lose their membrane integrity and release substances such as bactericidal permeability increasing protein (BPI) into the plasma. BPI was found in all units of packed red cells tested at concentrations up to 15 times preoperative plasma levels in patients.
- However, the issues are complex. For example, one study [23] has found a greater increase in cytokine concentration after autologous blood transfusion

than after allogeneic blood transfusion. The lower response in the latter may result from transfusion-induced suppression of cellular immunity.

Transmission of infection by blood transfusion

- Direct transmission of infection via contaminated blood is small but still possible.
- Human immunodeficiency virus (HIV). This risk is associated with the donation of blood during the immunologically silent "window period" of infection prior to the host antibody response. The current risk is estimated to be extremely low.
- Hepatitis B. The risk of transfusion-associated hepatitis B has fallen dramatically since routine surface antigen testing (1975) and is expected to fall further as the use of the hepatitis B vaccine becomes increasingly widespread. The current risk is between 1 in 30,000 and 1 in 250,000 unit transfusions and accounts for about 10% of all posttransfusion hepatitis [24].
- Transfusion is becoming an increasingly rare cause of hepatitis C infection, possibly as a result of HIV high-risk donation exclusion but with a high associated morbidity.
- Transmission of other viruses such as Parvovirus and West Nile Fever have been reported in the literature but are rare.
- Bacteria contamination of stored blood is related to the length of storage but is associated with a high mortality. Transmission rates of other quoted transfusion-associated non-viral infections such as Plasmodium and Trypanosoma cruzi are vanishingly small.
- The potential for transmission by blood products of protein containing prion particles such as those responsible for human variant Creutzfeldt Jacob Disease (vCJD) represents an unknown risk. There has been 1 case of blood donation from someone carrying the vCJD prion resulting in the later death from vCJD of both the donor and the recipient. The UK Government has recently banned the donation of blood by anyone who has received a blood transfusion since 1980 (to limit donation to those who received transfusion prior to the assumed introduction of the Bovine Spongiform Encephalopathy prion into the UK food chain). A screening test for vCJD prion in blood donors is also being developed. Additional attempts to minimise transmission of vCJD by blood products include the purchasing of plasma products from the USA and the universal leucodepletion of blood components (at a cost of £85 million/year).

Immunosuppressive effects of blood transfusion

The immunosuppressive effects of allogenic blood transfusion are well established [25]. The clinical relevance primarily revolves around two areas of concern:

Postoperative infection

The effects of blood-transfusion-induced immunosuppression have been thought to increase the risk of postoperative infection including wound infections. Many studies have suggested such an increased infection rate in patients undergoing colorectal, orthopaedic, gynaecological, trauma and CABG surgery. Much of the evidence is retrospective and some reports have shown no effect of transfusion on postoperative infection rates:

- A retrospective study of post CABG patients, showing that the age of the stored blood was associated with the chance of developing pneumonia [18], has already been highlighted.
- A further study from Spain [26] examined risk factors from nosocomial pneumonia in cardiac surgery patients and concluded that there was a significant association between the transfusion of four or more units of blood products and the chance of developing nosocomial pneumonia.

Cancer recurrence

Much data exists to support the concept of increased tumour recurrence in patients who have received perioperative transfusion whilst undergoing potentially curative surgery for colorectal, breast, lung, sarcoma, hepatic and head and neck cancers.

Vamvakas [27] disputes much of the evidence for infection and tumour recurrence, stating that most is retrospective and that analysis of prospective, randomised, controlled trials show very little difference between those transfused and those not transfused. He suggests that differences are due to retrospective trial design and that immunosuppression may occur secondary to the variables that lead to the transfusion and not as a result of the transfusion itself.

Leucodepleted blood transfusion

The evidence from RCTs of infection and recurrence rates comparing allogenic with either leucodepleted or autologous blood are, as yet, inconclusive:

- Leucodepletion reduces the levels of BPI and other substances in stored blood [28].

- The use of leukoreduced blood was associated with a decrease in the post-operative length of stay in a study of cardiac surgery patients [29].
- Canada has recently introduced a universal leucoreduction programme. A retrospective "before and after" study of hip fracture patients, cardiac surgery patients and surgical and trauma admissions to ICU (in other words not all types of ICU patients) has shown reduced in-hospital mortality rates but no decrease in serious nosocomial infections [30]. The frequency of posttransfusion fever and antibiotic use also decreased significantly following leukoreduction.
- However, the most recent meta-analysis found a weak association between leucodepletion and a reduction in infection risk but no effect on overall mortality [31].

Since 1999 all blood for transfusion in the UK has been leucodepleted thus rendering much of the above debate academic.

Transfusion and outcome in ICU

Current recommendations re-transfusion practice apply to the broadest spectrum of pathology and pathology severity. Often no mention is made of the critically ill in whom metabolic demands and cardiorespiratory physiology are altered in the extreme.

However, a few studies have looked at the impact of transfusion strategy on outcome in ICU patients:

- In a combined retrospective and prospective cohort study of 4470 general ICU patients, Hebert [32] found that non-survivors had lower Hb and had received more transfused red cell units than survivors. From their data the authors concluded that anaemia increases the risk of death in critically patients with cardiac disease and that blood transfusion of up to 6 units will reduce this risk by 40%.
- The most significant study on this issue, from the same group, has been the Transfusion Requirements in Critical Care (TRICC) study [33]. This Canadian multicentre, prospective, randomised study compared a restrictive with a liberal transfusion strategy in 838 general ICU patients. Those in the restrictive strategy group were transfused at an Hb <7 g/dl with packed red cells to maintain their Hb at 7–9 g/dl. Those in the liberal strategy group were transfused with packed red cells at an Hb <10 g/dl to maintain their Hb at 10–12 g/dl. In those patients with an acute physiology and chronic health evaluation (APACHE) score <20 and in patients aged <55 years the 30-day survival and overall

hospital mortality was significantly better in those randomised to the restrictive transfusion strategy. Amongst patients with cardiac disease the 30-day mortality was reduced, but not significantly so, if allocated to the restrictive strategy. This groundbreaking trial – the first large, prospective study of blood transfusion strategy on outcome in ICU – also showed a significant decrease in organ dysfunction and cardiac complications in the restrictive strategy group.

- Later subgroup analysis of critically ill patients with cardiac disease confirmed that a restrictive RBC transfusion strategy generally appears safe with the possible exception of patients with acute myocardial infarcts and unstable angina [34].
- A similar negative effect of transfusion on outcome was demonstrated in patients having coronary artery bypass surgery [35]. They also demonstrated a significantly increased risk of left ventricular dysfunction and mortality in the high and medium Hct groups compared to the low Hct group. The authors proposed that increased blood viscosity may require increased myocardial work while reducing coronary flow.
- A contrary view comes from a retrospective study of data on 78,974 Medicare beneficiaries 65 years old or older who were hospitalised with acute myocardial infarction. Blood transfusion is associated with a lower short-term mortality rate among elderly patients with acute myocardial infarction if the hematocrit on admission is 30% or lower [8].
- In a study from a major US Trauma Centre, blood transfusion seems to be an independent predictor of mortality, need for ICU admission and ICU and hospital length of stay (even after controlling for severity of shock and injury) [36].

Transfusion and mechanical ventilation

Anecdotal reports exist of successful weaning after transfusion to an Hb higher than that which would now normally be desired in critically ill patients:

- Schonhofer et al [37] demonstrated a decreased work of breathing and decreased minute ventilation in anaemic patients with chronic obstructive pulmonary disease (COPD) when transfused from an Hb of 8–9 g/dl to an Hb of >12 g/dl. This seemed to be primarily through a decrease in tidal volumes with a resultant slight rise in PCO_2 levels. A similar effect was not seen in anaemic patients without COPD who were transfused with an identical strategy.
- This work complements case reports by the same authors concerning six patients successfully weaned after transfusion to Hb >12 g/dl. All patients had failed several attempts to wean over several weeks at much lower Hb [38]. Anecdotal

though this is, it supports a strategy used by many intensivists in which anaemic patients, who are proving difficult to wean, are transfused to a "normal" Hb.

- A further subgroup analysis of the TRICC study, however failed to demonstrate any benefit in terms of shortened duration of IPVV in patients in the liberal transfusion strategy group [39]. However, this was not a study of specific weaning problem patients.
- Complementing the work on increase in infections associated with transfusion of allogenic blood comes a large study strongly suggesting that transfusion is associated with an increase in the risk of developing ventilator associated pneumonia [40].

It may be that getting the balance right is important with transfusion being potentially of benefit to patients who are a problem to wean (and possibly patients with cardiac disease) while being detrimental to other patients!

Reducing the need for blood transfusion

General

A major trend in recent years has been a greater reluctance to expose patients to the problems associated with allogenic blood transfusion. This in part reflects greater understanding of these problems but also a realisation that beneficial effects of transfusion are less apparent in many groups of patients. Requirement for allogenic blood transfusion can be reduced by:

- Accepting the appropriateness of a restrictive transfusion strategy for most patients.
- Other methods of combating the development of anaemia in ICU patients mentioned previously especially, perhaps for the future, the role of EPO.
- Increased use perioperatively of predonation and other forms of autologous blood transfusion.

Blood substitutes

Interest continues in the use of blood substitutes to reduce the need for allogenic blood transfusion. In general, there may be toxicity relating to the cell debris contained within preparations of Hb – chiefly renal toxicity. Another source of concern in early studies of free Hb in solution was a marked vasopressor effect probably related to scavenging of the endogenous vasodilator, nitric oxide. This in itself may be harmful for trauma patients in the field if it encourages further bleeding.

There are several main areas of research:

- Diasprin cross linked haemoglobin (DCLB). Recent multicentre trials show some effect in limiting the transfusion of allogenic blood. However, two large multicentre trials have now been terminated early owing to safety concerns. Interest in this product thus seems to have waned.
- Polymerised human Hb. Seems to be free of significant side effects and early reports regarding efficacy are encouraging.
- Bovine Hb. Has been used successfully in surgery associated with major blood loss but there are concerns related to increase blood pressure and production of antibodies. Nevertheless, a commercial product has been approved for use in South Africa.
- Human recombinant Hb. Likely to be expensive but may prove useful in the future.
- Perfluorocarbons carry increased oxygen in solution but have a requirement for a high FiO_2. Early trials suggest a reduction in the requirement for transfusion of allogenic blood.

Practical approach

Recommendations by the ASA Task Force on Blood Component Therapy [41] state that transfusion is:

- "rarely required above an Hb of 10 g/dl",
- "almost always indicated when Hb is <6 g/dl".

Current evidence supports a restrictive strategy for transfusion in ICU with some evidence to support a more liberal strategy in patients with cardiac disease and possibly patients who are proving difficult to wean from intermittent positive pressure ventilation (IPPV).

FURTHER READING

An entire recent supplement issue of *Critical Care Medicine* has been devoted to the subject of anaemia and transfusion practices in critically ill patients. *Critical Care Medicine* 2003; 31(Suppl 12).

REFERENCES

1. Vincent JL, Baron JF, Reinhart K, Gattinoni L et al. Anemia and blood transfusion in critically ill patients. *J Am Med Assoc* 2002; 288: 1499–507.

2. Nguyen BV, Bota DP, Melot C, Vincent JL. Time course of hemoglobin concentrations in nonbleeding intensive care unit patients. *Crit Care Med* 2003; 31: 406–10.

3. Von Ahsen N, Muller C, Serke S, Frei U, Eckardt K. Important role of non-diagnostic blood loss and blunted erythropoietic response in the anaemia of medical intensive care patients. *Crit Care Med* 1999; 27: 2630–9.

4. Eddleston JM, Pearson RC, Holland J, Tooth JA et al. Prospective endoscopic study of stress erosions and ulcers in critically ill adult patients treated with either sucralfate or placebo. *Crit Care Med* 1994; 22: 1949–54.

5. Cutts MW, Thomas AN, Kishen R. Transfusion requirements during continuous venovenous haemofiltration: the importance of filter life. *Intens Care Med* 2000; 26: 1694–7.

6. Carson JL, Duff A, Poses R et al. Effect of anaemia and cardiovascular disease on surgical mortality and morbidity. *Lancet* 1996; 348: 1055–9.

7. Carson JL, Noveck H, Berlin JA, Gould SA. Mortality and morbidity in patients with very low postoperative Hb levels who decline blood transfusion. *Transfusion* 2002; 42: 812–18.

8. Wu WC, Rathore SS, Wang Y, Radford MJ, Krumholz HM. Blood transfusion in elderly patients with acute myocardial infarction. *New Engl J Med* 2001; 345: 1230–6.

9. van Iperen CE, Gaillard CA, Kraaijenhagen RJ, Braam BG et al. Response of erythropoiesis and iron metabolism to recombinant human erythropoietin in intensive care unit patients. *Crit Care Med* 2000; 28: 2773–8.

10. Corwin HL, Gettinger A, Pearl RG, Fink MP et al. Efficacy of recombinant human erythropoietin in critically ill patients: a randomized controlled trial. *J Am Med Assoc* 2002; 288: 2827–35.

11. Shapiro MJ, Gettinger A, Corwin HL, Napolitano L et al. Anemia and blood transfusion in trauma patients admitted to the intensive care unit. *J Trauma* 2003; 55: 269–73.

12. Dietrich KA, Conrad SA, Hebert CA et al. Cardiovascular and metabolic response to red blood cell transfusion in critically ill volume-resuscitated nonsurgical patients. *Crit Care Med* 1990; 18: 940–5.

13. Casutt M, Seifert B, Pasch T, Schmid ER et al. Factors influencing the individual effects of blood transfusions on oxygen delivery and oxygen consumption. *Crit Care Med* 1999; 27: 2194–200.

14. Conrad SA, Dietrich KA, Hebert CA, Romero MD. Effect of red cell transfusion on oxygen consumption following fluid resuscitation in septic shock. *Circ Shock* 1990; 31: 419–29.

15. Steffes CP, Bender JS, Levison MA. Blood transfusion and oxygen consumption in surgical sepsis. *Crit Care Med* 1991; 19: 512–17.

16. Williamson LM, Lowe S, Love EM, Cohen H et al. Serious hazards of transfusion (SHOT) initiative: analysis of the first two annual reports. *Br Med J* 1999; 319: 16–19.

17. Purdy FR, Tweeddale MG, Merrick PM. Association of mortality with age of blood transfused in septic ICU patients. *Can J Anaesth* 1997; 44: 1256–61.
18. Vamvakas EC, Carven JH. Transfusion and postoperative pneumonia in coronary artery bypass graft surgery: effect of the length of storage of transfused red cells. *Transfusion* 1999; 39: 701–10.
19. Vamvakas EC, Carven JH. Length of storage of transfused red cells and postoperative morbidity in patients undergoing coronary artery bypass graft surgery. *Transfusion* 2000; 40: 101–9.
20. Zallen G, Offner PJ, Moore EE, Blackwell J et al. Age of transfused blood is an independent risk factor for postinjury multiple organ failure. *Am J Surg* 1999; 178: 570–2.
21. Zallen G, Moore EE, Ciesla DJ, Brown M et al. Stored red blood cells selectively activate human neutrophils to release IL-8 and secretory PLA2. *Shock* 2000; 13: 29–33.
22. Fransen E, Maessen J, Dentener M, Senden N et al. Impact of blood transfusions on inflammatory mediator release in patients undergoing cardiac surgery. *Chest* 1999; 116: 1233–9.
23. Avall A, Hyllner M, Bengtson JP, Carlsson L et al. Postoperative inflammatory response after autologous and allogeneic blood transfusion. *Anesthesiology* 1997; 87: 511–16.
24. Schreiber GB, Busch MP, Kleinman SH, Korelitz JJ. The risk of transfusion-transmitted viral infections. *New Engl J Med* 1996; 334: 1685–9.
25. Landers DF, Hill GE, Wong KC, Fox IJ. Blood transfusion-induced immunomodulation. *Anesth Analg* 1996; 82: 187–204.
26. Leal-Noval SR, Marquez-Vacaro JA, Garcia-Curiel A, Camacho-Larana P et al. Nosocomial pneumonia in patients undergoing heart surgery. *Crit Care Med* 2000; 28: 935–40.
27. Vamvakas EC. Transfusion-associated cancer recurrence and postoperative infection: meta-analysis of randomised, controlled clinical trials. *Transfusion* 1996; 36: 175–86.
28. Fransen EJ, Rombout-Sestrienkova E, van Pampus EC, Buurman WA et al. Prestorage leucocyte reduction of red cell components prevents release of bactericidal permeability increasing protein and defensins. *Vox Sang* 2002; 83: 119–24.
29. Fung MK, Rao N, Rice J, Ridenour M et al. Leukoreduction in the setting of open heart surgery: a prospective cohort-controlled study. *Transfusion* 2004; 44: 30–5.
30. Hebert PC, Fergusson D, Blajchman MA, Wells GA et al. Clinical outcomes following institution of the Canadian universal leukoreduction program for red blood cell transfusions. *J Am Med Assoc* 2003; 289: 1941–9.
31. Vamvakas EC. White blood cell-containing allogeneic blood transfusion, postoperative infection and mortality: a meta-analysis of observational "before-and-after" studies. *Vox Sang* 2004; 86: 111–19.
32. Hebert PC, Wells G, Tweeddale M et al. Does transfusion practice affect mortality in critically ill patients? *Am J Respir Crit Care Med* 1997; 155: 1618–23.
33. Hebert PC, Wells G, Blajchman MA et al. A multicentre, randomised, controlled clinical trial of transfusion requirements in critical care. *New Eng J Med* 1999; 340: 409–17.

34. Hebert PC, Yetisir E, Martin C, Blajchman MA et al. Is a low transfusion threshold safe in critically ill patients with cardiovascular diseases? *Crit Care Med* 2001; 29: 227–34.

35. Speiss BD, Ley C, Body SC et al. Haematocrit value on intensive care unit entry influences the frequency of Q-wave myocardial infarction after coronary artery bypass grafting. *J Thorac Cardiovasc Surg* 1998; 116: 460–7.

36. Malone DL, Dunne J, Tracy JK, Putnam AT et al. Blood transfusion, independent of shock severity, is associated with worse outcome in trauma. *J Trauma* 2003; 54: 898–905.

37. Schonhofer B, Wenzel M, Geibel M, Kohler D. Blood transfusion and lung function in chronically anaemic patients with severe chronic obstructive pulmonary disease. *Crit Care Med* 1998; 26: 1824–8.

38. Schonhofer B, Bohrer H, Kohler D. Blood transfusion facilitating difficult weaning from the ventilator. *Anaesthesia* 1998; 53: 169–84.

39. Hebert PC, Blajchman MA, Cook DJ, Yetisir E et al. Do blood transfusions improve outcomes related to mechanical ventilation? *Chest* 2001; 119: 1850–7.

40. Shorr AF, Duh MS, Kelly K, Kollef MK. Red blood cell transfusion and ventilator associated pneumonia: A potential link? *Crit Care Med* 2004; 32: 666–74.

41. ASA Task Force on Blood Component Therapy. Practice guidelines for blood component therapy. *Anesthesiology* 1996; 84: 732–47.

7

Nutrition

S. Wiggans

Nutrition

Appropriate nutrition is vital in the critically ill patient. In its absence there will be:

- Muscle atrophy and weakness.
- Decrease in immune function.
- Decrease in wound healing.
- Impaired weaning off intermittent positive pressure ventilation (IPPV).
- Gut mucosal atrophy.

In the critically ill patient who is markedly catabolic the above may occur in a few days. Nutritional support improves nutritional status but there is little concrete evidence for a beneficial effect on survival. However, promoting ongoing mal-nourishment must be detrimental to the patient. Certainly more than 10,000 kcal negative caloric balance is associated with a poor outcome in intensive care unit (ICU) patients [1]. There is little evidence that nutritional support can reverse the negative nitrogen balance or catabolism which occurs in the critically ill patient. In which case the purpose of support is to *minimise* the negative nitrogen balance.

In simple starvation (i.e. non-physiologically stressed), the energy requirements in the first week are chiefly met by protein breakdown to amino acids and subsequent glucose formation via gluconeogenesis. The body adapts to a protein sparing metabolism in starvation, but these changes are absent or opposed in the ICU patient.

In addition:

- Sepsis results in a preferential metabolism of fat rather than glucose partly due to inhibition of the enzyme complex pyruvate dehydrogenase.

- Despite increased protein synthesis for
    (i) inflammatory response,
    (ii) wound healing and
    (iii) acute phase proteins; protein breakdown is accelerated leading to a net negative nitrogen balance – the acute catabolic state.
- Catecholamines, stress response hormones and cytokines (especially tumour necrosis factor (TNF)) are responsible for the changes compared to starvation.
- Reversal of these obligatory catabolic changes is not possible during severe physiological stress [2] – only reversed when the cause of the hormonal release is removed (i.e. resolution of the underlying condition).
- Gluconeogenesis cannot be inhibited completely by provision of adequate substrate in severe catabolism [3].
- Growth hormone administration to stimulate a positive nitrogen balance seemed promising in early studies but later studies were stopped due to an excess mortality in study group.
- Muscle wasting from catabolic changes is compounded by prolonged immobilisation.
- "Overfeeding" [4] will not promote a positive nitrogen balance until the underlying condition resolves *and* the patient is mobilising. Body weight may increase but this is mainly fat and total body protein still falls.
- When the patient is recovering *and* mobilising, energy and protein intake should be increased to allow weight gain.

Reasons for feeding the critically ill patient

- To minimise the net negative balance and breakdown of the body's tissues.
- To provide precursors for the immune response, wound repair and hepatic protein synthesis.
- Provision of nutritional support may increase the protein synthesis rate even if it does not decrease the catabolic rate.
- Glucose administration is partly protein sparing [5], but this effect is blunted by sepsis.
- Even low rates of enteral feeding limit gut mucosal atrophy.

Nutritional status

Nutritional status prior to critical illness is important because:

- Protein reserves are called upon in critical illness. Reserves are low in the malnourished patient.

- Low body mass index (BMI) (not high BMI) is an independent risk factor for increased mortality in ICU [6].
- ICU patients lose 1% of lean body mass per day – mainly muscle.
- *Sarcopenia* (literally means "lack of muscle") describes both atrophy and reduction in the number of muscle fibres. Incidence increases with age – as high as 50% in the over 80s [7].
- Muscle mass represents a major store of protein and therefore sarcopenia weakens the metabolic defence to illness. High incidence of sarcopenia in the elderly is thought to be a major factor in the poor outcome of this group.
- BMI can predict the degree of sarcopenia [8].

Assessment of nutritional status

Malnutrition is very common in hospital patients:

- Common sense clinical examination will be helpful, for example, history of weight loss and food intake, measured versus usual weight, specific features (e.g. of vitamin deficiencies and signs of muscle weakness and atrophy). Measured height and weight should be compared to standard tables.
- Anthropometric measurements, for example Triceps skin-fold thickness and mid-arm muscle circumference are crude, occasionally useful but are operator dependent to some degree and may not be reproducible.
- Albumin as an index of visceral protein mass is useful in pure malnutrition. However, in ICU, influences of decreased synthesis due to liver disturbances and loss due to capillary leak confuse the picture (see Chapter 5 on fluid therapy).
- Serum transferrin has been suggested as a better index of body proteins as it has a longer circulating half-life and is not an acute phase protein.
- Lymphocyte count and skin tests for common allergens (an index of immune competence which is depressed in malnutrition) are useful in pure malnutrition but, again, are less useful in ICU.
- Of experimental interest at present are accurate measurements from bioelectrical impedance, which quantitatively measures lean body mass.

In summary, there are no simple tests appropriate for assessing acute malnutrition in critically ill patients. Clinical impression and serial estimations of weight compared to premorbid weight are probably as useful as more complex tests [9].

Timing of initiation of feeding

- Although many patients may seem to tolerate a short period of low or no caloric intake, the greater the degree of catabolism, the less the period of hypocaloric intake should be.
- Enteral nutrition (EN) should be attempted within 24–48 h if there are no contraindications, due to the rapid onset of gut mucosal atrophy.
- If EN is not possible, total parenteral nutrition (TPN) should be commenced as soon as the patient is haemodynamically stable.
- Occasionally TPN will be started at the same time as EN in an attempt to maximise caloric intake. A systematic review has concluded that, in critically ill patients who are not malnourished and have an intact gastrointestinal (GI) tract, starting TPN at the same time as EN provides no benefit over EN alone [10].

TPN

- Only indicated if unable to feed the patient via the enteral route.
- Gut mucosal atrophy still occurs.
- More expensive.
- More metabolic problems.
- Requires dedicated central venous access (with all its complications).
- Incidence of infectious complications related to the care of the site rather than the type of site (e.g. tunnelled versus non-tunnelled).
- Usually administered as a 2.5 or 3 l "big bag" feed with all the nutritional components mixed in pharmacy in a laminar flow cabinet under strict aseptic conditions.

Enteral nutrition

- Eating is normal. The gut is not designed to be rested.
- Mucosal atrophy is rapid.
- Requires a functioning GI tract. Bowel sounds not essential for absorption.
- NG used most commonly, but gastric atony can be a problem. Placement of the tube distal to the stomach (duodenum or jejunum) is advantageous.

- Prokinetic drugs (metoclopramide and erythromycin) are useful in improving gut motility and absorption [11]. Although withdrawn in the UK, cisapride is also used [12].
- Supports normal gut flora.
- Possibly reduces GI bleeding from stress ulcers.
- Decreases infective complications in surgical patients [13].
- May preserve the gut barrier and prevent bacterial or endotoxin translocation.
- Reduced incidence of acalculous cholecystitis.
- Many commercial preparations. All approximately 1 kcal/ml.
- Cheaper than TPN and with less metabolic and infectious complications.
- Elemental, that is predigested feeds only necessary in short bowel syndrome following small bowel resection.
- No need for "starter" diluted feeds. If problems occur, start at lower rate rather than diluting the feed.
- A 4-h rest period during the night is often recommended. Stomach acidity during this period may limit bacterial growth in the stomach.
- Continuous pump feeding better than intermittent bolus feeding – less risk of aspiration.
- Fine bore tubes are difficult to aspirate from, block easily and have few advantages in the critically ill patient.

There is uncertainty from animal studies as to whether enteral feeding promotes a better outcome or whether TPN promotes a worse outcome due to higher rates of complications.

Complications of enteral nutrition

- Aspiration – watch for large residual volumes. Large residual volumes are probably a factor in the development of nosocomial pneumonia.
- Infection/contamination – feeds are excellent bacteria growth media.
- Blockage of tubes – flush all medications with H_2O.
- Malposition of tubes – check with chest X-ray.
- Constipation – often due to inadequate H_2O intake or possibly lack of fibre.
- Diarrhoea – very common. Check for antibiotics and other medications as causes of diarrhoea. *Clostridium difficile* infection must always be excluded. In the absence of these causes treat symptomatically rather than automatically stopping the feed. Fibre may be important.

Nutritional composition

In the last 15 years there have been three major trends in ICU nutrition:

- A shift from parenteral to EN (see above).
- A decrease in the total quantity of calories administered.
- An improvement in the *quality* of nutrients administered (i.e. novel substrates).

Energy and protein requirements

Formulae (e.g. Harris Benedict) *estimate* the basal energy expenditure (BEE) based on patient age, weight and sex. Studies have shown that the mean metabolic rate, and therefore caloric requirement, approximates to BEE + 30%. Adjustments are often made as percentage increases based on the degree of "stress" and activity [14]. For clinical purposes 25–30 kcal/kg/day is sufficient. It has been suggested, however, that caloric requirements may be much higher (50–60 kcal/kg/day) in the second week after an episode of severe sepsis or trauma [15]. Fear of hyper- or hypo-nutritional states have lead to the use of indirect calorimetry. Indirect calorimetry *measures* energy expenditure based on measurements of oxygen consumption and CO_2 production. The aim is to tailor nutritional needs on a daily basis, thus avoiding hyper- or hypo-nutritional states. This may be useful but:

- Errors, for example, from leaks are a problem especially when the patient is on a high inspired O_2 concentration.
- Once daily "spot check" measurements may be inappropriately extrapolated to the whole 24 h day.
- Marked differences have been reported from different studies of similar groups of patients.
- One review [16] concluded "At present indirect calorimetry may be better viewed as an investigative tool than a necessary part of routine patient care".
- With refinement of techniques, this may be a routine measurement in the future.

Protein losses can be measured but in practice 1–1.5 g/kg/day are required. Alternatively, protein intake can be assessed on the basis of a ratio of 150:1 of non-protein calories to nitrogen (approximately 6 g protein = 1 g nitrogen).

When calculating requirements, an admission "dry weight" should be used as most ICU patients gain weight as metabolically inactive oedema fluid during their illness.

Composition of non-protein calories

There is still controversy over the ratio of fat to carbohydrate (CHO) intake in the critically ill patient.

> Pro fat: Lipid preferentially metabolised in sepsis especially medium chain fatty acids (MCFA).
> Lipid is non-irritant to veins and theoretically can be given via a peripheral vein.
> Fat gives more calories per gram compared to glucose (nine compared to four).
> Requirement for essential fatty acids.
> Con fat: Lipid particles may be taken up by the reticulo endothelial system.
> > Long chain fatty acid (LCFA) metabolism impaired in sepsis (due to a deficit of intracellular carnititne).
> > Fat possesses little or no protein sparing effect.
> > Hyperlipidaemia may impair oxygenation but changes are small and probably of little clinical significance.
> Pro CHO: Some protein sparing effect especially if lipid is also given.
> > Some glucose intake probably essential.
> Con CHO: Hyperglycaemia (see below).
> > Limit to utilisation – maximum uptake 4–6 mg/kg/min.
> > Excess CHO leads to hepatic steatosis.
> > Caution in respiratory failure (see below).

Most authorities recommend approximately 50% of non-protein calories be administered as fat.

Note: If propofol is infused for sedation one must remember that this is dissolved in a fat emulsion equivalent to 10% intralipid.

Other nutritional requirements

- H_2O and standard electrolytes need to be supplied. Magnesium and phosphate supplements may be required.
- Vitamins, both fat and H_2O soluble should be supplied in the form of a commercial multivitamin preparation. Requirements are mainly not known with certainty in the critically ill patient and are often extrapolated from normal requirements. Water-soluble vitamins should be administered every day. Fat-soluble vitamins are required at least twice a week. In the long term: vitamins

B12, K and folate supplements may be required. Currently there is great interest in the role of vitamins C and E as antioxidants.

- Specific elemental requirements (e.g. zinc and manganese may also be supplied commercially). Trace elements with lesser or unknown requirements can be assumed to be supplied as contaminants of other fluids and in blood transfusions [17].
- Commercially produced EN preparations are generally balanced nutritional sources.

Hyperglycaemia

- Common in the critically ill patient due to hormonal changes and insulin resistance. May be related more to increased production from gluconeogenesis rather than decreased utilisation (unless septic).
- Assess whether intake is too high prior to prescribing insulin.
- High levels should *not* be viewed as innocuous. Associated with osmotic diuresis and increased infections.
- Evidence suggests that a very tight control of blood sugar improves outcome in critical illness [18].

Nutrition in respiratory failure

Malnutrition impairs respiratory muscle strength. On the other hand, glucose and amino acid infusions increase VO_2. Glucose oxidation produces more CO_2 per gram than fat and, therefore, excess supply of glucose may increase CO_2 production, work of breathing and impair ability to be weaned from mechanical ventilation. Enteral feeds with an increased proportion of fat to CHO may reduce CO_2 production and allow easier weaning [19], although this is still controversial. It is possible that avoiding excess calories may be as important in this matter as the source of the calories.

Novel nutritional substrates

The exact mechanism of action of novel substrates is controversial as many have multiple physiological actions. It has been suggested that some directly "boost" the immune system – immunonutrition (see below).

It should be emphasised that in many instances the administration of these novel substrates is supported by, at best, circumstantial evidence. Few are supported by adequate controlled studies.

Note: Remember to ensure that sufficient amounts of "conventional" nutrients are supplied before becoming overconcerned with novel substrates [20].

MCFA versus LCFA

(Refers to the position of the first double bond in the carbon chain – LCFA usually ω 6, MCFA usually ω 3 – "fish oils".)

LCFA may affect the immune system as can enter arachidonic acid pathways, for example forming prostaglandins, platelet activating factor and leukotrienes. MCFA are utilised solely for energy and not metabolised to active products. MCFA in some studies may have beneficial effects on protein balance and may have no adverse effect on lung function.

Branched chain amino acids

Branched chain amino acids (BCAA) (leucine, isoleucine and valine) are metabolised in skeletal muscle and, in theory, should decrease muscle protein breakdown if preferentially administered. In the body their main role may be to generate glutamine and alanine. Routine use at present is unsubstantiated.

Glutamine

- Not an essential amino acid, that is the body should be able to synthesise sufficient glutamine from other essential amino acids.
- Despite this, it has been suggested that the synthesis of glutamine is inadequate in critical illness (i.e. a *conditional* essential AA).
- The role of BCAA to provide glutamine has led to interest in administering glutamine itself.
- An essential fuel for bowel mucosal cells (may protect bowel mucosa) and for fibroblasts, lymphocytes and macrophages.
- Forms approximately 50% of the body's amino acid pool.
- Plasma and muscle glutamine levels fall after burns, trauma and major surgery [21].
- Not included in standard formulations of TPN as is relatively unstable in solution.
- Can be supplied via enteral supplements.

Arguably, of all the novel supplements, the strongest evidence supports glutamine. Supplementation has been shown to lessen the negative nitrogen balance after injury and major surgery [22]. A study in a heterogenous group of ICU patients found a significant improvement in outcome in those patients who received glutamine supplements [23].

Arginine

- Technically another non-essential amino acid.
- Important for wound healing, collagen deposition and immune function.
- Stimulates growth hormone, glucagon and insulin secretion.
- Stimulates T-cell function.
- Precursor of nitric oxide. May have a role in preventing ischaemia/reperfusion injury [24].

Nucleotides

- May stimulate the immune system.
- Absent in standard TPNs.

Immunonutrition

The concept of certain nutrients (e.g. ω 3 MCFA, nucleotides and arginine) directly stimulating the immune system in critically ill patients and therefore reducing infectious complications and improving outcome is potentially useful.

- One study compared a standard enteral feed with a preparation (Impact®, Sandoz nutrition) containing the so-called immunonutrients found a reduced length of stay on average and a decrease in infectious complications in the immunonutrient group [25].
- The same immune stimulating feed has been shown to improve various indices of immune status in ICU patients [26].
- A more recent study of major GI surgery found a reduced incidence of late complications in the study group with the same preparation [27]. Analysis showed substantial savings in the Impact group because of the reduced complications despite the greater comparative cost of this preparation.
- Immunonutrition strategies have been shown to decrease multiple organ factor (MOF) scores, length of stay (LOS) and duration of IPPV if started early [28, 29].

- However, an interim analysis of a multicentre randomised trial comparing an immune enhancing enteral feed (not Impact®) with TPN in patients with severe sepsis resulted in the trial being stopped. Mortality in those patients given the enteral feed was higher than in those given TPN [30]. It has been postulated that Arginine, being a precursor of nitric oxide, may increase the mortality in septic patients.
- This study has raised many issues not least being a lone modern voice recommending TPN over EN!

Fibre

- Many believe that fibre should be added routinely as part of an enteral feed regime. Short chain fatty acids produced by its breakdown by gut bacteria are essential nutrients for the colon. It may support normal gut flora, bind bile salts, absorb water, reduce gram negative bacteria overgrowth and improve glucose intolerance.
- Reduces enteral feeding associated diarrhoea in non-critically ill patients but there are no studies showing definite benefit in ICU patients [31].

FURTHER READING

Biolo G, Grimble G, Preiser J-C et al. Metabolic basis of nutrition in intensive care unit patients: ten critical questions. *Intens Care Med* 2002; 28: 1512–20.

Gramlich L, Kichian K, Pinilla J, Rodych NJ et al. Does enteral nutrition compared to parenteral nutrition result in better outcomes in critically ill adult patients? A systematic review of the literature. *Nutrition* 2004; 20: 843–8.

Heyland DK, Dhaliwal R, Drover JW, Gramlich L et al. Canadian clinical practice guidelines for nutrition support in mechanically ventilated, critically ill adult patients. *J Parent Enter Nutr* 2003; 27: 355–73.

REFERENCES

1. Bartlett RH, Allyn PA, Medley T. Nutritional therapy based on positive caloric balance in burn patients. *Arch Surg* 1977; 112: 974–80.
2. Long CL, Schiller WR, Geiger JW. Gluconeogenic response during glucose infusions in patients following skeletal trauma or sepsis. *J Parent Enter Nutr* 1978; 22: 619–25.
3. Elwyn DH, Kinney JM, Jeevanandam M. Influence of increasing carbohydrate intake on glucose kinetics in injured patients. *Ann Surg* 1977; 190: 170–5.

4. Streat SJ, Beddoe AH, Hill GH. Aggressive nutritional support does not prevent protein loss despite fat gain in septic intensive care patients. *J Trauma* 1987; 27: 262–6.

5. Long JM, Wilmore DW, Mason AD. Effect of carbohydrate and fat intake on nitrogen excretion during total intravenous feeding. *Ann Surg* 1977; 185: 417–22.

6. Tremblay A, Bandi V. Impact of body mass index on outcomes following critical care. *Chest* 2003; 123: 1202–7.

7. Baumgartner RN, Koehler KM, Gallagher D et al. Epidemiology of sarcopenia among the elderly in New Mexico. *Am J Epidemiol* 1998; 147: 755–63.

8. Iannuzzi-Sucich M, Prestwood KM, Kenny AM. Prevalence of sarcopenia and predictors of skeletal muscle mass in healthy, older men and women. *J Gerontol A Biol Sci Med Sci* 2002; 57: 772–7.

9. Baker JP, Detsky AS, Wesson DE. Nutritional assessment: a comparison of clinical judgement and objective measurement. *New Engl J Med* 1982; 306: 969–72.

10. Dhaliwal R, Jurewitsch B, Harrietha D, Heyland DK. Combination enteral and parenteral nutrition in critically ill patients: harmful or beneficial? A systematic review of the evidence. *Intens Care Med* 2004; 30: 1661–71.

11. Jooste CA, Mustoe J, Collee G. Metoclopramide improves gastric motility in critically ill patients. *Intens Care Med* 1999; 25: 464–8.

12. Spapen HD, Duinslaeger L, Diltoer M, Gillet R, Bossuyt A et al. Gastric emptying in critically ill patients is accelerated by adding cisapride to a standard enteral feeding protocol: results of a prospective, randomized, controlled trial. *Crit Care Med* 1995; 23: 481–5.

13. Moore FA, Feliciano DV, Andrassy RJ, McArdle AH et al. Early enteral feeding, compared with parenteral, reduces postoperative septic complications. The results of a meta-analysis. *Ann Surg* 1992; 216: 172–83.

14. Schofield WN. Predicting basal metabolic rate, new standards and review of previous work. *Human Nutr Clin Nutr* 1985; 39C(Suppl 1.5): 41.

15. Uehara M, Plamk LD, Hill GL. Components of energy expenditure in patients with severe sepsis and major trauma: a basis for clinical care. *Crit Care Med* 1999; 27: 1295–302.

16. Christman JW, McCain RW. A sensible approach to the nutritional support of mechanically ventilated critically ill patients. *Intens Care Med* 1993; 19: 129–36.

17. Berger MM, Cavadini C. Unrecognised intake of trace elements in polytraumatised and burnt patients. *Ann Francaises Anesth reanim* 1994; 13: 289–96.

18. Van den Berghe G, Wouters P, Weekers F et al. Intensive insulin therapy in critically ill patients. *New Engl J Med* 2001; 345: 1359–67.

19. Al-Saady NM, Blackmore CM, Bennett ED. High fat, low carbohydrate, enteral feeding lowers $PaCO_2$ and reduces the period of ventilation in artificially ventilated patients. *Intens Care Med* 1989; 15: 290–5.

20. Griffiths RD. Feeding the critically ill – should we do better? *Intens Care Med* 1997; 23: 246–7.

21. Askanazi J, Carpentier YA, Michelsen CB. Muscle and plasma amino acids following injury: influence of intercurrent infection. *Ann Surg* 1980; 192: 78–82.

22. Stehle P, Zanders J, Mertes N, Albers S et al. Effect of parenteral glutamine peptide sup-
    plements on muscle glutamine loss and nitrogen balance after major surgery. *Lancet*
    1989; 1: 231–3.

23. Griffiths RD, Jones C, Palmer TEA. Six-month outcome of critically ill patients given
    glutamine supplemented parenteral nutrition. *Nutrition* 1997; 13: 295–302.

24. Roth E. The impact of L-arginine-nitric oxide metabolism on ischaemic/reperfusion
    injury. *Curr Opin Clin Nutr Metab Care* 1998; 1: 97–9.

25. Bower RH, Cerra F, Bershadsky B, Licar JJ et al. Early enteral administration of a for-
    mula (Impact®) supplemented with arginine, nucleotides and fish oil in intensive care
    patients: results of a multicentre, prospective, randomised clinical trial. *Crit Care Med*
    1995; 23: 436–49.

26. Kemen K, Senkal M, Homann HH, Mumme A et al. Early postoperative enteral nutri-
    tion with arginine, omega-3 fatty acids and ribonucleic acid supplemented diet versus
    placebo in cancer patients: an immunologic evaluation of impact®. *Crit Care Med*
    1995; 23: 6542–9.

27. Senkal M, Mumme A, Eickhoff U, Geier B et al. Early postoperative enteral immunonu-
    trition: clinical outcome and cost-comparison analysis in surgical patients. *Crit Care
    Med* 1997; 25: 1489–96.

28. Atkinson S, Sieffert E, Bihari D. A prospective, randomized, double-blind, controlled
    clinical trial of enteral immunonutrition in the critically ill. *Crit Care Med* 1998; 26:
    1164–72.

29. Weimann A, Bashau L, Bischoff WE et al. Influence of arginine, omega-3 fatty acids
    and nucleotide-supplemented enteral support on systemic inflammatory response
    syndrome and multiple organ failure in patients after severe trauma. *Nutrition* 1997;
    14: 165–72.

30. Bertolini G, Iapichino G, Radrizzani D, Facchini R et al. Early enteral immunonutrition
    in patients with severe sepsis: results of an interim analysis of a randomized multicen-
    tre clinical trial. *Intens Care Med* 2003; 29: 834–40.

31. Dobb G, Towler S. Diarrhoea during enteral feeding in the critically ill: a comparison of
    feeds with and without fibre. *Intens Care Med* 1990; 16: 252–5.

8

Non-invasive mechanical ventilation

D. Kelly

As critical care consumes increasing amounts of health care budgets globally there is an increasing demand for interventions that are clinically effective in the sense that they reduce patient length of stay, reduce complications and are less demanding of medical and nursing resources:

- However, the evidence base for critical care interventions is very narrow and it is often very difficult to find any intervention that meets the above criteria.
- Non-invasive ventilation (NIV) comes close if applied to patients with the appropriate indications [1].
- Like all interventions, if used indiscriminately these benefits are lost and it is the purpose of this chapter to give the reader some insight into how best to apply this technology to achieve the best outcomes.

Definition

NIV is the application of bi-level airway pressure support using a nasal or full face mask as the patient interface:

- The lower level of support will be referred to as expiratory positive airway pressure (EPAP) and the upper level as inspiratory positive airway pressure (IPAP).
- If the IPAP is set on zero then the patient will be receiving what is conventionally known as constant positive airway pressure or CPAP as it is better known.
- NIV and CPAP as terms are often used interchangeably but they should be regarded as two quite separate forms of airway support.

It should be remembered that the gas flow that generates the EPAP has another function. It helps to clear the CO_2 and reduce rebreathing.

History

NIV was initially used to support individuals with neuromuscular disease to avoid hypoventilation during sleep. It has become the ventilatory support of choice for all patients at risk of hypercapnia due to neuromuscular disease, chest wall deformity or impaired respiratory drive. Its use in the acute care setting began with trials on patients admitted in acute hypercapnic respiratory failure with chronic obstructive pulmonary disease (COPD) [2].

Machines

When the priorities and market lay in the community the development of NIV ventilators focused on ease of use and minimal reliance on gas supplies. Once it became adopted by the critical care community for the treatment of acute respiratory failure in the hospital setting the specifications changed and became more sophisticated.

There is a huge variety of ventilators to choose from. The range includes:

- Relatively simple flow generators which can be used at home to support hypoventilation in compliant patients who are sleeping.
- Sophisticated intensive therapy unit (ITU) ventilators that have a numbers of ventilator modes to choose from and can be used in a critical care setting to support a hypoxic, hypercapnic patient.

It is essential when reading the literature that one is very clear exactly which type is being used and in what mode, as success or failure with the technique may depend on using the correct type in the right mode for the appropriate patient.

Definitions

One must be familiar with the following definitions to interpret the published information.

CPAP

This refers to the technique of respiratory support that provides a CPAP throughout the whole of the respiratory cycle. It will allow higher FiO_2 than conventional face mask oxygen, recruits collapsed lung and will reduce the work of breathing. Many NIV ventilators will function in this mode but it is not NIV although the two techniques are often referred to interchangeably.

Controlled mechanical ventilation

No patient effort is required. Either the inflation pressure or the tidal volume is set. There are numerous ways to refine these settings further but it is rarely used as a NIV mode.

Assist/control ventilation

Like controlled mandatory ventilation (CMV), the pressure or volume is set by the operator, as are the number of breaths per minute. Patient triggering can also cycle the ventilator although the breath delivered is identical to a mandatory breath. If patient triggering subsequently delays a mandatory breath then the mode is said to be synchronised and is called synchronised intermittent mandatory ventilation (SIMV).

SIMV is a term familiar to critical care staff but is not generally used in NIV machines where it is more likely to be referred to as spontaneous/timed (S/T) or IE mode.

Assisted spontaneous breathing

In this mode the pressure is set and the volume delivered depends on:

- the resistance and compliance of the patient: ventilator system,
- the respiratory rate of the patient,
- their compliance with this mode of ventilation,
- the presence or absence of any leaks and their magnitude.

This mode is better known to critical care staff as pressure support. In addition because it depends on patient triggering there is often the option to set a backup mandatory ventilator rate in case of apnoea.

In some machines it is known as the S/T mode and the pressure set is the IPAP pressure.

Bi-level pressure support

This refers to the technique that combines CPAP with pressure support. The CPAP pressure is set when the EPAP level is adjusted and the pressure support when the IPAP level is adjusted.

Patient ventilator interface

These depend on the circumstances. There are mouth pieces, nasal masks and face masks:

- The biggest problem is with leaks. As you tighten the mask to reduce the leak you increase the pressure effects on the face and it is usually the nose that bears the brunt of this leading in some cases to full thickness erosion of the skin on the bridge of the nose.
- In many of the early trials of NIV in critical care, conventional intensive care ventilators were used. As these were relatively intolerant of leaks good mask fit was essential and pressure effects were more of a problem.
- Nasal masks are preferred when possible as they allow the patient to communicate, eat and drink as required and are less claustrophobic. Gas leaks through the mouth can be a problem and chin straps can be helpful.
- Face masks are more useful in the hypoxaemic patient as they tend to be mouth breathers in the acute phase of their illness. In some circumstances the dead space of the mask can become significant and can be the reason why the CO_2 fails to fall in a hypercapnic patient despite apparently adequate ventilation.

Compliance with the technique is sometimes helped if the patient is allowed to settle on a mouthpiece first before switching to a face mask [3].

Humidification

This is generally not regarded as a major problem as the upper airways are not bypassed. The addition of humidification to a circuit may increase the work of breathing so must not be done without a thorough consideration of the risks involved. In some machines expiratory valves are used to ensure CO_2 elimination. Any additional moisture in the circuit can impair the function of these valves leading to an increase in circuit dead space.

Indications

There are many case reports anecdotally recounting the successful use of NIV in circumstances where intubation and ventilation would previously have been the only option. Its growing popularity reflects the advantages that it confers as well as the disadvantages of conventional ventilation that it avoids.

The advantages include:

- speech is retained,
- eating and drinking are possible,
- it can be delivered intermittently,
- normal humidification mechanisms are retained,
- patients do not require sedation,
- respiratory defences against infection are not breached,
- the patients retain mobility,
- monitoring is usually less invasive as a consequence further promoting mobility,
- once stable the patients are less nurse dependent.

It avoids:

- intubation of larynx and trachea, and inevitable trauma,
- immobility,
- haemodynamic compromise of sedation and ventilation.

These reasons alone probably explain the three key benefits seen if NIV is used:

- shorter intensive care unit (ICU) stay,
- shorter hospital stay,
- reduced morbidity particularly from infectious complications of conventional ventilation such as ventilator acquired pneumonia, sinusitis and line sepsis [4].

It was certainly true in one study of NIV that the NIV group of patients had fewer lines and catheters [5].

Contraindications

There are very few absolute contraindications especially if NIV is commenced in an environment where immediate intubation and ventilation is available. If this is not the case and NIV is commenced in a ward-based setting then the contraindications acquire more strength. The safe choice then depends on the experience of the practitioners involved in the initiation of the therapy and the subsequent degree of supervision.

Most people would agree that the following probably constitute the absolute contraindications:

- facial burns or trauma,
- obstruction of the upper airway,
- coma,
- haemodynamic instability.

Relative contraindications exist but it may acceptable to use NIV despite these if NIV is used as a trial and is to be the ceiling on treatment. Some of them exist because they herald failure and would be more safely managed by immediate intubation. These include:

- inability to protect the airway,
- agitation or confusion,
- copious respiratory secretions,
- reduced conscious level,
- life threatening hypoxaemia.

Some however exist because NIV under these circumstances would lead to patient compromise:

- recent upper gastrointestinal surgery,
- obstructed bowel,
- vomiting.

The list of conditions or clinical circumstances when NIV may be used is growing everyday but level I evidence of benefit is harder to find. There are however a number of conditions where there is sufficient evidence now to make judgements about the effectiveness or otherwise of NIV.

COPD

Severe exacerbations of COPD are the commonest respiratory cause for emergency admission in the UK. Overall mortality rates can be as high as 14%. The risk of death is increased if intubation and ventilation are required [6]. NIV has been studied extensively as an alternative means of support and it has been demonstrated that it confers the following advantages if applied to the subgroup who present with $PaCO_2$ greater than 6 kPa:

- lower mortality,
- reduction in need for intubation,
- shortened hospital stay.

As this can be achieved in ward-based settings and admission to intensive care averted this technique is a very cost effective intervention that reduces total costs whilst reducing mortality at the same time.

Cardiogenic pulmonary oedema

Whilst the use of CPAP is established as a successful support mode in cardiogenic pulmonary oedema the use of NIV is less certain. One study had an increase in myocardial infarction in the NIV groups [7]. NIV should only be considered if CPAP fails despite full medical therapy.

Neuromuscular disorders and chest wall deformities

NIV was well established in the community to support individuals who required mechanical support to avoid hypercapnia because of chest wall deformity or neuromuscular disease before it was used in the acute sector. Consequently there have been no randomised controlled trials in these settings. It remains the support of choice when these individuals develop decompensation due to acute on chronic respiratory failure usually as a result of acquired infection. These individuals praise their ability to communicate very highly and fear intubation and tracheostomy as much as their attendants who are only too aware of the weaning difficulties they will face even with an early tracheostomy.

Haematological disorders and immunosuppression

Any patient with a haematological disorder who presents with acute hypoxaemic respiratory failure that requires intubation and ventilation has a greater than 70% mortality [8]. Pneumocystis pneumonia in acquired immune deficiency syndrome (AIDS) leading to intubation and ventilation carries a mortality of approximately 60%. By avoiding ventilator acquired pneumonia and sepsis secondary to invasive monitoring NIV should improve these figures and recent studies confirm that NIV should be considered as an alternative to intubation and ventilation [8].

These considerations have prompted its use in any patient whose immune system is so compromised that nosocomial infection constitutes a serious risk and these include:

- following lung transplantation,
- following any transplantation surgery of any kind,
- reversible insults such as retinoic acid syndrome.

Acute hypoxaemic respiratory failure

Although it is tempting to avoid intubation in conditions such as pneumonia and acute respiratory distress syndrome (ARDS) from any cause there are some hazards that must be considered:

- the failure rate is high;
- secretions can be hard to clear especially if a full face mask is required;
- delaying intubation may mean that the subsequent intubation is much more hazardous because of life threatening hypoxaemia.

There is now a consensus developing that any condition that is slow to develop and slow to resolve like pneumonia is less likely to benefit from NIV. Although the improvement in oxygenation can be life saving it is not the sole reason for resolution of the presenting complaint and these other factors soon determine whether or not the condition resolves. For example in one recent study of NIV in acute renal failure (ARF) due to pneumonia all but one of the failures had developed bacteraemia [9].

Thoracic trauma

Although CPAP is safe and a well-recognised treatment in conjunction with effective epidural analgesia the role of NIV is less clear. If epidural analgesia is not possible or there are injuries that are not covered then NIV will allow high-dose opioid analgesia without the inevitable hypercapnia due to respiratory depression. However, there is an increased risk of pneumothorax that must be managed.

Postoperative weaning

It is not always easy to predict a successful wean and NIV allows trials of extubation and reduces the incidence of reintubation. This applies to cardiothoracic surgery as well as abdominal surgery. This is particularly true in those patients who have preoperative morbidities such as COPD or obesity.

Diagnostic bronchoscopy

Just as the development of cheap ultrasound devices have revolutionised the placement of central venous catheter (CVC) lines and redefined the gold standard of safe practice the newer generation of NIV machines have allowed diagnostic bronchoscopy in patients who would otherwise have deemed to be too hypoxic. It is now possible to support patients through the procedure by NIV application before, during and after the procedure. This is particularly important if bronchoalveolar lavage is required as this inevitably leads to a short-term decrease in an already low PaO_2 [10].

There are machines which are designed to tolerate large leaks and these are ideal for the procedure allowing ventilation even when the bronchoscope is in situ in the trachea.

Monitoring

Appropriate monitoring will depend on the environment.

In order to choose appropriate monitoring it is essential to be aware of the signs of impending failure of the technique so that these can be picked up in a timely fashion. Clinically the patient should have:

- improved chest wall movement,
- good coordination with the ventilator,
- a reduction in accessory muscle use,
- a reduction in heart rate,
- reduced respiratory rate,
- be more comfortable,
- be more awake.

Physiological improvement must include:

- reduction in CO_2,
- improvement in PaO_2,
- resolution of acidosis,
- these changes are usually seen within 1 h and must certainly be evident at 4 h otherwise failure is to be expected.

Routine assessment 1 h after commencement should include blood gas analysis. Thereafter continuous oximetry with 6 hourly gas analysis should suffice. The intensity of monitoring will be determined by the progress of the patient and the environment in which the therapy is instituted.

The reasons for failure can be as much to do with flaws in the application of the technique as it can be to do with the patient and the following should be considered:

- Is medical treatment suboptimal.
- Have complications developed (e.g. pneumonia).
- Too much oxygen leading to hypercapnia.
- Too much leak.
- Circuit problems leading to rebreathing or leaks.
- Can one improve patient acceptability.
- Is support adequate.

Weaning from NIV

The patient should be ventilated for as long as they will tolerate initially. Signs of improvement include:

- heart rate below 110 beats/min,
- respiratory rate less than 24/min,
- SpO_2 above 90% on FiO_2 less than 4 l/min,
- compensated pH greater than 7.35.

Sometimes the patient will be aware of when they are ready to begin weaning. Weaning should begin first during awake periods. Weaning periods when asleep should then follow.

NIV facilities

There is a consensus developing about the appropriate setting for the provision of NIV. The British Thoracic Society Guidelines on NIV (see Further reading) suggest the following:

- Ward-based NIV is appropriate if there is a designated location in the hospital, appropriately trained staff to manage it and a system in place that ensures that the right patients get referred in a timely manner.
- Ward-based services should have a designated lead clinician with overall responsibility for the service.
- Sicker patients who would be intubated if NIV fails, should be managed in a critical care area.

- Patients with conditions such as pneumonia or ARDS should be managed in a critical care area unless NIV is the limit to the treatment on offer. This applies to any condition where the role of NIV has not clearly been established.

FURTHER READING

British Thoracic Society. Non-invasive ventilation in acute respiratory failure. *Thorax* 2002; 57: 192–211.

Evans TW. International Consensus Conferences in Intensive Care Medicine: non-invasive positive pressure ventilation in acute respiratory failure. *Intens Care Med* 2001; 27: 166–78.

NHS Modernisation Agency. *Critical Care Programme: Weaning and Long Term Ventilation.* NHS Modernisation Agency, London, 2002.

REFERENCES

1. Plant PK, Owen JL, Parrott S, Elliot MW. Cost effectiveness of ward based non-invasive ventilation for acute exacerbations of chronic obstructive pulmonary disease: economic analysis of randomised controlled trial. *Br Med J* 2003; 326: 956–8.

2. Bott J, Carroll MP, Conway JH et al. Randomised controlled trial of nasal ventilation in acute ventilatory failure due to chronic obstructive airways disease. *Lancet* 1993; 341: 1555–7.

3. British Thoracic Society. Non-invasive ventilation in acute respiratory failure. *Thorax* 2002; 57: 192–211.

4. Antonelli M, Conti G, Bufi M et al. Non-invasive ventilation for treatment of acute respiratory failure in patients undergoing solid organ transplantation: a randomised trial. *J Am Med Assoc* 2000; 283: 235–41.

5. Confalonieri M, Calderini E, Terraciano S et al. Non-invasive ventilation for treating acute respiratory failure in AIDS patients with pneumocystis carinii pneumonia. *Intens Care Med* 2002; 28: 1233–8.

6. Seneff MG, Wagner DP, Wagner RP, Zimmerman JE et al. Hospital and 1-year survival of patients admitted to intensive care units with acute exacerbations of chronic obstructive pulmonary disease. *J Am Med Assoc* 1995; 274: 1852–7.

7. Mehta S, Jay GD, Woolard RH et al. Randomized prospective trial of bilevel versus continuous positive airway pressure in acute pulmonary edema. *Crit Care Med* 1997; 25: 620–8.

8. Kroschinsky F, Weise M, Illmer T et al. Outcome and prognostic features of intensive care unit treatment in patients with haematological malignancies. *Intens Care Med* 2002; 28: 1294–1300.

  9. Domenighetti G, Gayer R, Gentilini R. Noninvasive pressure support ventilation in non-COPD patients with acute cardiogenic pulmonary oedema and severe community-acquired pneumonia: acute effects and outcome. *Intens Care Med* 2002; 28: 1226–32.
 10. Antonnelli M, Conti G, Riccioni L, Meduri GU. Non-invasive positive pressure ventilation via face mask during bronchoscopy with bronchoalveolar lavage in high risk hypoxaemic patients. *Chest* 1996; 110: 724–8.

9

Principles of IPPV

I. McConachie

Mechanical ventilation, especially intermittent positive pressure ventilation (IPPV) is the mainstay of modern intensive care practice and of fundamental importance to intensive care unit (ICU) therapy.

Care of the ventilated patient

General issues

- *Airway*. Access via cuffed tracheal tube or tracheostomy. *Secure* the tube. Do not overinflate the tracheal cuff. Cuff pressure should be regularly measured, even in tubes with a high-volume/low-pressure cuff.
- Provide adequate humidification and clearance of secretions. The absence of humidification will encourage heat loss and dehydration of the upper respiratory tract. This can cause upper airway epithelial damage, and difficulties with clearance of dry secretions. Conversely, excess heat and/or humidification can cause problems.
- Routine nursing care including care of the unconscious patient.
- Monitor appropriately. In view of the unpredictable and complex effects of IPPV on the circulation be prepared to monitor the central vascular pressures and cardiac output (CO). An arterial line is mandatory to facilitate blood gas sampling for all but the shortest periods of ventilation.
- Nasogastric (N/G) tube to relieve gastric distension and permit administration of medications and nutrition.
- Ensure patient comfort as far as possible. See Chapter 14, Sedation, Analgesia and Neuromuscular Blockade.
- Ensure adequate nutrition and hydration.

Specific issues

Deep vein thrombosis prevention

Deep vein thrombosis (DVT) is common among patients requiring prolonged mechanical ventilation in the ICU setting despite the use of prophylaxis measures. Pharmacological prophylaxis is commonly used but mechanical devices may also be effective and preferred where the risk of bleeding is high. Alternatively, low molecular weight heparins are associated with less bleeding (and less heparin induced thrombocytopenia) than standard heparin.

Coagulopathy negates the need for DVT prophylaxis and many hold the administration of heparin if the International Normalisation Ratio (INR) >1.5:

- In an early study there was a 12% incidence of DVT as documented by duplex ultrasonography [1]. Ninety-two per cent of patients had received DVT prophylaxis. Twelve patients (12%) were documented to have DVT by venous duplex scans. The incidence of DVT in those patients without signs or symptoms of DVT was only 3.6%. However, there was a poor correlation between leg swelling and DVT.
- In a more recent study of patients ventilated for >7 days, 23.6% were shown to have a DVT by the use of duplex ultrasonography [2]. *All patients had received prophylaxis.* However, there were no statistically significant differences in hospital mortality or lengths of stay in the hospital and ICU for patients with and without DVT.
- Perfusion problems have led to the questioning of the appropriateness of the subcutaneous route in critically ill patients. A recent study in ICU patients has shown significantly lower anti-Xa levels in response to a single daily dose of subcutaneous enoxaparin compared with medical non-ICU patients [3].

Pressure area care

In a recent study [4] the risk of developing pressure ulcers in ICU was associated with the following:

- noradrenaline infusion,
- high acute physiology and chronic health evaluation II (APACHE II) score,
- faecal incontinence,
- anaemia,
- long length of stay.

The usefulness of the commonly used waterlow pressure sore risk (PSR) scale in the ICU has been established [5]. In that study, when a patient had a PSR score >25 on admission, the risk of developing a pressure sore was significantly increased.

The prevalence of pressure ulcers in Dutch ICUs has been shown to be 28% [6]. Specialised support systems were only in use in 60% of patients at high risk of ulcers. Worse, only 37% of patients for whom regular turning was appropriate were actually being turned. There is no reason to presume these problems are specific to Dutch ICUs.

Eye care

Eye problems especially microbial keratitis can have devastating effects on vision in survivors from ICU. The incidence and prevalence is unknown. Pseudomonas is commonly the reported infecting organism.

In a small study [7], 60% of ventilated patients receiving sedation for more than 48 h had developed corneal erosion when assessed using the ocular slit lamp especially in those patients who were unable to close their eyes. Protective eyelid taping was effective in preventing and treating the corneal erosion.

The use of an algorithm has been proposed [8] to reduce the incidence of these problems revolving around:

- *Lids closed*: no specific treatment.
- *Conjunctive exposed*: use of 4 hourly lubricants.
- *Cornea exposed*: use of tape over eyes + 4 hourly lubricants.
- *Prone position*: use of tape over eyes + 4 hourly lubricants.

One must not forget to administer chronic eye medications to ventilated patients, especially medication for glaucoma. It is important to be aware that other medications may affect intraocular pressures. For example, the use of dopamine is associated with increased intraocular pressures in critically ill patients [9]. This may not be a problem in normal patients but may represent a significant risk in patients with glaucoma.

Daily assessment and management planning (courtesy Dr DR Kelly)

The ventilated patient should receive a full clinical examination each day with special focus on the cardiopulmonary system. In addition a suggested structured programme for assessment and management planning is as follows:

(1) Is the diagnosis secure?
(2) If not, what investigations are necessary?

(3) Are the treatments correct?

Right dose?

Right duration?

Secure from allergy or toxicity?

Effect of renal or liver dysfunction?

(4) Consider the supportive therapy:

Are they on appropriate dose of inotrope?

Are they too vasoconstricted?

Stress ulcer prophylaxis?

DVT prophylaxis?

(5) Consider the haemodynamics:

Adequate organ perfusion?

Adequate filling?

Appropriate haematocrit?

Adequate monitoring?

Signs of myocardial or other ischaemia?

Antifailure medication optimal?

(6) Consider the ventilation:

Is the tidal volume (TV) appropriate? Low enough?

Adequate positive end expiratory pressure (PEEP) to keep lung open?

Are recruitment manoeuvres necessary?

Appropriate mode?

(7) Consider the lungs:

Are they draining? Are secretions changing?

Does the airway resistance or lung compliance indicate bronchodilators or steroids?

Pneumothorax?

Plugging/inspissation?

Appropriate humidification?

Are they head up?

(8) Can they wean? If not, why not?

(9) Can they be mobilised to a chair? If not, why not?

(10) Is sedation appropriate? What is depth? Is it stopped daily?

(11) Check parameters of liver and renal function. Is renal support required?

(12) Is the gut working? Gut protection prescribed? Prokinetics? Enteral nutrition? Diarrhoea or constipation?

(13) Adequate calorie intake? Adequate non-protein calories? Novel substrates?

(14) What bacteriological evidence is there for antibiotics?

(15) What specimens have been sent? When? Need repeating?

(16) Any evidence for line sepsis? How old are lines?

(17) Is the white cell count (WCC) rising/falling? Temperature?

(18) Have you checked for focal neurological signs?

(19) Have specialist referrals been done?

(20) Do relatives need counselling?

Airway management

The choice is between oral tracheal tubes, nasal tracheal tubes and tracheostomy tubes. Each have their advantages, disadvantages and complications.

General disadvantages include:

- bypassing upper airway defences against infection;
- loss of humidification of inspired gases;
- less effective cough;
- long term damage to airway;
- increased work of breathing due to increased airway resistance.

Oral tubes

Advantages	Usually smooth atraumatic insertion
	Easy suction of secretions
	Familiarity
Disadvantages	Patient discomfort
	Obstruction by bite
	Problems with oral hygiene and mouth care
	Laryngeal damage if cuff overinflated (reduced by low-pressure cuffs)
	Occasionally difficult to secure (e.g. patients with beards)
	Dental trauma on insertion
	Moulding at body temperature and movement within the oropharynx

Nasal tubes

Advantages	Better comfort (i.e. less sedation requirements)
	Easy fixation
	Less oropharyngeal movement

Disadvantages   Sinusitis as occult source of sepsis
                False passages created during insertion
                Bacteraemia on insertion
                Nasal erosions
                Epistaxis on insertion
                Difficult for suction
                Laryngeal damage, as for above
                Longer than oral tubes, slightly increased work of breathing

Overall, most would agree that oral tracheal tubes are preferred to nasal tracheal tubes for most situations in the adult ICU.

The role of chest X-rays

All new admissions to ICU will need a chest X-ray (CXR), even if only as a baseline. In the past it was considered important to perform CXR daily on ventilated patients. European legislation mandates us to reduce, where possible, patients' exposure to ionising radiation leading to a re-examination of this practice:

- Studies show us that clinical examination can effectively predict the need for radiography [10].
- The most recent study of the value of routine daily CXR found that this practice was not associated with a reduction in ICU or hospital length of stay or mortality [11].
- Radiological changes may lag behind clinical changes.

Thus CXRs should be performed largely on the basis of clinical change in the patient's condition. In particular, regular CXRs performed on patients who are rapidly improving seem pointless.

Exceptions to the above are CXRs following central venous pressure (CVP) placement or following intubation; that is, those circumstances where clinical assessment of placement position may be unreliable. In addition, many would still argue for occasional "screening" CXRs to be performed in long stay ventilated patients, that is, to assess resolution of fibrosis or early detection of new infiltrates.

Principles of ventilatory support

- IPPV should only be used where there is a reasonable chance of survival.
- It should not be used as the last therapeutic act in a dying patient purely because it is available if it will only prolong the act of dying and the relatives' distress. Patients who are clearly dying should be allowed to do so without a period of inappropriate therapy on a ventilator. This is explored in Chapter 16, Withholding and Withdrawing Therapy in ICU.

The prime indication for IPPV outside of the operating theatre is respiratory failure but modern ICU practice recognises the value of early ventilation as part of organ support in other critically ill patients, especially in the presence of shock or cardiac failure.

Indications

Indications in the ICU include:

- *Postoperative management*: for example, patients with morbid obesity, postoperative hypothermia, preexisting lung disease, cardiac surgery and gross abdominal distension.
- *Respiratory disease*: for example, pneumonia, lung contusion, asthma and other chronic obstructive respiratory diseases and acute respiratory distress syndrome (ARDS).
- *Chest wall disease*: for example, patient with "flail chest" following trauma.
- *Neuromuscular disease*: for example, Guillain–Barre syndrome, myasthenia, etc.
- *Central nervous system (CNS) impairment*: for example, drug overdose, trauma, status epilepticus, cerebral haemorrhage, tetanus.
- *Cardiovascular disease*: for example, cardiac arrest, severe shock of any aetiology, pulmonary oedema.
- To provide organ support prior to organ donation in patients fulfilling appropriate criteria.

Protecting the airway against aspiration strictly only requires tracheal intubation or tracheostomy, not IPPV, but the clinical circumstances nearly always require IPPV as well as intubation.

The difficult decision is often not whether to ventilate a patient but more often *when* to ventilate a patient (apart from acute emergencies, e.g. cardiac arrest). This is difficult to be precise about and experience is often the deciding factor:

- Certainly gross hypoxia: for example, PO_2 <8 kPa on 60% concentration of inspired oxygen is a strong indication if there are no contraindications.
- Similarly, worsening hypercarbia and respiratory and or metabolic acidosis are highly significant.
- Often trends of physical and physiological variables are more useful than absolute values.
- In accepting this one must not forget that hypercarbia usually develops relatively slowly whereas acute hypoxia can be lethal within minutes. It is better to intubate early rather than too late!
- General condition of the patient, for example, presence of exhaustion, sweating, increasing restlessness or an inability to clear sputum is important in indicating need for ventilatory support.

Contraindications to IPPV

The decision to withhold IPPV in patients with chronic respiratory failure is difficult and requires the judgment of experienced practitioners. Ideally, the family and other professionals involved in caring for the patient should be involved in this decision. The patient's wishes should be paramount but unfortunately when the situation arises the patient is often unable to become rationally involved due to their illness.

   In general, it may be appropriate to avoid IPPV (and possibly try non-invasive ventilation) in patients with one or more of the following:

- Severe chronic respiratory disease with severe dyspnoea. Such patients are often receiving domiciliary oxygen.
- No identifiable reversible features. In addition, certain precipitating conditions, for example, heart failure or pneumonia in chronic obstructive pulmonary disease (COPD) patients also predict a poor outcome and reduced life expectancy [12].
- Poor quality of life (e.g. housebound, wheelchair bound). Take care, as this is highly subjective! Functional measures; for example, ability to walk unaided are more objective and also may have prognostic significance [13] (in e.g. COPD).
- Previous objective respiratory measurements may be helpful (e.g. documented functional expiratory volume 1 (FEV1) <0.75) [13].
- If the patient has established or chronic multiple organ failure it may not be appropriate to offer IPPV if respiratory failure supervenes.

The situation is further complicated by the more widespread use of non-invasive forms of respiratory support which, indeed, are now the respiratory support mechanism of choice in exacerbations of COPD. Two points are worth noting:

- A failed trial of non-invasive support does not necessarily mean that IPPV is inappropriate.
- However, just because a patient is considered suitable for a trial of non-invasive support does not automatically mandate invasive ventilation if it fails, especially if IPPV had been originally requested by the referring team and declined.

Physiological effects of IPPV

Cardiovascular effects

The two main effects of IPPV are:

(1) Lung volumes are increased, often significantly compared to spontaneous ventilation:
   – Large TVs causes a rise in pulmonary vascular resistance (PVR) which may lead to pulmonary hypertension and right ventricular (RV) compromise. This is due to the over inflated alveoli causing compression of the alveolar blood vessels. (Conversely shallow breathing, e.g. during weaning can also increase PVR, partly by collapsing alveoli causing a fall in diameter of extra alveolar pulmonary blood vessels and partly by development of hypoxic pulmonary vasoconstriction.)
   – In addition, large TV leading to hyperinflation releases factors into the circulation depressing the blood pressure. Animal studies suggest these to be prostaglandins.
   – Hyperinflation can occasionally "squeeze" the heart in the cardiac fossa causing falls in CO analogous with cardiac tamponade. This is occasionally seen in severe asthma or emphysemas.
(2) Intrathoracic pressure (ITP) is increased at all points in the respiratory cycle, compared to the "negative" pressures generated during spontaneous ventilation:
   – The heart operates as a "pressure chamber within a pressure chamber" (as described by Pinsky, see Further reading) and it is therefore not surprising that changes in ITP affect cardiac function.

- – Thus changes in ITP are transmitted to the cardiac chambers during ventilation.
- – Inspiration during IPPV increases ITP and therefore increases right atrial (RA) pressure relative to atmospheric pressure leading to a decreased gradient for venous return, reduced RV filling and reduced RV stroke volume. In addition the increased ITP decreases the gradient across the left ventricle (LV) that the LV has to work against, this is one aspect of afterload. In other words decreased transmural pressure decreases LV afterload. Both of these effects tend to reduce intrathoracic blood volume.
- – Conversely, with decreased ITP, as occurs with spontaneous breathing during inspiration, the opposite is achieved; for example, decreased RA pressure, increased gradient for venous return, increased RV stroke volume, increased LV transmural pressure and increased LV afterload. The combined effect is to increase intrathoracic blood volume.
- – The decreased venous return and therefore decreased CO with IPPV is the major haemodynamic effect of ventilation in most patients. As it is related to ITP it is worse if the ventilator is set to provide either a high TV (high-peak ITP) or a prolonged inspiratory time (high-mean ITP). PEEP also exacerbates the fall in venous return.
- – Venous return and CO can be restored by either fluid infusion or sympathetic drugs both of which restore the gradient for venous return despite further increases in RA pressure.

Thus increased ITP reduces venous return (preload) but also reduces afterload on the heart due to effects on transmural pressure. Which effect predominates depends on several factors; for example, presence of hypovolaemia and, most importantly, the state of the heart. Any beneficial effect on afterload in the normal heart is limited by the fall in venous return. In the failing heart the CO is relatively insensitive to changes in preload (flat part of the Starling curve) but exquisitely sensitive to small reductions in afterload. Thus in heart failure there may be beneficial effects on CO from increases in ITP with ventilation. In addition it will be crucial in the failing heart to avoid large falls in ITP as may occur during laboured spontaneous breathing as this can dramatically increase both preload and afterload producing pulmonary oedema.

With high ITP, RV afterload usually increases due to increasing PVR and development of pulmonary hypertension. Thus, high thoracic pressures can reduce LV filling due to RV distension pushing the septum to the left to reduce LV chamber size (known as interventricular independence). This effect of excessive high thoracic pressure can counteract the beneficial effects on LV afterload.

Thus the cardiovascular consequences of IPPV are complex and vary in differing disease states.

Respiratory effects

- IPPV causes a potential increase in ventilation and perfusion (V/Q) mismatch due to preferential ventilation of the non-dependant, poorly perfused lung regions. PEEP in general will improve oxygenation by recruitment of poorly ventilated lung regions [14].
- In the supine position functional residual capacity (FRC) will be reduced due in part to upward displacement of the abdominal contents. This contribute to an increase in micro atelectasis.
- Decreased pulmonary perfusion if CO falls with IPPV causes an increase in alveolar dead space.
- Surfactant secretion is also reduced by prolonged IPPV.

Other effects

- Humoral effects include an increase in antidiuretic hormone (ADH), renin–angiotensin and atrial natriuretic peptide leading to an overall retention of sodium and water.
- The oedema, particularly in the upper body, seen with prolonged IPPV is also promoted by inhibition of lymph and venous drainage from the upper body.
- The inhibition of venous drainage from the head may also result in a rise in intracranial pressure (ICP).

Beneficial effects

There is a considerable reduction in work of breathing and proportion of CO and VO_2 going to the lungs and diaphragm with a resultant increase in available CO and VO_2 elsewhere.

There are some who think this may be the only definite beneficial effect of IPPV

Other beneficial effects include:

- Improvement in alveolar expansion particularly where there is lobar collapse often secondary to progressive hypoventilation and exhaustion.
- Recruitment of collapsed lung units.

- Oxygenation usually does increase but not necessarily in severe pulmonary disorders (e.g. ARDS).
- Secretions are easily removed by suction or bronchoscopy.
- It is often only with IPPV support that adequate analgesia can be given to some patients (e.g. with multiple injuries).

Limitations of IPPV

- In general IPPV does not reverse any intrinsic lung problem and is rarely curative.
- The ventilator should be viewed as adjunctive rather than primary support.

From the moment a patient is connected to the ventilator the goal should be to remove him from it as soon as it is safe to do so:

- The results of ventilation are best when it is given as pure temporary support of a patient with a relatively healthy lung (e.g. drug overdose, hypothermia, post-operative patient).
- Results are not so good for patients with intrinsic lung disease especially if this is longstanding as there may not be any improvement possible in the long term. The aim is such patients therefore is to support respiration while allowing time for other measures to be effective (e.g. antibiotics in infection, steroids in asthma).
- The results are worst when IPPV is instituted in conditions for which there is *no* specific therapy for the underlying problem (e.g. ARDS).

Goals of ventilatory support

- Maintain oxygenation. The two main determinants of arterial oxygenation are the inspired oxygen concentration (obviously) and the mean airway pressure. This was first observed in neonates undergoing IPPV but was later observed in adult patients with ARDS [15]. Arguably, all other manipulations known to increase oxygenation, for example, increased TV, PEEP, inverse ratio ventilation exert their beneficial effect secondary to an increase in mean airway pressure. However, not all methods of increasing airway pressure may be of equal bene-fit to the patient (e.g. a minimum level of PEEP may be crucial).
- Recruit alveoli, that is, open lung units and then keep them open. A low level of PEEP and a low TV avoids overdistension while preventing derecruitment of alveoli.
- Control PCO_2.

- Reduce work of breathing.
- Achieve patient/ventilator synchrony by use of more flexible modes and/or by use of sedation.
- Minimise complications of IPPV.

Initial ventilator settings

- Set inspired oxygen concentration. Hundred per cent initially is sensible if there is doubt regarding the adequacy of oxygenation. This may avoid the patient suffering a period of ongoing hypoxia while waiting for arterial blood gas (ABG) analysis.
- Adjust inspired oxygen according to ABGs. Accept PaO_2 >10 for most patients or oxyhaemoglobin saturations >92%. Patients with severe lung injury may tolerate a lower PaO_2 ("permissive hypoxaemia") so as to limit the dangers from excessive TVs or airway pressures [16].
- Set TV at 6–10 ml/kg. Current research supports TVs at the lower end of this scale (see below).
- Set rate at 10–14 breaths/min. Lower rates may be appropriate in severe asthma or ARDS ("permissive hypercapnia").
- Set PEEP. Almost without exception patients benefit from at least 5 cm PEEP if only to limit the required inspired oxygen concentration and prevent "low level barotrauma", see below. The full recruitment effect may not be seen for several hours.
- Usual inspiratory:expiratory (I:E) ratio 1:2. Patients with ARDS are discussed elsewhere but they may need a longer inspiratory time setting. Care should be taken if the patient is at risk of air trapping.
- Usual inspiratory flow rate of approximately 50–100 l/min.
- Continuous ventilation usually initially with pressure support if not deeply sedated. It is considered desirable to set the ventilator as soon as possible so as to allow the patient to maintain spontaneous respiratory efforts in order to limit respiratory muscle wasting and shorten the duration of ventilatory support [17].
- Set volume and pressure alarms.
- Set reasonable trigger sensitivity so as to be able to initiate spontaneous breaths if appropriate but so as to avoid too sensitive a trigger which may trigger related to oscillations in the cardiac cycle.

All must be adjusted according to clinical response and frequent assessment. Lung protective strategies (e.g. permissive hypercapnia are more fully discussed in the next chapter).

Complications of IPPV

- Cardiac and fluid retention problems as mentioned above.
- Ventilator induced lung injury (VILI).
- Nosocomial pneumonia (see Chapter 13, Infection and Infection Control).
- Stress ulceration (see Chapter 25, The Patient with Gastrointestinal Problems).
- Complications of airway management.
- Complications associated with ventilator malfunction or human error.

VILI

- Barotrauma strictly refers to any complication of ventilation related to thoracic pressures and could therefore include the cardiac effects but most limit barotrauma to pneumothorax, pneumomediastinum, subcutaneous emphysema and the rare occurrence of systemic air embolus.

  The mechanism is probably related to alveolar and bronchiolar distension leading to eventual airway disruption and interstitial gas formation. It is generally accepted that high levels of PEEP, endobronchial intubation and unilateral lung disease increase the incidence of barotrauma. Many now recommend that plateau airway pressures be maintained, where possible, below 35 cmH$_2$O [18].

  It has become accepted in recent years that "low level barotrauma" can occur. Here, in the absence of PEEP, repetitive opening and closure of alveoli cause damage from shearing forces [19].
- It is now believed that in many acute lung disorders, especially ARDS, the disease process is non-homogenous; that is, there are small, relatively normal areas of lung in conjunction with areas of diseased lung (known as the "baby lung" concept). Put another way, in any one patient there will probably be areas of lung which cannot be recruited for gas exchange, areas which can be recruited with large TV and pressure and areas of normal lung already recruited for gas exchange. If sufficiently high TV are used to recruit the diseased areas which can be recruited then the normal areas will be overdistended and damaged. Thus conventional IPPV may contribute to further parenchymal lung damage.
- The term "volutrauma" itself was coined to emphasise the role of excessive inflation volumes in secondary lung damage. Confusion arose because most early animal studies of barotrauma raised the airway pressure by increasing TV. A very elegant study examined pressure and volume truly independently for the first time (using a veterinary "iron lung" to generate volume without increasing

pressure and thoracoabdominal binding to increase thoracic pressures without altering TV). The authors clearly showed that histological lung damage only occurred in the high-volume group [20]. Hyperinflation may also place the inspiratory muscles at a disadvantage by flattening the diaphragm.
• High TVs in critically ill patients cause the release of inflammatory mediators into the circulation. A recent study [21] of patients with acute lung injury demonstrated that low PEEP/high TV mechanical ventilation was associated with cytokine release into the circulation within 1 h. This could be avoided by application of a lung protective strategy of high PEEP/low TV. It is uncertain why ventilating patients with normal lungs in a similar manner does not result in a similar release of inflammatory mediators. For example, during elective major thoracic or abdominal surgery, IPPV with low TV/PEEP or high TV/no PEEP did not result in different levels of inflammatory mediators [22].

IPPV and the kidney

The retention of sodium and water mentioned above tend to promote a reduction in urine volumes. In addition, IPPV often leads to reductions in glomerular filtration rate at the kidney. There are several mechanisms for this:

• decrease CO;
• redistribution of intrarenal blood flow;
• stimulation of sympathetic and hormonal pathways;
• release of inflammatory mediators (discussed above). It is of note that the ARDS net study discussed in the Chapter 24, Acute Lung Injury and ARDS found that high TVs were associated with an increased rate of renal failure.

FURTHER READING

Artigas A, Bernard GR, Carlet J, Dreyfuss D et al. The American–European Consensus Conference on ARDS, Part 2. Ventilatory, pharmacologic, supportive therapy, study design strategies and issues related to recovery and remodeling. *Intens Care Med* 1998; 24: 378–98.
Pinsky MR. The hemodynamic consequences of mechanical ventilation: an evolving story. *Intens Care Med* 1997; 23: 493–503.
Slutsky AS, Imai Y. Ventilator-induced lung injury, cytokines, PEEP, and mortality: implications for practice and for clinical trials. *Intens Care Med* 2003; 29: 1218–21.

REFERENCES

1. Marik PE, Andrews L, Maini B. The incidence of deep venous thrombosis in ICU patients. *Chest* 1997; 111: 661–4.
2. Ibrahim EH, Iregui M, Prentice D, Sherman G et al. Deep vein thrombosis during prolonged mechanical ventilation despite prophylaxis. *Crit Care Med* 2002; 30: 771–4.
3. Priglinger U, Delle Karth G, Geppert A, Joukhadar C et al. Prophylactic anticoagulation with enoxaparin: Is the subcutaneous route appropriate in the critically ill? *Crit Care Med* 2003; 31: 1405–9.
4. Theaker C, Mannan M, Ives N, Soni N. Risk factors for pressure sores in the critically ill. *Anaesthesia* 2000; 55: 221–4.
5. Weststrate JT, Hop WC, Aalbers AG, Vreeling AW, Bruining HA. The clinical relevance of the waterlow pressure sore risk scale in the ICU. *Intens Care Med* 1998; 24: 815–20.
6. Bours GJ, De Laat E, Halfens RJ, Lubbers M. Prevalence, risk factors and prevention of pressure ulcers in Dutch intensive care units. Results of a cross-sectional survey. *Intens Care Med* 2001; 27: 1599–605.
7. Imanaka H, Taenaka N, Nakamura J, Aoyama K et al. Ocular surface disorders in the critically ill. *Anesth Analg* 1997; 85: 343–6.
8. Suresh P, Mercieca F, Morton A, Tullo AB. Eye care for the critically ill. *Intens Care Med* 2000; 26: 162–6.
9. Brath PC, MacGregor DA, Ford JG, Prielipp RC. Dopamine and intraocular pressure in critically ill patients. *Anesthesiology* 2000; 93: 1398–400.
10. Krivopal M, Shlobin OA, Schwartzstein RM. Utility of daily routine portable chest radiographs in mechanically ventilated patients in the medical ICU. *Chest* 2003; 123: 1607–14.
11. Bhagwanjee S, Muckart DJ. Routine daily chest radiography is not indicated for ventilated patients in a surgical ICU. *Intens Care Med* 1996; 22: 1335–8.
12. Hudson L. Survival data in patients with acute and chronic lung disease requiring mechanical ventilation. *Am Rev Respir Dis* 1989; 140: S19–24.
13. Menzies R, Gibbons W, Goldberg P. Determinants of weaning and survival among patients with COPD who require mechanical ventilation for acute respiratory failure. *Chest* 1989; 95: 398–405.
14. Ralph DD, Robertson HT, Weaver LJ. Distribution of ventilation and perfusion during positive end-expiratory pressure in the adult respiratory distress syndrome. *Am Rev Resp Dis* 1985; 131: 54–60.
15. Marini JJ, Ravenscraft SA. Mean airway pressure: physiologic determinants and clinical importance – Part 2: Clinical implications. *Crit Care Med* 1992; 20: 1604–16.
16. Bugge JF. Pressure limited ventilation with permissive hypoxia and nitric oxide in the treatment of adult respiratory distress syndrome. *Eur J Anaesthesiol* 1999; 16: 799–802.
17. Putensen C, Zech S, Wrigge H, Zinserling J, Stuber F et al. Long-term effects of spontaneous breathing during ventilatory support in patients with acute lung injury. *Am J Respir Crit Care Med* 2001; 164: 43–9.

18. Slutsky AS. American College of Chest Physicians' Consensus Conference on Mechanical Ventilation. *Chest* 1993; 104: 1833–59.

19. Muncedere JG, Mullen JBM, Gan AS, Slutsky AS. Tidal ventilation at low airway pressures can augment lung injury. *Am J Resp Crit Care Med* 1994; 149: 1327–34.

20. Dreyfuss D, Soler G, Basset G, Saumon G. High inflation pressure pulmonary oedema – respiratory effects of high airway pressure, high tidal volume, and positive end-expiratory pressure. *Am Rev Respir Dis* 1988; 137: 1159–64.

21. Stuber F, Wrigge H, Schroeder S, Wetegrove S et al. Kinetic and reversibility of mechanical ventilation-associated pulmonary and systemic inflammatory response in patients with acute lung injury. *Intens Care Med* 2002; 28: 834–41.

22. Wrigge H, Uhlig U, Zinserling J, Behrends-Callsen E et al. The effects of different ventilatory settings on pulmonary and systemic inflammatory responses during major surgery. *Anesth Analg* 2004; 98: 775–81.

10

Modes of ventilation and ventilatory strategies

P. Nightingale

This chapter will review:

- lung protective ventilator strategy,
- ventilatory techniques,
- ventilator modes and adjuncts.

Lung protective ventilator strategy

Mechanical ventilation may produce lung damage due to:

- high end-inspiratory lung volume,
- repeated collapse and reopening of distal airways.

In adult respiratory distress syndrome (ARDS) some lung units remain relatively normal (typically 30%) while others are collapsed, consolidated or fluid filled. The lung is actually small and not merely stiff. With volume-controlled ventilation (VCV) using large tidal volumes the relatively normal areas may be over distended leading to barotrauma.

Modern ventilatory management follows that of the ARDS Network study [1] and adopts a lung protective ventilatory strategy:

- low tidal volume;
- increasing levels of positive end expiratory pressure (PEEP) to maintain oxygenation (see Table 10.1).

This is based on the concepts of keeping the lung open with PEEP, but avoiding over distension by limiting tidal volume and so end-inspiratory pressure.

Table 10.1. Aspects of a lung protective ventilator strategy

Maintain spontaneous ventilation wherever possible
Initial alveolar recruitment manoeuvres:
• Positional changes (including the prone position)
• Periodical sustained lung inflation (e.g. 35 cmH$_2$O for 30 s) [2]
Adequate levels of PEEP to prevent alveolar collapse
Keep above lower inflection point on the static pressure–volume curve:
• Measure PEEPi
• Avoid 100% oxygen; may prevent reabsorption atelectasis
Avoid alveolar over distension
Keep below upper inflection point on the static pressure–volume curve:
• Limit tidal volume (6–8 ml/kg)
• Limit inspiratory pressure (end-inspiratory plateau <30 cmH$_2$O)
Permissive hypercapnia:
• Allow PaCO$_2$ to rise if there are no contraindications

This strategy can use either pressure-controlled ventilation (PCV) or VCV. Modern ventilators may now have modes that combine elements of both techniques.

However, monitoring the static pressure–volume curve to determine the upper and lower inflection points is not routine in most intensive care units (ICUs), although some newer ventilators are able to produce a quasi-static curve automatically, for example, the Hamilton Galileo. The role of the dynamic pressure–volume curve remains unclear.

There have been criticisms of the ARDS Network study:

• the inappropriately high tidal volume in the control group (12 ml/kg);
• the safety of very low tidal volumes.

A number of centres have not adopted the protocol fully [3]. The ARDS Network have also shown that the level of PEEP is not critical in ARDS when ventilating patients with 6 ml/kg tidal volume and a plateau-pressure limit of 30 cmH$_2$O [4].

With a lung protective ventilatory strategy, even if respiratory rate is increased, effective alveolar minute volume is likely to fall and hypercapnia will develop.

This so-called permissive hypercapnia is also seen in severe acute asthma where low ventilatory rates (<6 breaths/min) may be needed to allow sufficient time for expiration to occur:

• Although there are some potential cardiac and cerebral problems with permissive hypercapnia, at moderate levels (8–10 kPa) it appears well tolerated [5].

- The acute respiratory acidosis does not require bicarbonate therapy.
- Interestingly, there is some evidence that hypercapnia may be beneficial in acute lung injury [6].

Ventilatory techniques

VCV

VCV with external PEEP has been the traditional mode of ventilation, and is still used in many ICUs. Tidal volume and ventilator rate are preset and expiration is time cycled. Inspiratory flow rate is usually preset ($\sim$60 l/min) and constant, although it may be possible to set a decelerating waveform. Tidal volume is guaranteed in the absence of leaks in the respiratory system, even if there are changes in airway resistance or total thoracic compliance, although high airway pressures may be produced. The realization that high airway pressures were associated with barotrauma led to a degree of pressure regulation by setting an upper pressure alarm limit above which the inspiration was terminated.

PEEP

When airway pressure in the ventilator system has not returned to atmospherical at the onset of inspiration then, by definition, there is PEEP present. This may be set externally (usually in the range 5–15 cmH$_2$O), but intrinsic PEEP (PEEPi) may also be present. PEEPi occurs when there is expiratory flow obstruction, for example, asthma, chronic obstructive pulmonary disease (COPD), or when expiratory time is too short, for example, a rapid respiratory rate, prolonged inspiratory time. Newer ventilators usually have a means of checking the PEEPi level. It is important to note that the value on the pressure dial of a ventilator during expiration does not reflect the level of PEEPi.

When beneficial, PEEP increases functional residual capacity by alveolar recruitment. This reduces pulmonary venous admixture and increases PaO$_2$ at any given FiO$_2$. However, PEEP may produce unpredictable effects, especially if lung compliance is dyshomogenous, for example, consolidation in one lung. In VCV, PEEP will increase peak airway pressure and may cause over distension of lung units. Hence:

- Barotrauma is a risk.
- Compression of vessels around distended alveoli may divert blood to under ventilated regions; hence:
  - physiological dead space may be increased,

- shunt fraction may worsen,
- pulmonary vascular resistance may be increased.

The preset tidal volume must, therefore, be reduced appropriately.

Pressure control ventilation (PCV)

With this technique combinations of rate, inspiratory time or inspiratory:expiratory (I:E) ratio and pressure level can be set, according to the type of ventilator. Initially, the pressure is set ~25 cmH$_2$O and I:E ratio ~1:2 or 1:1 in the patient with acute lung injury. Adjustments are then made according to achieved tidal volume. Small air leaks are compensated for and excessive airway pressure is avoided, but tidal volume will vary with changes in respiratory mechanics. Improvements in compliance can lead to increases in tidal volume. This can be missed since not all ventilators have a high tidal volume alarm. In PCV, PEEP will lead to a fall in tidal volume. Hence, preset pressure or inspiratory time must be increased to compensate for this.

There are some theoretical advantages to PCV when compared with VCV. These include:

- regional over distension/high regional PEEPi is avoided,
- peak airway pressure is lower for the same mean airway pressure,
- decelerating flow rate may be less injurious,
- alveolar ventilation may be improved.

Inverse ratio ventilation

In this mode the usual set I:E ratio of 1:2 or 1:3 is adjusted by prolonging inspiration so that the ratio becomes 1:1, or greater. This theoretically allows for more even distribution of inspired gas to lung units with longer time constants. As expiration is usually not complete before the next inspiration commences, air trapping occurs and PEEPi develops:

- Inverse ratio ventilation (IRV) can be produced in VCV by an end-inspiratory pause or use of a slow or decelerating inspiratory flow rate, but there is still a danger of an excessively high airway pressure developing.
- IRV is often used with PCV by prolonging the inspiratory time. This may be safer than using VCV since high pressures cannot be developed.

Independent lung ventilation

By using a double-lumen tube it is possible to ventilate each lung separately, using different modes and ventilator settings as appropriate. This may be useful in unilateral lung disease, for example, the presence of one-sided aspiration, infection or broncho-pleural fistula. The ventilators do not have to be synchronized.

Modes of ventilation

Although a large number of different modes of ventilation are available, it is difficult to show that any one is superior to the rest. Any mode that allows the patient to breathe spontaneously, and which minimize further lung damage, should produce the best outcome.

Triggering

Ventilator manufacturers are continually striving to improve the patient – machine interface in order to reduce any imposed work of breathing. Patient – ventilator asynchrony has typically centred on sensitivity of triggering and timeliness of gas delivery; this may, or may not, be obvious clinically. Flow triggering is preferred because of the slightly faster response, especially where there is a continuous background flow of gas through the breathing system. With pressure triggering, there is a delay before the expiratory valve closes whilst a negative pressure is created in the breathing system. When there is PEEPi, an inspiratory effort by the patient may fail to pressure trigger the ventilator; the PEEPi has to be overcome first before a pressure drop occurs at the ventilator. A new method of triggering which utilizes changes in the shape of the expiratory flow curve could be useful in these circumstances. So far, this method (AutoTrak™ sensitivity) has only been used in a non-invasive ventilator made by Respironics.

Often less well recognized is cycle asynchrony. During controlled ventilation, the inspiratory time is fixed and there may be failure of the ventilator to end inspiration at the appropriate time in relation to patient effort. The patient may still be breathing in when the ventilator switches to expiration, or be starting to breath out whilst the ventilator is continuing to inflate their lungs. Although under appreciated, this occurs frequently and can also lead to patient discomfort and fatigue. By using an "active exhalation valve" it is now possible for ventilators to let the patient breathe spontaneously even during prolonged inspiratory periods. This appears to improve patient discomfort and allows a reduction in sedation and avoidance of neuromuscular blocking drugs.

Even during pressure support ventilation (PSV), when cycling to expiration is not time related but rather when inspiratory flow falls to a certain level, asynchrony occurs frequently. The slope or rise time of the ventilator pressure must be fast enough to support the inspiratory effort the patient makes, but not so fast that overshoot occurs; it is possible to set the rise time manually on some ventilators. Unfortunately, patient demand is variable, as are lung mechanics due to secretions, position changes, etc. However, some ventilators can now automatically set the flow.

Volume preset modes

Controlled mandatory ventilation

In this mode, all breaths are mandatory machine breaths and the set minute volume is delivered totally by the ventilator. The disadvantage of this technique is that if the patient tries to take a spontaneous breath or cough then not only is it very uncomfortable, but also surges in peak inspiratory pressure are produced.

Assist control

This term is used when the patient can trigger a mandatory machine breath.

Intermittent mandatory ventilation

This mode was introduced to allow the patient to breathe spontaneously between mandatory machine breaths. As the frequency of mandatory breaths were reduced it was thought that the patient could add extra spontaneous breaths to maintain minute volume. However, the rate and timing of mandatory breaths were fixed, and once commenced continued until the preset tidal volume had been delivered, with the potential for hyperinflation.

Synchronized intermittent mandatory ventilation

The technique IMV was further refined to allow mandatory mechanical breaths to be initiated by, and synchronized with, patient effort. This added considerably to patient comfort with less need for sedation and paralysis. A problem remained, however, since patients with poorly compliant lungs tend to breathe rapidly. The increase in physiological dead space commonly seen in these patients meant that dead space ventilation tended to increase even though minute volume was maintained. Work of breathing could actually be increased if the ventilator was not able to respond fast enough to the patient's effort, see section Triggering in this chapter.

Mandatory minute volume ventilation

If, during spontaneous breathing, the set minute volume was not going to be reached, machine breaths were given. Unfortunately, when first introduced, the ventilator was not able to recognize the presence of rapid shallow breathing, and ventilation remained inefficient despite the set minute volume being reached.

Pressure preset modes

PSV

When the patient takes a spontaneous breath a variable flow inspiratory pressure is applied to the respiratory system by the ventilator. The level of pressure support should be set ($\sim$20 cmH$_2$O initially) so as to give an appropriate tidal volume. Usually, airway pressure is maintained at the preset level until inspiratory flow starts to fall, at which point the expiratory phase commences. On some ventilators the level at which this occurs can be adjusted:

- This mode is now frequently used with synchronized IMV (SIMV) as the mode of first choice for initiating mechanical ventilation.
- As with all triggered modes, it is vital that the response time of the ventilator is rapid or the patient's work of breathing can be increased dramatically.
- Newer ventilators have more rapid response times, often using flow-triggering, and the ability to control the rate of increase of airway pressure ("rise time"), thus reducing the patient's work of breathing.

PCV

A preset pressure that is maintained within the respiratory system throughout inspiration; expiration is time cycled. Flow rate is determined by algorithms in the ventilator, and is initially high in order to pressurize the respiratory system and then decelerates:

- In clinical practice, for those patients with the most severe forms of respiratory failure, PCV is frequently used to produce PEEPi by prolonging the inspiratory time.
- Extrinsic PEEP is still required ($\sim$8 cmH$_2$O), to stabilize the remaining relatively normal lung units.

- Unless the patient is on a ventilator that allows spontaneous breaths, this mode of ventilation is uncomfortable and this should be taken into account when prescribing sedation and muscle relaxants.

Airway pressure release ventilation

This mode of assisted ventilation utilizes a high level of constant positive airway pressure (CPAP) with the ventilator falling to a lower level ("release") at a set time. The patient can breathe spontaneously at both CPAP levels, but the release of CPAP from a supra-ambient level to a lower level augments alveolar ventilation and hence CO_2 clearance:

- Typical initial values would be low pressure ~8 cmH$_2$O, high pressure 20 cm H$_2$O and I:E ratio of 1:2.
- Tidal volume is adjusted by varying the pressure range.

Biphasic positive airway pressure

This mode is very similar to airway pressure release ventilation (APRV). Switching between high and low pressures can be synchronized with patient effort, and inspiratory efforts pressure supported. Essentially, this mode is PCV but allowing unimpeded spontaneous breathing at all times [7]. (Biphasic positive airway pressure (BiPAP) is a trademark under license to Dräger and should not be confused with the Respironics BiPAP non-invasive pressure support ventilator.)

Mixed modes

Electronic control of the ventilators has become extremely sophisticated and this has allowed a number of other modes to be developed. They all have the same underlying philosophy, which is to minimize airway pressure while ensuring an adequate tidal volume. It is now possible for ventilators to calculate the optimum ventilator settings and then allow breath-by-breath alterations in ventilatory support, during both controlled and spontaneous breathing.

These modes include:

- Adaptive support ventilation (ASV) and adaptive pressure ventilation (APV) (Hamilton Galileo ventilator).
- Pressure augment maximum (PAM) (Bear 1000 ventilator).

- Pressure regulated volume control (PRVC), volume support (VS) and Automode® (Siemens SV 300 series).
- SIMV$^{AutoFlow®}$ (Dräger Evita series).
- Variable pressure support/variable pressure control (VPS/VPC) (Kontron Venturi ventilator).
- Volume assured pressure support (VAPS) (Inter7 ventilator).

As rapid advances in developing ventilator technology, the reader is advised to become familiar with each ventilator in use on their ICU by reading the manufacturer's literature and undergoing appropriate training.

Other modes

Proportional assist ventilation

In this mode neither flow, pressure, nor volume are set by the clinician! A positive gain control is adjusted to determine what proportion of the patient's inspiratory effort (inspiratory flow and volume) is supported by the ventilator. However, to do this it is necessary to measure respiratory elastance and resistance. This is technologically very demanding and there is a risk of "run away" ventilation; this mode has yet to achieve any sort of popularity. The term proportional pressure support (PPS) is used by Dräger in the Evita series.

High-frequency techniques

These are arbitrarily subdivided into high frequency positive pressure ventilation, high frequency jet ventilation (HFJV) and high-frequency oscillation. The rate varies from 60 to as high as 3000 ventilatory cycles/min. Since gas distribution may relate to airways resistance rather than compliance, it is possible to ventilate areas with both low and high compliance that are adjacent, for example, a patient with ARDS and a broncho-pleural fistula [8]. Newer machines are capable of providing better humidification, and are powerful enough to maintain lung volume in patients with ARDS.

Non-invasive techniques

The use of non-invasive ventilation is increasing in hospital practice, particularly in areas such as the Emergency Department, Coronary Care Unit and in Chest

Medicine as well as on the high dependency unit (HDU) and ICU. Developments in non-invasive ventilators mean that these now rival traditional ventilators in their versatility. This is further discussed in Chapter 8.

Mask ventilation

There have been significant improvements in mask design. As well as nasal and traditional face masks there are now full-face masks and hoods, which are much more comfortable that previously and allow non-invasive ventilation to be used in a wider range of patients. However, patient selection is vital, especially the ability to maintain upper airway protective reflexes. Typical uses include acute left ventricular failure, acute exacerbations of COPD, postoperative atelectasis and acute lung injury. The evidence for a trial of non-invasive ventilation in an acute exacerbation of COPD is now compelling. On the ICU non-invasive ventilation is frequently used as a weaning aid although a large multicentre study has shown no benefit [9].

External negative pressure ventilation

External negative pressure ventilation (historically provided by an iron lung) may be performed by applying a cuirass device to the chest wall. The Hayek oscillator maintains a negative baseline pressure to increase lung volume and oscillates around this [10]. There is a built in physiotherapy mode to aid removal of secretions.

Adjuncts

Tracheal gas insufflation

Oxygen is delivered to just above the carina ($\sim 4\,l/min$) by catheter either continuously or intermittently during expiration. The effect is to reduce anatomical dead space and increase CO_2 clearance [11]. The effect is more marked when there is permissive hypercapnia but there is obviously the possibility of excessive pressure developing in the lungs.

Automatic tube compensation

It is possible to estimate tracheal pressure based on the length and diameter of the tracheal tube and gas flow. By increasing ventilator pressure during inspiration the resistance of the tracheal tube can be overcome and flow improved; this will reduce the imposed work of breathing. Similarly, if ventilator pressure is decreased during expiration expiratory flow will be enhanced and PEEPi reduced. Clinical trials suggest that automatic tube compensation (ATC) has significant advantages [12] over simply increasing PSV, particularly by minimizing PEEPi during spontaneous breathing. ATC is available on a number of ventilators including the Drager Evita 4 and Puritan Bennett 840.

FURTHER READING

Branson R. Understanding and implementing advances in ventilator capabilities. *Curr Opin Crit Care* 2004; 10: 23–32.

Brochard L. Intrinsic (or auto-) PEEP during controlled mechanical ventilation. *Intens Care Med* 2002; 28: 1376–8.

REFERENCES

1. The Acute Respiratory Distress Syndrome Network. Ventilation with lower tidal volumes as compared with traditional tidal volumes for acute lung injury and the acute respiratory distress syndrome. *New Engl J Med* 2000; 342: 1301–8.

2. Brower RG, Morris A, MacIntyre N et al. Effects of recruitment maneuvers in patients with acute lung injury and acute respiratory distress syndrome ventilated with high positive end-expiratory pressure. *Crit Care Med* 2003; 31: 2592–7.

3. Young MP, Manning HL, Wilson DL, Mette SA, Riker RR, Leiter JC, Liu SK, Bates JT, Parsons PE. Ventilation of patients with acute lung injury and acute respiratory distress syndrome: has new evidence changed clinical practice? *Crit Care Med* 2004; 32: 1260–5.

4. Brower RG, Lanken PN, MacIntyre N et al. Higher versus lower positive end-expiratory pressures in patients with the Acute Respiratory Distress Syndrome. *New Engl J Med* 2004; 351: 327–36.

5. Feihl F, Perret C. Permissive hypercapnia: how permissive should we be? *Am J Respir Crit Care Med* 1994; 150: 1722–37.

6. Laffey JG, O'Croinin D, McLoughlin P, Kavanagh BP. Permissive hypercapnia – role in protective lung ventilatory strategies. *Intens Care Med* 2004; 30: 347–56.

7. Hormann C, Baum M, Putensen C, Mutz NJ, Benzer H. Biphasic positive airway pressure (BIPAP) – a new mode of ventilatory support. *Eur J Anaesthesiol* 1994; 11: 37–42.

8. Venegas JG, Fredburgh JJ. Understanding the pressure cost of ventilation: why does high-frequency ventilation work? *Crit Care Med* 1994; 22: S49–57.

9. Esteban A, Frutos-Vivar F, Ferguson ND et al. Noninvasive positive-pressure ventilation for respiratory failure after extubation. *New Engl J Med* 2004; 350: 2452–60.

10. Petros AJ, Fernando SSD, Shenoy VS, Al-Saady NM. The Hayek oscillator. *Anaesthesia* 1995; 50: 601–6.

11. Avi Nahum. Tracheal gas insufflation. *Crit Care* 1998; 2: 43–7.

12. Fabry B. Breathing pattern and additional work in spontaneous breathing patients with different ventilatory demands during inspiratory pressure support and automatic tube compensation. *Intens Care Med* 1997; 23: 545–52.

Weaning and tracheostomy

J. Cupitt

The key points of this chapter are as follows:

- Mechanical ventilation (MV) is a life-saving procedure but it can also be harmful. Some of the side effects are related to the presence of an endotracheal tube.
- Separating the critically ill patient from the ventilator is referred to as "weaning".
- It is crucial to discontinue ventilatory support and extubate at the earliest opportunity that a patient can sustain spontaneous ventilation safely.
- Over 40% of the time that a patient receives MV is spent in weaning.
- The most important indicator of readiness for weaning is resolution of the acute event which necessitated ventilation.

For the majority of patients, especially those requiring short-term respiratory support, MV can be removed safely and easily. However, in those recovering from serious illness or respiratory failure, discontinuation may be associated with considerable difficulty. Few guidelines exist for the optimal approach to this problem.

Before attempting the weaning process, it is important to satisfy various pre-conditions related to the patient's general state:

- absence of major organ or system failure, in particular, a stable cardiovascular system;
- no severe abdominal distension;
- absence of fluid, acid-base or electrolyte imbalance;
- adequate nutrition;
- correction of pain and anaemia;
- cooperative patient with minimal sedation.

Prediction of successful weaning

Various criteria have been suggested that predict the readiness, and likelihood of success, of weaning:

- vital capacity 10–15 ml/kg,
- tidal volume >5 ml/kg,
- spontaneous MV <12 l/min,
- respiratory rate <35 breaths/min,
- peak negative inspiratory pressure >-20 cmH$_2$O,
- PaO$_2$ >8 kPa on fraction of inspired oxygen (FiO$_2$) <0.4,
- pH >7.3.

A recent evidence-based medicine review of weaning parameters concluded that these predictors had only limited utility in predicting weaning outcome [1]. It has been shown that a subjective process of patient assessment, independent of weaning indices, yields a satisfactory outcome in the majority of patients [2]. Some have even questioned whether strict adherence to weaning parameters may even prolong ventilatory support.

An important study [3] examined various physiological predictors of the likelihood of successful weaning. Various indices related to oxygenation or the ability to generate pressures or volume were not useful. They found that the best predictor was the ratio of respiratory rate to tidal volume (f/V_T) index. Normally this ratio is <30. The study found that <80 predicted success whereas >100 predicted failure in 95% of patients. Unfortunately the findings have not been confirmed by other investigators [4, 5].

Spontaneous breathing trials

One important strategy used to reduce the duration of both MV and weaning is to identify, as soon as possible, which patients are capable of breathing spontaneously. This is by means of spontaneous breathing trials. There is little risk in performing a closely observed trial to assess the patient's ability to sustain spontaneous breathing. This is a simple and reliable method to identify which patients can be safely extubated without a formal trial of weaning.

Spontaneous breathing trials can be performed via a T-piece, constant positive airway pressure (CPAP) circuit or pressure support ventilation (PSV, levels up to 10 cmH$_2$O) [6]. The duration of a trial has been set at 2 h but the optimal duration is unknown. Recent studies suggest it can be reduced without an increased risk of reintubation [7, 8].

Weaning techniques

Around 20% of patients receiving MV pose difficulties in weaning. Factors influencing the length and difficulty in weaning include advanced age, prolonged ventilatory support and chronic obstructive pulmonary disease (COPD).

There are three main methods available for discontinuing MV:

- *T-piece*: The oldest method. Represents the only method with no additionally imposed work of breathing (WOB) in that neither ventilator valves nor circuits are involved. The only factor which can increase the resistive WOB is the endotracheal tube. This method allows periods of rest when the patient is reconnected to the ventilator between periods of spontaneous breathing. Progressive ventilatory withdrawal is designed to restore muscle function by brief periods of fatiguing stress followed by longer periods of rest [9]. Particularly useful following brief periods of intermittent positive pressure ventilation (IPPV).
- *Synchronised intermittent mandatory ventilation (SIMV)*: This method is supposed to prevent a patient from "fighting" the ventilator and reduce respiratory muscle fatigue. The patient is allowed to breathe between machine breaths and the frequency of machine breaths is reduced as weaning progresses. Unfortunately intermittent mandatory ventilation may contribute to respiratory muscle fatigue.
- *PSV*: This ventilatory mode allows patients to retain nearly complete control over respiratory rate and timing, inspiratory flow rate and tidal volume. An increase in the level of pressure support leads to a reduction in the WOB and a decrease in oxygen consumption of the respiratory muscles. The amount of pressure support is reduced until the patient is doing virtually all the work. A low level of PSV will counteract the extra WOB via the ventilator circuit and endotracheal tube [10].

Two important studies have compared the various weaning techniques [11, 12]. The study by Brochard et al found that PSV was the best method to separate patients from the ventilator whilst Esteban et al found the T-piece to be superior. Both studies concluded that SIMV was the least efficient method of weaning and may prolong the time to extubation. The most important message is probably that a weaning method which encourages spontaneous breathing is likely to be appropriate.

Automatic tube compensation

Various modern ventilators have the option to automatically compensate for the presence of the tube be it a oral tube or a tracheostomy tube. Preliminary work suggests that such a facility may improve the ability to successfully extubate patients following spontaneous breathing trials [13].

Weaning protocols

Using protocols to wean patients instead of the traditional practice based on physician preference and experience can reduce the duration of MV and weaning.

Nurses using protocol guidance wean patients more quickly than a medical team following the common practice of physician-directed weaning [14]. It is likely that when a weaning protocol does not exist, physicians adopt a conservative approach by reducing support gradually.

Weaning difficulties

There are many factors that may be involved in failure to wean:

- *Increased WOB* due to poor compliance (e.g. obesity, stiff lungs, bronchospasm).
- *Unrecognised sepsis*, especially nosocomial pneumonia.
- *Decreased ventilatory reserve* (e.g. muscle wasting and fatigue, negative nitrogen balance, electrolyte imbalance).
- *Disuse atrophy and fatigue* of the respiratory muscles, especially of the diaphragm.
- *Neurological causes* of muscle weakness in intensive care unit (ICU) patients may be a factor in the requirement for prolonged ventilatory support.
- *Increased ventilatory requirements,* for example, increased dead space, increased carbon dioxide (CO_2) load due to burns, fever or over feeding with carbohydrate and increased VO_2 (e.g. shivering).
- *Psychological dependence.*
- *Abnormal cardiac function* (see below).
- *Airway factors.* Small diameter tracheal tubes increase WOB as do dried secretions in the tube lumen. Adequate humidification is essential during weaning.

- *Ventilators.* WOB is increased by demand and expiratory valves, tubing, etc., especially with SIMV. Also inability of the ventilator to provide peak inspiratory flow rates on demand. Older ventilators may have an inadequate response time for cycling when the spontaneous rate >30/min.

Correction of the above problems where possible may help the weaning process but failure to wean from IPPV is a difficult problem with no simple solution. The weaning process may be helped by using non-invasive positive pressure ventilation (NPPV) or tracheostomy.

Cardiac problems during weaning

The beneficial effects of IPPV on cardiac function have been alluded to. Spontaneous ventilation is exercise and it can place an excessive burden on the heart, induce myocardial ischaemia and promote cardiogenic shock. Much of the evidence for this is indirect, that is, adverse effects of discontinuing IPPV on cardiac function:

- Patients with left ventricular failure (LVF) and COPD may develop pulmonary oedema when IPPV is weaned with increases in pulmonary capillary "wedge" pressure (PCWP) from 8 ± 5 to 25 ± 13 mmHg [15].
- Cardiac ischaemia, manifested by electrocardiographical (ECG) changes or thallium scanning defects, can occur during weaning [16].
- A study of patients with COPD but no identifiable heart disease demonstrated reductions in left ventricle (LV) fraction in all patients during spontaneous ventilation which was not apparent in those patients on PSV [17].

The mechanisms proposed for these observations include:

- Increases in LV afterload with the decreases in intrathoracic pressure. It is recognised that positive pressure unloads the heart and may result in improved LV systolic function compared to the negative pressure inspiratory cycles of extubated breathing.
- Increases in intrathoracic blood volume as venous return increases with the falls in intrathoracic pressure. The act of spontaneous inspiratory efforts can precipitate LV dilation.
- Release of catecholamines during spontaneous breathing.

- Increases in the WOB, myocardial work and myocardial oxygen requirements. The increased oxygen demand during weaning is met by increasing cardiac output and/or oxygen extraction. The presence of an increased arterio-venous O_2 difference implies occult cardiovascular insufficiency and suggests that weaning trials may fail [18].
- Increases in pulmonary vascular resistance (PVR) with rapid, shallow breathing.

Thus diuretics, nitrate infusions and/or angiotensin converting enzyme (ACE) inhibitors may all be temporarily required during weaning. Inotropic support for the heart may be beneficial. In many patients the cardiac status is the main limiting factor for successful weaning.

Non-invasive ventilation

NPPV (Non-invasive ventilation) has been shown to be more successful for weaning than a conventional approach in certain patient groups [19]. Mehta et al demonstrated a reduced WOB using NPPV [20].

The use of NPPV for weaning might allow extubation much earlier than usually assumed and it might help to reduce weaning failure rates and episodes of reintubation.

Patient selection is important, as are the potential side effects, for example, risk of aspiration.

Iatrogenic ventilator dependency

A tracheal tube increases WOB. Generating pressure to "trigger" the ventilator during spontaneous breathing requires "work". It has been suggested that a too cautious approach to weaning may result in "nosocomial respiratory failure" [21], that is, tachypnoea during weaning may represent imposed work rather than patient WOB, and is thus not always a sign of respiratory fatigue. If inadequately managed, the patient's ventilatory support will be increased rather than the correct response which is to extubate the patient.

A high index of suspicion will help to avoid this situation and performing a spontaneous breathing trial will assist in the decision of whether to extubate.

Failed extubation

Failed extubation is distinct from failed weaning. The former is an inability to tolerate removal of the tracheal tube whereas the latter is an inability to tolerate spontaneous breathing without ventilatory support.

Pathophysiology of extubation failure is distinct from weaning failure and includes upper airway obstruction, inadequate cough, excess respiratory secretions, encephalopathy, etc. These become apparent only after removal of the tracheal tube.

Extubation failure is highest amongst medical, paediatric and multidisciplinary patients [22].

Risk factors for extubation failure (and thus need for reintubation) include:

- neurological impairment,
- older age,
- prolonged duration of ventilation prior to extubation,
- anaemia,
- severity of illness at time of extubation.

Extubation failure prolongs the duration of MV, increases length of hospital and ICU stay, increases need for tracheostomy and is associated with higher hospital mortality.

Tests designed to assess upper airway obstruction, secretion volume and effectiveness of cough may help predict extubation outcome. Certainly, after patients recovering from respiratory failure have successfully completed a trial of spontaneous breathing, cough strength and amount of endotracheal secretions are important predictors of extubation outcome [23].

Tracheostomy

A tracheostomy offers a number of practical advantages compared to conventional endotracheal intubation:

- Decrease of airway resistance and dead space (and therefore reduced WOB).
- Easy airway suctioning.
- Improved patient comfort and tolerance.
- Avoidance of laryngeal and vocal cord injury.

- Allows reduction in sedation and awake patients are able to communicate easier using lip reading.
- Fewer accidental extubations compared with oral tubes.

Potential disadvantages include:

- The surgical technique requires transfer to theatre.
- Early (insertion) complications, for example, bleeding, misplacement creating false passage, posterior tracheal wall damage (especially percutaneous technique), pneumothorax/pneumomediastinum.
- Late complications, for example, mucosal ulceration, erosion into innominate artery or oesophagus, tracheal stenosis.
- Accidental removal may be life threatening until track is well established (~48 h).

Indications for tracheostomy are controversial and include:

- To assist in difficult weaning problems.
- Timing in relation to prolonged oral intubation and MV (see below).
- Laryngeal incompetence (e.g. after cerebrovascular accidents (CVA)).
- Reduced level of consciousness (e.g. after head injury).
- Problems with sputum retention.
- Airway obstruction (e.g. after trauma, may be an indication for an emergency tracheostomy).

Percutaneous tracheostomy

Percutaneous tracheostomy is a technique that can be safely and easily performed at the bedside. It avoids the delays and costs of theatre time. The technique involves insertion of a needle and guidewire into the trachea followed by progressive or one-step dilatation of the resultant tract.

Many centre routinely perform this procedure with the aid of bronchoscopic guidance [24]. This is safe, helps identify needle insertion in the midline of the trachea, helps avoid damage to the posterior tracheal wall and confirms final tube placement.

Four different types of percutaneous tracheostomy technique based on commercially available kits are commonly used (though others are available):

- Ciaglia set (Cook) – increasing sizes of dilators.
- Portex set (Portex) – specially designed forceps for dilatation.

- Ciaglia Blue Rhino set (Cook) – single conical (horn) shaped dilator.
- Fantoni translaryngeal set (Mallinkrodt) – specially designed cannula consisting of a flexible plastic cone with a pointed metal tip at its end to enter and dilate the trachea from its inner lumen outwards.

Many comparative studies have now been performed both between open and percutaneous tracheostomy, and between different techniques of percutaneous tracheostomy. Evidence shows a low incidence of late complications and improved cosmetic results of percutaneous compared with surgical tracheostomy [25, 26]. A recent meta-analysis of these studies suggests potential advantages of percutaneous compared with open techniques including ease of performance and lower incidence of early bleeding and postoperative infection [27].

Although it appears that the percutaneous technique is becoming the first line method in intensive care patients, one should be aware that a lower risk does not imply a less serious consideration of indications. Percutaneous techniques are certainly more cost effective [28].

Timing of tracheostomy

The optimal timing of tracheostomy remains controversial. A tracheostomy need not be performed at 2 weeks if the patient will be extubated successfully in the subsequent few days. Conversely, an early tracheostomy should be performed in a patient requiring long-term ventilation, for example, Guillain–Barré syndrome. Early tracheostomy avoids the complications arising from prolonged endotracheal intubation and might also reduce ventilator days [29], rates of reintubation and ICU, and hospital stay.

A recent randomised study [30] of medical ICU patients compared tracheostomy performed at 48 h with tracheostomy performed at days 14–16. The early group showed significantly less mortality, pneumonia and accidental extubations compared with the prolonged intubation group. Time on the ventilator and in ICU was also reduced.

A major multicentre UK study (Tracman) may help resolve this issue.

Decannulation

When the patient's condition improves, and as part of the over all weaning process, the initial cuffed tracheostomy tube can be exchanged for a uncuffed tube with or without fenestrations. The latter allow for improved translaryngeal airflow and reduce the WOB and allow the patient to speak. Laryngeal competence should be tested before removing a cuffed tracheostomy tube as even brief periods of endotracheal intubation have been shown to disrupt the upper airway reflexes. The stoma should be covered by a dry, occlusive dressing and allowed to heal spontaneously. Note that decannulation results in an increase in dead space which can increase the WOB by more than 30% [31].

Minitracheostomy

A small diameter uncuffed tube inserted percutaneously via the cricothyroid membrane. Allows for tracheobronchial suction in patients with poor cough and sputum retention. Routinely used in some centres to aid sputum clearance following thoracic surgery [32]. Can also be used to administer oxygen, particularly in the emergency situation.

FURTHER READING

Ely EW, Meade MO, Haponik EF, Kollef MH et al. Mechanical ventilator weaning protocols driven by nonphysician health-care professionals: evidence-based clinical practice guidelines. *Chest* 2001; 120: 454S–63S.

Friedman Y. Indications, timing, techniques and complications of tracheostomy in the critically ill patient. *Curr Opin Crit Care* 1996; 2: 47–53.

Friedman Y, Mizock BA. Percutaneous versus surgical tracheostomy: procedure of choice or choice of procedure. *Crit Care Med* 1999; 27: 1684–5.

MacIntyre NR, Cook DJ, Ely EW, Epstein Jr SK et al. Evidence-based guidelines for weaning and discontinuing ventilatory support: a collective task force facilitated by the American College of Chest Physicians; the American Association for Respiratory Care; and the American College of Critical Care Medicine. *Chest* 2001; 120: 375S–95S.

Manthous CA, Schmidt GA, Hall JB. Liberation from mechanical ventilation: a decade of progress. *Chest* 1998; 114: 886–901.

REFERENCES

1. Meade M, Guyatt G, Cook D et al. Predicting success in weaning from mechanical ventilation. *Chest* 2001; 120: 400S–4S.

2. Leitch EA, Moran JL, Grealy B. Weaning and extubation in the intensive care unit. Clinical or index-driven approach? *Intens Care Med* 1996; 22: 752–9.

3. Yang KL, Tobin MJ. A prospective study of indexes predicting the outcome of trials of weaning from mechanical ventilation. *New Engl J Med* 1991; 324: 1445–50.
4. Lee KH, Hui KP, Chan TB, Tan WC, Lim TK. Rapid shallow breathing (frequency–tidal volume ratio) did not predict extubation outcome. *Chest* 1994; 105: 540–3.
5. Epstein SK. Aetiology of extubation failure and the predictive value of the rapid shallow breathing index. *Am J Respir Crit Care Med* 1995; 152: 545–9.
6. Esteban A, Alia I, Gordo F et al. Extubation outcome after spontaneous breathing trials with T-tube or pressure support ventilation. *Am J Respir Crit Care Med* 1997; 156: 459–65.
7. The Spanish Lung Failure Collaborative Group. Multicentre, prospective comparison of 30 and 120 minute trials of weaning from mechanical ventilation. *Am J Respir Crit Care Med* 1997; 155(4): A20.
8. Perren A, Domenighetti G, Mauri S, Genini F, Vizzardi N. Protocol-directed weaning from mechanical ventilation: clinical outcome in patients randomised for a 30-min or 120-min trial with pressure support ventilation. *Intens Care Med* 2002; 28: 1058–63.
9. Aldrich TK, Karpel JP, Uhrlass RM, Sparapan MA, Earmo D, Ferranti R. Weaning from mechanical ventilation: adjunctive use of inspiratory muscle resistive training. *Crit Care Med* 1989; 17: 143–7.
10. Brochard L, Rua F, Lorino H et al. Inspiratory pressure support compensates for the additional work of breathing caused by the endotracheal tube. *Anaesthesiology* 1991; 75: 739–45.
11. Brochard L, Rauss A, Benito S et al. Comparison of three methods of gradual withdrawal from ventilatory support during weaning from mechanical ventilation. *Am J Respir Crit Care Med* 1994; 150: 896–903.
12. Esteban A, Frutos F, Tobin MJ et al. A comparison of four methods of weaning patients from mechanical ventilation. *New Engl J Med* 1995; 332: 345–50.
13. Haberthur C, Mols G, Elsasser S, Bingisser R et al. Extubation after breathing trials with automatic tube compensation, T-tube, or pressure support ventilation. *Acta Anaesthesiol Scand* 2002; 46: 973–9.
14. Kollef MH, Shapiro SD, Silver P et al. A randomised, controlled trial of protocol-directed versus physician-directed weaning from mechanical ventilation. *Crit Care Med* 1997; 25: 567–74.
15. Lemaire F, Teboul JL, Cinotti L et al. Acute left ventricular dysfunction during unsuccessful weaning from mechanical ventilation. *Anaesthesiology* 1998; 69: 171–9.
16. Hurford WE, Favorito F. Association of myocardial ischaemia with failure to wean from mechanical ventilation. *Crit Care Med* 1995; 23: 1475–80.
17. Richard CH, Teboul JL, Archambaud F et al. Left ventricular function during weaning of patients with chronic obstructive pulmonary disease. *Int Care Med* 1994; 20: 181–6.
18. Jubran A, Mathru M, Dries D, Tobin MJ. Continuous recordings of mixed venous oxygen saturation during weaning from mechanical ventilation and the ramifications thereof. *Am J Respir Crit Care Med* 1998; 158: 1763–9.

19. Nava S, Ambrosini N, Clini E et al. Noninvasive mechanical ventilation in the weaning of patients with respiratory due to chronic obstructive pulmonary disease. *Ann Intern Med* 1998; 128: 721–8.

20. Mehta S, Nelson DL, Klinger JR, Buczko GB, Levy MM. Prediction of post-extubation work of breathing. *Crit Care Med* 2000; 28: 1341–6.

21. Civetta JM. Nosocomial respiratory failure or iatrogenic ventilator dependency. *Crit Care Med* 1993; 21: 171–3.

22. Epstein SK. Decision to extubate. *Intens Care Med* 2002; 28: 535–46.

23. Khamiees M, Raju P, DeGirolamo A, Amoateng-Adjepong Y et al. Predictors of extubation outcome in patients who have successfully completed a spontaneous breathing trial. *Chest* 2001; 1262–70.

24. Hinerman R, Alvarez F, Keller CA. Outcome of bedside percutaneous tracheostomy with bronchoscopic guidance. *Intens Care Med* 2000; 26: 1850–6.

25. Hill BB, Zweng TN, Maley RH, Charash WE, Toursarkissian B, Kearney PA. Percutaneous dilational tracheostomy: report of 356 patients. *J Trauma* 1996; 40: 238–43.

26. Fischler MP, Kuhn M, Cantieni R, Frutiger A. Late outcome of percutaneous dilatational tracheostomy in intensive care patients. *Int Care Med* 1995; 21: 475–81.

27. Freeman BD, Isabella K, Lin N, Buchman TG. A meta-analysis of prospective trials comparing percutaneous and surgical tracheostomy in critically ill patients. *Chest* 2000; 118: 1412–8.

28. Grover A, Robbins J, Bendick P, Gibson M et al. Open versus percutaneous dilatational tracheostomy: efficacy and cost analysis. *Am Surg* 2001; 67: 297–301.

29. Lesnik I, Rappaport W, Filginiti J, Witzke D. The role of early tracheostomy in blunt, multiple organ trauma. *Ann Surg* 1992; 58: 346–9.

30. Rumbak MJ, Newton M, Truncale T, Schwartz SW et al. A prospective, randomized, study comparing early percutaneous dilational tracheotomy to prolonged translaryngeal intubation (delayed tracheotomy) in critically ill medical patients. *Crit Care Med* 2004; 32: 1689–94.

31. Chadda K, Louis B, Benaissa L et al. Physiological effects of decannulation in tracheostomised patients. *Intens Care Med* 2002; 28: 1761–7.

32. Bonde P, Papachristos I, McCraith A, Kelly B et al. Sputum retention after lung operation: prospective, randomized trial shows superiority of prophylactic minitracheostomy in high-risk patients. *Ann Thorac Surg* 2002; 74: 196–202.

12

Vasoactive drugs

V. Godbole

Inotropes and vasopressors

Support of the cardiovascular system forms a cornerstone in the management of the critically ill patient:

- Therapy is directed towards optimising cardiac output, organ blood flow and organ perfusion pressure. This in turn leads to improved oxygen delivery.
- The drugs used to achieve these goals work primarily on receptors found throughout the cardiovascular system. Other agents act by inhibiting catecholamine metabolism.

Receptor physiology

- Adrenoceptors form an integral part of the sympathetic nervous system. They are acted upon by noradrenaline released from nerve terminals, and by circulating adrenaline. The receptors are divided into α and β subgroups:
  - α_1 receptors are found primarily in blood vessels. Stimulation of these receptors leads to contraction of vascular smooth muscle with subsequent vasoconstriction.
  - α_2 receptors are located at pre-synaptic nerve terminals. They have a role in negative feedback, stimulation inhibiting further noradrenaline release.
  - β_1 receptors are located in the heart and intestinal smooth muscle. Noradrenaline and adrenaline are equipotent at these sites. Stimulation results in positive inotropy and chronotropy. Intestinal smooth muscle is relaxed.
  - β_2 receptors are found in bronchial, uterine and vascular smooth muscle, and stimulation results in muscle relaxation. This leads to bronchodilation

and vasodilation. β_2 receptors are more sensitive to adrenaline, suggesting they act primarily as hormonal receptors.

- The normal heart contains both β_1 and β_2 receptors in a ratio of 3:1. This may change to 3:2 in severe heart failure due to downregulation of β_1 receptors.
- The effects at adrenoceptors are mediated via second messenger systems involving G-proteins, coupled to either adenylate cyclase (β receptors) or phospholipase C (α_1 receptors). Phosphorylation of intracellular proteins then effects the response to stimulation.
- The natural ligands at adrenoceptors are initially derived from the amino acid phenylalanine. Hydroxylation of dopamine forms noradrenaline, which is the immediate precursor of adrenaline.
- Generally speaking, stimulation of β_1 receptors leads to an increase in cardiac output whilst activity at α_1 receptors will increase blood pressure.

Dopaminergic receptors

- There are two main sub-types of dopaminergic receptors – D_1 and D_2. Both are present in the central nervous system (CNS), where dopamine is an important neurotransmitter, and at peripheral sites:
  - D_1 receptors are found in vascular and mesenteric smooth muscle – stimulation leads to relaxation and subsequent vasodilation.
  - D_2 receptors are believed to have a role in pre-synaptic inhibition.
- Stimulation of dopaminergic receptors found in the renal and splanchnic beds results in increased renal and splanchnic blood flow.

Vasoactive drugs may act upon the various receptors to differing degrees, resulting in a mixture of effects. This has led to the terms inodilator and inoconstrictor.

- An inodilator is a drug with positive inotropic and vasodilator effects (e.g. enoximone).
- An inoconstrictor has positive inotropic and vasoconstrictor effects (e.g. adrenaline).

The armamentarium of agents has changed little over the past few years although our understanding of the effects of these drugs on the various organ systems has improved.

Note: Catecholamines appear to modulate cytokine response and may improve outcome in patients receiving supranormal oxygen delivery for sepsis [1].

Individual drugs

Adrenaline (epinephrine)

Adrenaline is the body's natural sympathomimetic agent. It is active at all adreno-ceptors and an infusion will lead to an increase in cardiac output and blood pressure with an accompanying tachycardia.

The use of adrenaline as a single agent is attractive but there are serious side effects associated with its use:

- It has potent dysrhythmogenic effects. The increase in cardiac workload may result in myocardial ischaemia.
- In severe sepsis the use of adrenaline can reduce splanchnic blood flow [2]. A recent study compared the effects of adrenaline, noradrenaline and dopamine on the splanchnic circulation in septic shock [3]. Whilst there was no difference in blood flow between the agents in patients with moderate shock, in severe shock splanchnic blood flow was lower during infusion of adrenaline than with noradrenaline.
- Administration of adrenaline may lead to lactic acidosis in patients with severe infections [4]. It can be postulated that this is a reflection of reduced hepatic blood flow.
- Metabolic disturbances such as hyperglycaemia and hypokalaemia can occur.

Adrenaline remains the agent of choice in the cardiac arrest situation and in the treatment of anaphylaxis.

Noradrenaline (Norepinephrine)

This compound is predominantly used for its effects at α_1 receptors where stimulation results in vasoconstriction with a resultant increase in blood pressure. It also has activity at β_1 receptors.

Noradrenaline is usually the first-line vasopressor and is often used to counteract the vasodilatory effects of sedation.

The agent is widely used in the treatment of sepsis where vasodilation is a major component of the disease process. However, there have been concerns regarding its potentially detrimental effects on various regional circulations.

However:

- In the normal mammalian circulation noradrenaline infusion has been shown to improve renal and coronary blood flow [5].

- In severe sepsis the use of noradrenaline improves splanchnic blood flow (despite its vasoconstrictor properties), oxygen delivery and oxygen uptake [6].
- A commonly expressed fear is that use of noradrenaline may cause falls in cardiac output due to increases in afterload. In fact, adding noradrenaline to patients resistant to dobutamine commonly causes *increases* in cardiac output [7].

Why should noradrenaline, a vasoconstrictor seemingly have a more beneficial effect on splanchnic blood flow than adrenaline, another vasoconstrictor? One theory is that it relates to the different ways they may be used. Noradrenaline is often used in combination with dobutamine and its effects are titrated to reverse the abnormal degree of vasodilation while, hopefully avoiding actual vasoconstriction. If adrenaline, however, is used as a sole agent one cannot modify in the same way its potential to cause actual vasoconstriction.

Dobutamine

Dobutamine is a synthetic drug acting mainly at β receptors although it does possess some α activity. It is a potent inotrope and is the agent of choice in cardiogenic shock.

- The increase in cardiac output secondary to increased stroke volume may be due to improved ventricular compliance [8].
- Tachycardia may be troublesome.
- Dobutamine may improve renal function [9] probably as a result of improved cardiac output.
- When compared to dopamine, dobutamine improves gastric mucosal perfusion in septic patients [10]. This may be beneficial during the establishment of enteral feeding.

Dopamine

Dopamine acts at α, β and dopaminergic receptors. At low doses ($<5\,\mu g/kg/min$) the dopaminergic effects predominate leading to improved renal blood flow. The β and α effects, seen at concentrations of $5–10\,\mu g/kg/min$ and $>10\,\mu g/kg/min$, respectively, allow the drug to be used as an inotrope and a vasopressor.

However, individual variation does not allow for such easy prediction of effects at a given dose.

Renal dose dopamine

- It would seem logical to use dopamine at low doses for the prevention and treatment of acute renal failure.
- Both diuresis and natriuresis can be demonstrated following dopamine administration. The increase in urinary flow most likely results from improved renal blood flow secondary to an increased cardiac output, although activity at dopaminergic receptors may also play a part.
- Dopamine has direct effects on renal tubular cells. It inhibits Na/K ATPase, which results in decreased sodium reabsorption [11]. This in turn leads to a natriuresis.
- Despite these effects the evidence against dopamine as a renal-protective agent is substantial.
- A recent multi-centre trial randomised 328 patients with at least two criteria for systemic inflammatory response syndrome (SIRS) and evidence of early renal dysfunction, to receive either dopamine or placebo [12]. The primary endpoint was peak serum creatinine concentration during the infusion. There was no difference in endpoint between the two groups.
- Two recent meta-analyses have shown that dopamine has no renal-protective effect [13, 14].

Whilst dopamine increases renal blood flow it may have deleterious effects on splanchnic blood flow. In an animal model of haemorrhagic shock splanchnic ischaemia worsened during an infusion of dopamine at $2\,\mu g/kg/min$ [15]. Dopamine may also reduce gastric mucosal perfusion in septic patients [10].

Clearance of dopamine is reduced in the critically ill [16]. This makes predicting the correct dose for a given effect even more difficult and increases the risk of adverse events.

Other suggested problems are the following:

- The commonest side effects of dopamine are tachycardia and arrhythmias.
- There is evidence to suggest harmful effects of dopamine on neuro-endocrine function, with infusions inhibiting prolactin, growth hormone and thyroid-stimulating hormone (TSH) release [17].
- Dopamine disrupts immune function, one result being the inhibition of T-cell proliferation [18].

A recent review by Holmes and Walley concluded "there is no longer a justification for using low-dose dopamine in treating critically ill patients" [19].

Despite these adverse effects and the lack of any renal protection the use of dopamine remains widespread with many considering it to be a "safe" drug.

Dopexamine

This is a relatively new drug with mainly β_2 activity. It is a synthetic analogue of dopamine and also demonstrates agonism at dopaminergic receptors:

- Dopexamine increases renal and splanchnic blood flow. Concerns over the effects of dopamine have led to the use of dopexamine as an alternative.
- Many studies have looked at the use of dopexamine to optimise oxygen delivery in high-risk surgical patients. Wilson demonstrated reduced morbidity when dopexamine was administered preoperatively [20]. However in a multi-centre study involving 412 patients Takala et al were unable to show an improved outcome [21]. More recently Stone and colleagues failed to demonstrate any benefit in giving dopexamine intraoperatively [22].
- Dopexamine does not prevent the development of multi-organ failure in the critically ill when commenced after initial resuscitation [23].
- At doses of >1 μg/kg/min dopexamine exhibits an inhibitory effect on prolactin release, similar to that seen with dopamine [24].

Tachycardia may be pronounced during dopexamine administration.

Whilst the use of dopexamine may seem attractive its benefits are still being evaluated. The use of dopexamine as part of a perioperative optimisation strategy is fully explored in Chapter 17.

Enoximone

Enoximone is a phosphodiesterase III inhibitor and acts to reduce the breakdown of cyclic AMP. This leads to vasodilation and increased cardiac output (i.e. it is an inodilator).

The drug also exhibits lusitropy – enhancing ventricular relaxation allows increased coronary blood flow.

Its use is limited due to the significant hypotension that can occur.

Enoximone may have some beneficial effects on hepato-splanchnic function when compared to dobutamine [25].

Milrinone

This phosphodiesterase inhibitor has similar properties to enoximone.

Hypotension may be worse with milrinone and its use is restricted to the treatment of severe cardiac failure.

Phenylephrine

This agent is a potent α_1 agonist. It is used primarily in vasodilation unresponsive to noradrenaline.

Vasopressin

Vasopressin is a naturally occurring compound, which is synthesised in the hypothalamus and released from the posterior pituitary gland. It has both vaso-pressor and anti-diuretic activity, mediated via vasopressin receptors (V_1 and V_2). V_2 receptors are located in the renal-collecting tubules and stimulation promotes water reabsorption. V_1 receptors are expressed in vascular smooth muscle and are responsible for vasoconstriction:

- Studies have demonstrated that in early septic shock the level of circulating vasopressin rises.
- However during prolonged shock the level falls. This relative deficiency is seen in a third of patients and may contribute to refractory hypotension [26].
- A low-dose vasopressin infusion may have some benefit in these patients and allow withdrawal or reduction of catecholamines [27, 28]. Infusion is recom-mended at 0.02–0.04 units/min with adverse cardiac events seen at higher doses. This is not a titratable drug.
- Outcome studies in septic shock are still awaited.

The role of Vasopressin in cardiac arrest is discussed in Chapter 30.

General points for inotropes and vasopressors

- Positive inotropes increase cardiac output. Mean arterial pressure (MAP) will usually increase as a secondary effect.
- Vasoconstrictors will increase blood pressure.
- Fluid resuscitation should precede the start of cardiovascular support in the presence of hypovolaemia. Starting therapy in a "dry" patient may have disas-trous consequences.
- Severe metabolic derangements (e.g. hypophosphataemia), can impair car-diac function. They should be sought for and corrected.
- Catecholamines may affect blood glucose control and frequent measurements should be taken.
- Vasoactive drugs are rapidly acting with a short half-life. They are given by intravenous infusion that allows easy titratability to desired end points.

- Drugs with α effects should be given into a central vein as extravasation can lead to tissue necrosis.
- Ideally, appropriate monitoring should be in place prior to the commencement of any infusions.
- It is advisable to titrate specific drugs to specific effects; for example, dobutamine to improve cardiac output; noradrenaline to increase blood pressure in the presence of a normal cardiac output.
- It is becoming increasingly clear that one drug does not fit all.
- Some patients are exquisitely sensitive to any interruption of the infusion. In order to minimise these effects it is advisable to "piggy-back" syringes – starting the new infusion shortly before the near-empty syringe runs out.
- Whilst the data sheet advises infusion rates in μg/kg/min; in practice working in ml/hr to a desired clinical effect is often more manageable. Many patients will require infusion rates greater than the manufacturer's recommended maximum.
- Prolonged exposure (>72 h) to positive inotropes leads to a downregulation of β_1 receptors. This may result in the need to increase the rate of infusion, and does not herald a deterioration in the patient's condition.
- When using cardiac monitoring it should be remembered that systemic vascular resistance (SVR) is a derived variable. In the presence of an adequate cardiac output and MAP a low SVR should not be treated to "make the numbers better".

Hypotensive agents

- Occasionally it is necessary to lower a patient's blood pressure (e.g. the obstetric patient with pre-eclampsia).
- Acute uncontrolled hypertension requires rapidly acting agents to minimise end-organ damage.

The commonest drugs in use are briefly outlined below.

Directly acting vasodilators

- *Glyceryl trinitrate (GTN)*: Predominantly causes venodilation resulting in reduced pre-load. Useful in patients with myocardial ischaemia and ventricular failure. Given by intravenous (IV) infusion.
- *Hydralazine*: Direct arteriodilator. Can be given orally or administered IV as a bolus or infusion. Mainly used in the treatment of pregnancy-induced hypertension.

- *Sodium nitroprusside*: Arterio- and veno-dilator. Acts by stabilising smooth muscle membrane. Infusion leads to compensatory tachycardia. May cause cyanide toxicity.

Adrenergic receptor antagonists

- *Labetalol*: Acts at α_1 and β receptors, the latter predominating especially on intravenous administration. Useful in obstetric hypertensive emergencies.
- *Esmolol*: Rapidly acting, selective β_1 blocker. It has a short life (9 mins) making it eminently suitable for IV infusion.
- *Phentolamine*: Competitive α blocker used in the treatment of hypertension associated with phaeochromocytoma.

FURTHER READING

Holmes CL, Patel BM, Russell, JA, Walley KR. Physiology of vasopressin relevant to management of septic shock. *Chest* 2001; 120: 989–1002.

Insel PA. Seminars in medicine of the Beth Israel Hospital, Boston. Adrenergic receptors – evolving concepts and clinical implications. *New Engl J Med* 1996; 334: 580–5.

Lisbon A. Dopexamine, dobutamine, and dopamine increase splanchnic blood flow: what is the evidence? *Chest* 2003; 123: 460S–3S.

REFERENCES

1. Uusaro A, Russell JA. Could anti-inflammatory actions of catecholamines explain the possible beneficial effects of supranormal oxygen delivery in critically ill surgical patients? *Int Care Med* 2000; 26: 299–304.
2. Meier-Hellman A, Reinhart K, Bredle DL, Specht M, Spies CD, Hannemann L. Epinephrine impairs splanchnic perfusion in septic shock. *Crit Care Med* 1997; 25: 399–404.
3. De Backer D, Creteur J, Silva E, Vincent J-L. Effects of dopamine, norepinephrine, and epinephrine on the splanchnic circulation in septic shock: Which is best? *Crit Care Med* 2003; 31: 1659–7.
4. Day NP, Phu NH, Bethell DP, Mai NT, Chau TT, Hien TT, White NJ. The effects of dopamine and adrenaline infusions on acid–base balance and systemic haemodynamics in severe infections. *Lancet* 1996; 348: 219–223.
5. Di Giantomasso D, May CN, Bellomo R. Norepinephrine and vital organ blood flow. *Int Care Med* 2002; 28:1804–9.

6. Meier-Hellmann A, Specht M, Hannemann L, Hassel H, Bredle DL, Reinhart K. Splanchnic flow is greater in septic shock treated with norepinephrine than in severe sepsis. *Int Care Med* 1996; 22: 1354–9.
7. Martin C, Viviand X, Arnaud S et al. Effects of norepinephrine plus dobutamine or norepinephrine alone on left ventricular performance of septic shock patients. *Crit Care Med* 1999; 7: 1708–13.
8. Pawha R, Anel R, Alahdad MT et al. Cardiovascular response to dobutamine in septic shock. *Crit Care Med* 1999; 27: A136.
9. Duke DJ, Briedis JH, Weaver RA. Renal support in critically ill patients: low-dose dopamine or low-dose dobutamine? *Crit Care Med* 1994; 22: 1893–4.
10. Neviere R, Mathieu D, Chagnon JL, Lebleue JN, Wattel F. The contrasting effects of dobutamine and dopamine on gastric mucosal perfusion in septic patients. *Am J Resp and Crit Care Med* 1996; 154: 1684–8.
11. Perdue PW, Balser JR, Lipsett PA, Breslow MJ. "Renal dose" dopamine in surgical patients. Dogma or science? *Ann Surg* 1998; 227: 470–73.
12. Bellomo R, Chapman M, Finfer S, Hickling K, Myburgh J. Low dose dopamine in patients with early renal dysfunction: a placebo-controlled randomised trial. Australian and New Zealand Intensive Care Society (ANZICS) Clinical Trials Group. *Lancet* 2000; 356: 2139–43.
13. Kellum JA, Decker JM. Use of dopamine in acute renal failure: a meta-analysis. *Crit Care Med* 2001; 29: 1526–31.
14. Marik PE. Low-dose dopamine: a systematic review. *Int Care Med* 2002; 28: 877–3.
15. Segal JM, Phang PT, Walley KR. Low-dose dopamine hastens onset of gut ischaemia in a porcine model of haemorrhagic shock. *J Appl Physiol* 1992; 73: 1159–64.
16. Juste RN, Moran L, Hooper J, Soni N. Dopamine clearance in critically ill patients. *Int Care Med* 1998; 24: 1217–20.
17. Van den Berghe G, de Zegher F. Anterior pituitary function during critical illness and dopamine treatment. *Crit Care Med* 1996; 24: 1580–90.
18. Devins SS, Miller A, Herndon BL, O'Toole L, Reisz G. Effects of dopamine on T-lymphocyte proliferative responses and serum prolactin concentrations in critically ill patients. *Crit Care Med* 1992; 20: 1644–9.
19. Holmes CL, Walley KR. Bad medicine: low-dose dopamine in the ICU. Chest 2003; 123: 1266–75.
20. Wilson J, Woods I, Fawcett J, Whall R, Dibb W, Morris C, McManus E. Reducing the risk of major elective surgery. A randomised controlled trial of preoperative optimisation of oxygen delivery. *Br Med J* 1999; 318: 1099–103.
21. Takala J, Meier-Hellmann A, Eddleston J, Hulstaert P, Sramek V. Effect of dopexamine on outcome after major abdominal surgery: a prospective randomized, controlled multicenter study. *Crit Care Med* 2000; 28: 3417–23.
22. Stone MD, Wilson RJT, Cross J, Williams BT. Effect of adding dopexamine to intraoperative volume expansion in patients undergoing major elective surgery. *Br J Anaesth* 2003; 91: 619–24.

23. Ralph CJ, Tanser SJ, Macnaughton PD, Sinclair DG. A randomised controlled trial investigating the effects of dopexamine on gastrointestinal function and organ dysfunction in the critically ill. *Int Care Med* 2002; 28: 884–90.

24. Schilling T, Strang CM, Wilhelm T, Moritz KU, Siegmund W, Grundling M, Haceknberg T. Endocrine effects of dopexamine vs. dopamine in high-risk surgical patients. *Int Care Med* 2001; 27: 1908–15.

25. Kern H, Schroder T, Kaulfuss M, Martin M, Kox WJ, Spies CD. Enoximone in contrast to dobutamine improves heptosplanchnic function in fluid-optimized septic shock patients. *Crit Care Med* 2001; 29: 1519–28.

26. Sharshar T, Blanchard A, Paillard M, Raphael JC, Gajdos P, Annane D. Circulating vasopressin levels in septic shock. *Crit Care Med* 2003; 31: 1752–8.

27. Malay MB, Ashton Jr RC, Landry DW, Townsend RN. Low-dose vasopressin in the treatment of vasodilatory septic shock. *J Trauma* 1999; 47: 699–703.

28. Patel BM, Chittock DR, Russell JA, Walley KR. Beneficial effects of short term vasopressin infusion during severe septic shock. *Anaesthesiology* 2002; 96: 576–82.

13

Infection and infection control

N. Randall

Infection is a common cause of admission to intensive care units (ICUs). In addition, around 30% of patients in ICUs will acquire infection (nosocomial infection) during their admission. The resulting increase in mortality is between 20 and 80% depending on site of infection and organism. The impact on length of stay and costs is substantial [1]. Increasing severity of illness is inevitably associated with more frequent infections.

Certain causes for admission are more commonly associated with infection:

- trauma,
- burns,
- following emergency surgery (particularly intra-abdominal).

Common intensive care interventions also increase nosocomial infections:

- tracheal intubation and ventilation,
- intravascular catheters,
- urinary catheters,
- drugs (sedatives, muscle relaxants, corticosteroids, antibiotics),
- blood transfusion.

Some patients are predisposed to infection:

- elderly,
- malnourished,
- high alcohol intake,
- heavy smoking,
- diabetes,
- neutropenia.

The EPIC study

Although 10-year old, the Early *Pseudomonas* Infection Control (EPIC) study [2] still gives a useful overview of infection in ICUs.

Causative organisms isolated in the EPIC study

- Enterobacter 34%.
- *Staphylococcus aureus* 30%, (60% MRSA) – probably now higher, with a greater proportion of MRSA.
- *Pseudomonas* 29%.
- *Staphylococcus epidemidis* 19%.
- *Candida* 17%.

The source of infection is evenly divided between the patients' bacterial flora and exogenous causes.

Site of infection in EPIC study

- All lower respiratory tract 65%.
- Urinary tract 17%.
- Blood 12%.

Pyrexia and leucocytosis are unreliable indicators of infection. C reactive protein trends are not specific. Although not well established, Procalcitonin shows promise as a more specific and sensitive indicator of developing infection [3]. However, any deterioration in the condition of a patient should stimulate a search for infection in each body system. Blood culture should always be part of the process. Chest and central vein catheter (CVC) infections are discussed below. In addition consider other sites:

- urine,
- abdomen including gall-bladder,
- surgical wounds,
- heart valves,
- nasal sinuses,
- central nervous system,
- prostheses (heart valves, vascular grafts, mesh implants, orthopaedic implants).

Appropriate and adequate cultures should usually be taken before antibiotics are started. If antibiotics are started empirically, microbiological results must be reviewed to check that the drug is appropriate. For patients on antibiotics who appear to be developing a secondary infection, it is preferable to stop antibiotics and take cultures after a 24–48 h antibiotic-free period.

After 48–72 h of treatment, the response should be assessed. If treatment seems to be unsuccessful, then further cultures should be taken.

The advice of a microbiologist is valuable.

Nosocomial respiratory infections [4, 5]

In the first 3 days of hospital admission, infections are usually community acquired. After 5 days, infections are usually hospital acquired. Between 3 and 5 days, both should be considered.

Hospital-acquired pneumonia (HAP) increases with:

- length of hospital stay,
- severity of underlying illness,
- presence of co-morbidities,
- immobility,
- abdominal distension,
- decreased cough reflex (debility, drugs, head injury).

Additionally, the following factors increase the risk of pneumonia while ventilated (ventilator-acquired pneumonia, VAP):

- endotracheal intubation,
- reintubation (following planned or unplanned extubation),
- sedation,
- supine position.

Keeping patients semi-recumbent (more than 30°) is the only measure shown to reduce VAP.

Choice of antacid treatment, oro- or naso-gastric tubes, enteral feeding, humidification, and suction management have not been shown to consistently affect VAP [6, 7]. Selective decontamination of the digestive tract (SDD) is discussed below.

The diagnosis of VAP depends on:

- Clinical features
  - white cell count (high or low),
  - pyrexia,

- increased and/or more purulent secretions,
- deterioration in oxygenation.
- Chest X-ray
  - new infiltrates (but these have to be distinguished from worsening acute respiratory distress syndrome (ARDS) or heart failure).
- Bacteriology
  - tracheal aspirates (poor sensitivity and specificity, both improved if cultures are *quantitative* rather than just *qualitative*),
  - invasive specimens (i.e. bronchoscopic, either by lavage or protected specimen brush (PSB) yielding >80% sensitivity and specificity),
  - non-bronchoscopic invasive techniques (blind PSB and mini-BAL, show some reduction in sensitivity and specificity compared with guided techniques).

Combining these factors into a score (clinical pulmonary infection score) has not been widely validated or adopted.

Other sites should be considered, as respiratory deterioration may be triggered by non-respiratory infection.

The *treatment* of VAP should be guided by bacteriological results. Empirical treatment will need to cover likely organisms:

- aerobic Gram-negative bacilli (including *Pseudomonas aeruginosa* and *Acinetobacter*),
- methicillin-resistant *S. aureus* (MRSA),
- *Candida* remains an under-diagnosed cause [6].

Local patterns of antibiotic resistance will guide the choice of drug.

Absence of clinical improvement by 72 h indicates the need for further investigation. At this point, ongoing antibiotic treatment seems to have less effect on bacteriological results, particularly on BAL specimens [4].

The *mortality* of VAP is 20–50%. How much of this is directly attributable to the VAP (rather than VAP identifying a group with worse survival) is debated.

CVC infections [8, 5, 9]

Routine cultures of CVCs removed from critical care patients will be positive in 15–40%. The incidence of bacteraemia from catheters is less common, at around 0.5% per 100 catheter days, occurring in between 3% and 7% of patients with CVCs. The attributable mortality is around 12%.

The morbidity results in an extra week in intensive care and an extra 2 weeks in hospital.

Colonization of the catheter occurs within a biofilm on the catheter. This is more commonly extra-luminal.

Bacteria may be carried into the subcutaneous tissue at the time of insertion, or may migrate along the CVC at a later time. Some infections are intraluminal, arising from CVC hub contamination. Infusates are exceptionally rare causes of infection. Administration sets are more likely to become infected if used for parenteral nutrition, blood, or several lots of fluid.

CVC infection should be a constant consideration in the management of critical care patients. The *diagnosis* of CVC infection is by culture of more than 15 colony forming units from a removed line.

CVC induced bacteraemia is confirmed by finding the same organism in peripheral blood and from no other site. The CVC remains the likely culprit even if the organism is found elsewhere, or if the patient's condition improves after catheter removal.

CVC infection can be reduced by the following:

- Experienced operator.
- Aseptic technique:
  - surgical scrub handwash,
  - hat, mask, gown, gloves,
  - 2% chlorhexidine antiseptic skin preparation,
  - wide sterile field.
- CVC care protocol:
  - non-occlusive dressing,
  - blood administration sets removed immediately after use,
  - other administration sets changed at 72 h,
  - aseptic technique when opening hubs, then new cap,
  - staff education programme.
- Subclavian route rather than jugular or femoral.
- Tunnelled lines (if femoral or jugular).
- Line replacement when clinically indicated. Guide wire exchange only in exceptional circumstances.
- Antiseptic impregnated catheters (and are probably cost-effective).
- Antibiotic impregnated catheters; effective but carry reservations over induction of bacterial resistance and drug allergy.

Antibiotic and antiseptic ointments at the puncture site have not consistently been shown to reduce CVC infection. Studies of antibiotic and anticoagulant luminal flush locks have also generated conflicting results (and studies are often in haematology patients).

The commonest organisms causing CVC infection are *S. epidermidis* and *S. aureus*. Less commonly, Candida and Gram-negative organisms are found.

Treatment is removal of the line. Removal should be for clinical reasons; scheduled removal after a fixed period does not reduce infection rates. It then follows that guide-wire exchange should only be used in exceptional circumstances.

This topic is also discussed in Chapter 4.

Specific nosocomial organisms

The risk factors (disease process, treatments, co-morbidities) for nosocomial infections have been listed above. The use of (broad spectrum) antibiotics results in certain organisms becoming more of a problem as an ICU admission lengthens.

MRSA [10]

MRSA is now endemic in many countries. An exception is the Netherlands, where strict antibiotic policies have controlled the incidence. ICUs often have the highest incidence in a hospital. High cephalosporin and quinolone usage correlates with increased MRSA colonization and infection.

MRSA carries significant attributable mortality, probably greater than that of methicillin-sensitive *S. aureus* (MSSA).

Treatment is by:

- vancomycin
- teicoplanin
- linezolid.

Vancomycin has to be administered slowly to avoid anaphylactoid reaction. Drug level monitoring is needed, particularly in renal impairment. Teicoplanin is less nephrotoxic but drug levels still need monitoring to ensure therapeutic levels as well as to avoid toxicity. Linezolid (see below) may be more effective than vancomycin [11] in treating MRSA pneumonia. Topical treatment of line sites, wounds, and nose and pharynx is usual.

Control of MRSA is difficult. In addition to general infection control measures (see below), routine screening and isolation of patients has not been widely adopted, although there is some evidence to support it [12].

Candidiasis

In the EPIC study [2], 17% of patients had a deep *Candida* infection, with significant morbidity and mortality. However, the spectrum of disease is wide:

- *Superficial*: Oropharyngeal, oesophageal, vaginal. Limited significance. Topical treatment.
- *Urinary*: In isolation, of limited significance. Change catheter, amphotericin bladder irrigation, with or without fluconazole. Recurrence may represent haematogenous spread from another more clinically significant site.
- *Deep infection*: Candidaemia, often from CVC infection. Pneumonia, difficult to diagnose. Tracheal aspirates may represent colonization rather than infection. Significant pneumonia may not release *Candida* in to bronchial secretions resulting in under-diagnosis [6]. Peritoneal *Candida* may also be missed; a cause of late recurrence of abdominal infection after a perforated viscus. Fundoscopy will identify retinal abscesses in 10% of disseminated *Candida* infection.

Treatment of deep infection [13]. *Candida albicans* remains widely sensitive to fluconazole; deep infections will need >6 mg/day and up to 10 mg/kg/day. In the unstable patient, amphotericin use should be considered (particularly in the absence of species identification or known sensitivity to fluconazole). Failure to respond to fluconazole should also lead to the consideration of amphotericin. In the critical care setting, one of the lipid-based formulations of amphotericin is usually more appropriate than the standard preparation. The possibility of non-*albicans Candida* would lead to an amphotericin formulation as first-line treatment. Sources of infection should be removed (CVCs, drainage of abdominal collection).

Prophylaxis (using fluconazole) for *Candida* has been suggested for critical care patients who have had a perforated viscus [14].

Two new anti-fungal agents are available. Caspofungin [15] is an echinocandin, fungicidal for *Candida* and *Aspergillus*. Voriconazole is a triazole related to fluconazole. Both have far fewer side-effects compared with amphotericin, but there is no evidence for improved efficacy [16].

Clostridium difficile (Cd)

This Gram-positive spore forming bacillus is widely present in the environment and is part of the bowel flora in 15–30% of patients. Prior exposure to antibiotics is usually required to precipitate a clinical problem. Third generation cephalosporins and clindamycin produce most Cd infections.

Clinical consequences are variable:

- colonization,
- diarrhoea (morbidity rather than mortality),
- pseudomembranous colitis (life threatening).

Diagnosis is by detection of the A and B toxin; this is more significant than culture of Cd.

Treatment is with metronidazole or oral vancomycin, for 10 days.

Vancomycin-resistant enterococci (VRE)

Two species of *Enterococcus, faecium* and *faecalis*, have a high level of resistance to vancomycin (Van A and Van B types).

Again, the consequences are variable:

- colonization,
- a range of infections, of gut, urine, blood, soft tissues, and CVCs,
- some excess morbidity and mortality.

There remains continuing concern about transmission of vancomycin resistance to *S. aureus*.

Extended spectrum beta-lactamase (ESBL) organisms

A range of Gram-negative organisms (*Pseudomonas, Acinetobacter, Serratia* and others) may acquire resistance to a wide range of antibiotics by the development or acquisition of beta-lactamases. These organisms may then be responsible for epidemics of infections in ICUs.

Control of infection [1, 17]

There are two broad strategies:

- prevention of spread of infection between patients,
- management of patients to reduce the incidence of infection.

Prevention of spread of infection

Spread is by contact or airborne. It can be reduced by the following:

- Unit design; size of bed space, "corridor" through unit, provision of cubicles, air-conditioning, provision of sinks, soap and alcoholic rub dispensers.

- Operational policies; staff and visitor access, clean/dirty utility rooms, cleaning and waste disposal.
- Clinical policies; nurse–patient staffing levels, staff clothing, hand-washing, use of gloves and aprons, tracheal suction.
- Microbiological policies; screening of admitted patients, epidemiology of unit infections.

Hand-washing (easier with alcohol rub preparations) and other basic clinical practices are at the core of infection control.

Patient management strategies

Those strategies related to respiratory infections and CVCs have been discussed above. In addition, two areas are of note; antibiotic management and SDD.

Antibiotic management

- Policies for choice of empirical antibiotics and drug change in response to microbiology results have been shown to improve outcome.
- Duration of antibiotic courses remains arbitrary [18] at between 5–10 days.
- Scheduled rotation of use of groups of antibiotics (antibiotic cycling) may reduce the emergence of resistant organisms.

SDD

SDD is a regimen of non-absorbable topically applied antibiotics (usually polymixin B, tobramycin, and amphotericin B) combined with a systemic broad-spectrum antibiotic (often cefotaxime). The objective is to decontaminate the upper gastro-intestinal tract and prevent nosocomial (mainly respiratory) infections. Anaerobic bacteria are preserved.

Meta-analyses [19] support the use of SDD, particularly in surgical and trauma patients. The benefits are reduction in episodes of infection and improved survival. Some studies [20] have shown additional benefits of reduced antibiotic use and less antibiotic resistance.

However, concerns remain regarding the lack of consistency in studies included in the meta-analyses as well as conflicting results. Areas at issue are the importance of the systemic component of the SDD, more antibiotic-resistant organisms (particularly Gram-positive ones), and whether there really is a beneficial effect on survival [21].

The context in which SDD is used is important; case-mix of patients, antibiotic usage, and prevalence of resistant organisms such as MRSA and VRE will change the risk/benefit of SDD [22].

SDD is also discussed in Chapter 25.

Antibiotic guidelines

The aim of such guidelines is to facilitate:

- effective treatment,
- reduce antibiotic side-effects,
- reduce antibiotic resistance.

This requires the following:

- Assessing the probability of infection, its source and likely organisms.
- Obtaining adequate specimens.
- Starting the most appropriate antibiotic(s) at the correct dose (considering body weight, renal function, and severity of infection).
- Reviewing treatment as results become available, trying to reduce the antibiotic spectrum of activity to a minimum.
- Critically assessing the response to treatment and changing therapy if it is failing.
- Limiting treatment courses to between 5 and 7 days (some exceptions).

The following table shows some antibiotic guidelines:

Infection	Treatment	Comment
Community-acquired pneumonia	Ceftriaxone ± erythromycin (or clarithromycin) or levofloxacin	Clarithromycin and rifampicin for *Legionella*, for 3 weeks
Hospital-acquired pneumonia	Piperacillin–tazobactam *or* ciprofloxacin	Gram-negative bacteria more common; consider anti-MRSA cover
ICU-acquired pneumonia	Ciprofloxacin *or* piperacillin–tazobactam *or* ceftazidime	ESBL cover needed; consider anti-MRSA cover
Abdominal sepsis	Cefuroxime + metronidazole	Initial treatment; poor response, consider

Infection	Treatment	Comment
		undrained infection, ESBL, MRSA or *Candida*
Pancreatitis		Antibiotics only if infection
Biliary tract infection	Cefuroxime *or* ciprofloxacin	
Renal tract	Cefuroxime *or* gentamicin	
Meningitis (adult)	Ceftriaxone *or* cefotaxime	Add in ampicillin in elderly (*Listeria* cover); acyclovir if encephalitis not excluded
Febrile neutropenic patients	Piperacillin–tazobactam	Cover may have to be extended for *S. epidermidis* and *Candida*

Practical points

- *Aminoglycosides*: efficacy dependent on high-peak concentrations. Higher peaks depress bacterial growth for longer (post-antibiotic effect). Nephrotoxicity related to high trough levels. Once-daily dosing is a useful strategy in ICU patients whose renal function and volume of distribution may be fluctuating. Trough drug levels may then be checked before each dose.
- *Cephalosporins*: renal excretion, but drugs vary; for example, ceftriaxone needs no reduction unless severe impairment; ceftazidime needs reduction at moderate renal impairment. Ceftazidime usually effective against *Pseudomonas*.
- *Quinolones*: ciprofloxacin usually effective against hospital-acquired Gram-negative organisms, including *Pseudomonas*. Levofloxacin has poorer Gram-negative cover, but better Gram positive, so useful for community-acquired pneumonia. All quinolones reduce seizure threshold and may precipitate fits. Ciprofloxacin increases theophylline levels.
- *Carbapenems*: Broad-spectrum cover, including ESBL organisms. Imipenem formulated with cilastatin to inhibit renal clearance. Convulsant metabolites may accumulate in renal failure. Meropenem does not have this problem.
- *Fluconazole*: useful anti-fungal, but dose at 5–10 mg/kg/day in serious infections. Decrease dose in renal impairment but double dose if haemofiltered.
- *Amphotericin*: 1 mg over 30 mins as test dose, then 0.5–0.7 mg/kg/day. Significant volume load. Hypokalaemia, hypomagnesaemia, renal and liver impairment are all common to varying extents. Colloidal and lipid-based preparations have fewer side-effects. Caspofungin is reported to have less renal toxicity than liposomal amphotericin [23].

- *Linezolid* [24]: from a new class of antibiotics, the oxazolidinones. Works by inhibiting the initiation of protein synthesis in the 50S sub-unit of bacterial ribosomes. Effective for Gram-positive organisms, including MRSA, VRE, *Listeria* and *C. difficile*. Particularly useful for pneumonia and soft tissue infections. An alternative for beta-lactam sensitive patients with pneumococcal pneumonia. Intravenous and oral (well absorbed) preparations. Enough liver metabolism (oxidation) for dosage adjustment not to be needed. Removed by haemodialysis. Few side-effects: reversible thrombocytopenia after long (>2 weeks) courses, weak monoamine oxidase inhibitor, not reported to be clinically significant.

FURTHER READING

Eggimann P, Pittet D. Critical care reviews: Infection Control in the ICU. *Chest* 2001; 120: 2059–93.

Hubmayr RD. Statement of the 4th International Consensus Conference in Critical Care on ICU-Acquired Pneumonia – Chicago, Illinois, May 2002. *Intens Care Med* 2002; 28: 1521–36.

Mouvillier B, Timsit JF. Management of catheter-related sepsis in the ICU. In Vincent JL (Eds), *Yearbook of Intensive Care and Emergency Medicine 2003*. Springer-Verlag, Berlin, 2003.

Vincent JL. Nosocomial infections in adult intensive care units. *Lancet* 2003; 361: 2068–82.

REFERENCES

1. Vincent JL. Nosocomial infections in adult intensive care units. *Lancet* 2003; 361: 2068–82.
2. Vincent JL, Bihari DJ, Suter PM et al. The prevalence of nosocomial infection in intensive care units in Europe. *J Am Med Assoc* 1995; 274: 639–44.
3. Harbarth S, Holeckova K, Froidevaux C et al. Diagnostic value of procalcitonin, interleukin-6, and interleukin-8 in critically ill patients admitted with suspected sepsis. *Am J Respir Crit Care Med* 2001; 164: 396–402.
4. Hubmayr RD. Statement of the 4th International Consensus Conference in Critical Care on ICU-Acquired Pneumonia – Chicago, Illinois, May 2002. *Intens Care Med* 2002; 28: 1521–36.
5. Mouvillier B, Timsit JF. Management of Catheter-Related Sepsis in the ICU. In Vincent JL (Eds), *Yearbook of Intensive Care and Emergency Medicine 2003*. Springer-Verlag, Berlin, 2003.
6. Lynch JP. Hospital – acquired pneumonia: risk factors, microbiology, and treatment. *Chest* 2001; 119: S373–85.
7. Collard HR, Saint S, Mathay MA. Prevention of ventilator-associated pneumonia: an evidence-based systematic review. *Ann Intern Med* 2003; 138: 494–503.

8. Fraenkel DJ, Rickard C, Lipman J. Can we achieve consensus on central venous catheter–related infections? *Anaesth Intens Care* 2000; 28: 475–90.

9. Eggimann P, Harbarth S, Constantin M-N et al. Impact of a prevention strategy targeted at vascular-access care on incidence of infections acquired in intensive care. *Lancet* 2000; 355: 1864–8.

10. Hardy KJ, Hawkey PM, Gao F, Oppenheim BA. Methicillin resistant *Staphylococcus aureus* in the critically ill. *Br J Anaesth* 2004; 92: 121–30.

11. Wunderink RG, Rello J, Cammarata SK et al. Linezolid vs vancomycin. Analysis of two double blind studies of patients with methicillin resistant *Staph. aureus* nosocomial pneumonia. *Chest* 2003; 124: 1789–97.

12. Chaix C, Durand-Zaleski I, Alberti C, Brun-Buisson C. Control of endemic methicillin resistant *Staphylococcus aureus*. A cost–benefit analysis in an intensive care unit. *J Am Med Assoc* 1999; 282: 1745–51.

13. Rex JH, Walsh TJ, Sobel JD et al. Practice guidelines for the treatment of Candidiasis. *Clin Infect Dis* 2004; 30: 662–78.

14. Eggimann P, Francioli P, Bille J et al. Fluconazole prophylaxis prevents intra-abdominal candidiasis in high-risk surgical patients. *Crit Care Med* 1999; 27: 1066–72.

15. Denning DW. Echinocandin antifungal drugs. *Lancet* 2003; 362: 1142–9.

16. Caspofungin and voriconazole for fungal infections. *Drug Therapeut Bull* 2004; 42: 7–8.

17. Eggimann P, Pittet D. Critical care reviews: infection control in the ICU. *Chest* 2001; 120: 2059–93.

18. Corona A, Bertolini G, Ricotta AM et al. Variability of treatment duration for bacteraemia in the critically ill: a multinational study. *J Antimicrob Chemother* 2003; 52: 849–52.

19. D'Amico R, Pifferi S, Leonetti C et al. Effectiveness of antibiotic prophylaxis in critically ill adult patients: systematic review of randomised controlled trials. *Br Med J* 1998; 316: 1275–85.

20. De Jonge E, Schultz MJ, Spanjaard L, Bossuyt PMM. Effects of selective decontamination of digestive tract on mortality and acquisition of resistant bacteria in intensive care: a randomised controlled trial. *Lancet* 2003; 362: 1011–16.

21. Kollef MH. Selective decontamination should not be routinely employed. *Chest* 2003; 123: S464–9.

22. Vincent JL. Selective digestive decontamination: for everyone, everywhere? *Lancet* 2003; 362: 1006.

23. Walsh TJ, Teppler H, Donowitz GR et al. Caspofungin versus liposomal amphotericin B for empirical antifungal therapy in patients with persistent fever and neutropenia. *New Engl J Med* 2004; 351: 1391–402.

24. Perry CM, Jarvis B. Linezolid: a review of its use in the management of serious Gram-positive infections. *Drugs* 2001; 61: 526–51.

14

Sedation, analgesia and neuromuscular blockade

N. Sharma and R. Morgan

Introduction

The two terms, sedation and analgesia, as used in the intensive care unit (ICU) setting, may be defined as follows:

- Sedation: for hypnosis and anxiolysis.
- Analgesia: for pain relief and suppression of respiratory drive.

In the 1980s ventilated patients were often deeply sedated and routinely paralysed with muscle relaxants.

In recent years many critically ill patients have come to be managed at much lighter levels of sedation, often without the coincident use of muscle relaxants [1] as a result of the following developments:

- Novel modes of mechanical ventilation which more readily complement and synchronise with the patient's own intrinsic respiratory pattern.
- A steady trend towards early percutaneous tracheostomy.
- Wider appreciation of the hazards and negative effects of excessive sedation and analgesia and the routine use of muscle relaxants.

Sleep, factual memory and amnesia

Patients in the ICU rarely have a normal sleep cycle [2]. They experience reduced rapid eye movement and slow wave sleep, both of which are important for the integration of factual memories [2, 3].

Complete amnesia results in fragmentation and distortion of patient's memory of their ICU stay in turn leading to delusional dreams with impairment of the experience and recognition of external reality [4]. This sequence of events has been postulated as a cause of anxiety, depression and later chronic stress disorders in some ICU patients [5].

Thus, complete amnesia with the total abolition of factual memories may not be appropriate for ICU patients, other than during periods of pharmacological muscle relaxation and for the facilitation of full intermittent positive pressure ventilation (IPPV) [6].

There is also evidence that hallucinations and delusions, coupled with sleep deprivation, may generate a state of paranoid delusions, hallucinations, panic and terror in ICU patients [7]. This transient psychosis may precipitate a withdrawn state, often mistakenly diagnosed as depression and treated with antidepressants rather than with anxiolytics.

However, whilst much can be achieved by explanation and reassurance, intubated patients undergoing mechanical IPPV generally benefit from a period of pharmacological sedation and analgesia, if only to facilitate "acclimatisation".

Indications for sedation

In addition to pain, patients in the critical care environment commonly experience fear and anxiety as a result of their "surfacing" in an alien and apparently hostile critical care environment. Many patients also experience profound apprehension upon coming to a realisation of the severity of their critical illness and of their consequent vulnerability.

Most patients appear to find the experience of tracheal intubation and positive pressure mechanical ventilation to be, at the very least, unpleasant.

Whilst alleviating overt distress, anxiety and pain, appropriately managed sedation and analgesia may also lead to a decrease in the work of breathing, myocardial and respiratory oxygen demand and a reduction in the level of metabolic and hormonal response to critical illness.

Sedation may also be indicated for the:

- control of agitation,
- control of intra-cranial pressure and seizures,
- patient's and health care professional's safety,
- facilitation of safe patient transport.

Therapeutic sedative agents

For patients undergoing Intermittent positive pressure ventilation (IPPV) there are several choices:

- *Midazolam*: Midazolam is administered by bolus (1–2 mg) or, more commonly, by infusion (1–5 mg/h). Concern has been expressed that this drug has the potential to accumulate in the critically ill patient with impaired hepatic and or renal function [8]. Midazolam is also extensively protein bound leading to a potential increase in depth of sedation and prolongation of action in hypo-albuminaemic critically ill patients.
- *Diazepam*: Diazepam is considered to have an unacceptably long, context sensitive half-life for intravenous use in ICU. It also generates pharmacologically active metabolites. Oral diazepam nevertheless does have a useful short-term role in the non-ventilated critical care patient suffering from severe acute anxiety.
- *Propofol*: Propofol may be administered by infusion at between 5 and 20 ml/h depending upon response. It results in much less hangover than other intra-venous hypnotic drugs and significantly shortens weaning time to ventilator independence [9] when compared with alternatives. Although propofol is expensive, it has been shown to be cost effective in terms of shorter weaning times after 5 day administration thus minimising undesirable delay between discontinuation of the drug and the regaining of consciousness [10].

  Despite its apparent ideal qualities the routine use of propofol may not be appropriate for every ventilated patient. It is principally indicated where short-term ventilatory support is expected (e.g. 24–48 h). Propofol may also be substituted for longer acting sedatives, after a prolonged period of IPPV, in order to allow those longer acting drugs to be cleared from the system whilst maintaining sedation control.

  In similar vein, propofol is a useful background sedative in cases of overdose with depressant drugs in order to maintain sedation control whilst the offending depressant drugs are metabolised and eliminated.
- *Haloperidol*: Some practitioners use major tranquilisers such as haloperidol [11] to control agitation in ventilated patients.
- *Clonidine*: Clonidine, a centrally acting α_2 agonist, in a dose of 50–250 µg IV, may be used to control agitation, delirium, anxiety and the coincident sympathetic hyperstimulation often associated with alcohol or opiate withdrawal [12, 13]. Clonidine also decreases the quantity of opioids required to achieve a given level analgesia with a corresponding reduction in hypotensive and respiratory depressant side effects.

- *Dexmedetomidine*: Dexmedetomidine, another α_2 agonist, when compared to propofol, provides an equivalent depth of sedation without increasing time to extubation. It also exhibits analgesic effects together with the capacity to attenuate the cardiovascular stress responses [14].
- *Temazepam*: Temazepam may be employed as an effective hypnotic in an effort to restore a "normal" sleep cycle.
- *Isoflurane*: Although an effective sedative at appropriate inhaled concentration, isoflurane is unsuitable for long-term ICU sedation on the grounds of cost and the requirement for efficient scavenging and vaporiser compatible ventilators.
- *Narcotic analgesics*: Intravenous opiates in general do also contribute to sedation, with the possible exception of alfentanil, which behaves almost as a pure analgesic respiratory depressant. Analgesia still remains the principle indication for the use of opiates along, with the facilitation of ventilator compliance through their respiratory suppressant effects.

Analgesia

Many patients in the ICU experience pain during their period of critical care [15, 16]:

- Postoperative surgical patients have painful wounds.
- Vascular cannulation, wound dressing, endotracheal and endobronchial suctioning, physiotherapy, etc. may also cause pain and discomfort.
- Uncontrolled pain frequently leads to agitation and anxiety in the ICU setting.

As previously noted, whilst the drive to breathe against IPPV may be reduced by appropriate selection of ventilator mode, constant "fighting" and failure to synchronise with mechanical IPPV may require pharmacological (opiate) therapy to suppress respiratory drive.

Therapeutic analgesic agents

- *Regional blockade*: The use of regional blockade, including epidural and interpleural local anaesthesia by continuous infusion, may be useful in specific circumstances (e.g. after thoracic injury or following major surgery). Epidural analgesia is discussed further in the chapter on the surgical patient.

Infiltration of local anaesthesia prior to vascular cannulation should always be considered even in the sedated patient.

- *Morphine*: Morphine by infusion (1–5 mg/h) is commonly used for analgesia in critical care causing few cardiovascular problems when given. Morphine and its pharmacologically active metabolites may, however, accumulate in patients suffering from renal failure [17].

- *Fentanyl*: Fentanyl at 1–5 μg/kg/h by infusion, is an alternative to morphine though more costly. Like morphine, fentanyl may accumulate with prolongation of action following long-term administration.

- *Alfentanil*: Alfentanil administered by 5 mg bolus followed by an infusion of 2–5 mg/h is a further alternative to morphine. Although costly, it is predictably short acting after brief administration. Long-term infusions of alfentanil may, however, also lead to prolongation of effect as a result of its context sensitive half-life and renal elimination.

- *Remifentanil*: Remifentanil at an infusion rate of 1–10 μg/kg/h is, by contrast, an ideal choice of analgesic for patients with renal failure [18]. This drug has a rapid onset of action (less than 60 s), a predictable metabolic profile and a relatively constant, context independent half-life of 2–3 min. It can therefore be used for long periods without the risk of accumulation.

Tolerance to opiate infusions is common in ICU. Discontinuing continuous infusions may prove challenging with some patients suffering from classical narcotic "withdrawal" (see later).

Whilst they are predictably effective analgesics, opiates alone cannot be relied upon to provide adequate sedation. The co-administration of an additional sedative such as midazolam is usually required although the absolute sedative dose requirement is often less in conjunction with opiates than when midazolam is administered alone.

Management of sedation and analgesia

It has been suggested that the goals of sedation and analgesia should be to achieve:

- a pain-free patient, who is clear, calm and cooperative during the day and has sufficient restful sleep at night;

- a patient who can be rapidly weaned from ventilatory support once sedation is switched off.

These goals may be difficult to achieve because of the following:

- the "ideal" drug does not exist;
- tolerance to pharmacological sedatives and analgesics is common;
- drug accumulation is common in the critically ill;
- whilst drug infusion rates are often increased during invasive procedures they may not be reduced again at procedural completion. This phenomenon may result in a "ratchet effect" leading to stepwise increases in drug plasma levels;
- critical care nursing and medical staff are sometimes inclined to accept an unresponsive patient who, though "flat", is also relatively "low maintenance".

Thus over sedation may be more common than under sedation and, on casual examination, less obviously a problem. Over sedation, however, should not be considered an acceptable substitute for inadequate levels of critical care staff. Sedation should be for the benefit of the patient and not for the convenience of medical and nursing staff.

The adverse consequences of over sedation include:

- cardiovascular and respiratory depression,
- decreased immune function,
- decreased cough reflex activity and strength,
- prolonged weaning with consequent increased risk of opportunist infection,
- suppression of neurological responses thus making assessment difficult and resulting in unnecessary diagnostic imaging,
- gastro-intestinal stasis, especially with opiates,
- increased risk of pressure sore development,
- increased risk of venous thrombo-embolism,
- development of physical and psychological drug dependence leading to withdrawal complications,
- increased risk of undesirable drug interactions,
- increased direct cost and secondary cost from increased length of stay in ICU.

There does, however, remain a group of patients who do need deep sedation whilst receiving muscle relaxants to permit optimal mechanical ventilation for the indications mentioned earlier.

The process of initiation and maintenance of sedation and analgesia in critical ill patients is as important as is the choice of individual sedative or analgesic drug. Agents should be individually titrated against definable end points appropriate to the given patient.

The monitoring of sedation through the use of target criteria can be effective in ensuring that individual goals are met.

The following approaches may help optimise sedation and analgesia in given patients:

- sedation scoring systems,
- guidelines for use in specific patient groups, for example renal and/or hepatic failure,
- nurse directed sedation protocols [19],
- daily interruption of sedation.

Numerous scoring systems have been developed suggesting that there is, as yet, no "ideal" system [20].

Sedation scoring system

Subjective scoring systems include the following:

- The Ramsay system scores comfort, sedation and agitation and, along with the Cook system, has been shown to have good reliability when scored at a single point in time [21]. System responsiveness and reliability when scored over a period of time, however, is either poor or has not been subject to analysis.
- The UK Intensive Care Society (ICS) has recommended the routine use of regular sedation scoring using the society's subjective criteria and numerical designations for different levels of sedation [22]. These ICS guidelines on sedation also include an operative flow chart for use with the scoring criteria.

Objective scoring systems are attractive in principle but difficult to apply in practice because of the following:

- Plasma drug concentration does not necessarily correspond with effector organ concentration.
- Frontalis muscle electro-myography and lower oesophageal sphincter contractions have low sensitivity and vary between individuals [23].
- Continuous electro-encephalography also varies between individuals and according to chosen sedative [23].
- The cerebral function and cerebral function analysing monitors are complex and difficult to interpret [24].
- Bi spectral index (BIS) varies between patients [25] and is affected by the use of opioids [26] becoming unreliable at deeper levels of sedation [27].

- Auditory evoked potentials (AEP) are not reliable at light levels of sedation and remain under evaluation [23].

Daily interruption of sedation

Daily interruption of sedation implies switching off sedative infusions completely every day in order to assess conscious level and minimise the risk of undetected drug accumulation.

Interrupted infusions are recommenced when necessary. Where there is no significant drug accumulation this may be almost immediately. Where accumulation has occurred the interrupted infusion(s) may not need recommencing for several hours allowing clearance of excess sedative agent and potentially shortening time to wean from ventilatory support [28].

Whilst daily awakening does not demonstrably contribute to the development of depression or post-traumatic stress disorder after ICU discharge [29], daily sedation holds may be counterproductive in some groups of patients, for example those with significant ischaemic heart disease.

Delirium in the intensive care patient

- Delirium is a manifestation of acute cerebral insufficiency accompanied by neurotransmitter abnormalities.
- It affects cognition, wakefulness and psychomotor behaviour.
- It may be manifest as extreme agitation or as quiet withdrawal.
- The onset of delirium may be sudden or occur more slowly over days. It typically fluctuates periodically with symptoms and signs often being more florid at night.
- The true overall incidence of delirium in critically ill patients is unknown (32–67%) being commonly misdiagnosed or unrecognised [30].
- Its incidence in surgical ICU patients is 40%, increasing to 60% in elderly.
- Whilst sometimes a consequence of haemodynamic and metabolic decompensation, delirium can also be caused by pain, anxiety and disruption of normal circadian rhythms.
- Delirium is also a common side effect of sedative and analgesic drugs themselves.

Agitation may make patients uncooperative, difficult to monitor and treat. Delirium and agitation can thus pose risks to both patients and carers.

The management of delirium and agitation includes:

- Sympathetic communication with the patient to calm him or her down.
- Identification and treatment of underlying remediable patho-physiological or pharmacological causes.
- The administration of pharmacological sedatives when no other remediable causative factors can be identified and treated [31].

Suitable sedatives include:

- *Butyrophenones*: Haloperidol works by preventing dopamine surges and is best used intravenously beginning with a low dose at which it may not cause significant sedation.
- *Benzodiazepines*: Longer acting agents such as lorazepam and diazepam may be given by intravenous bolus and shorter acting agents such as midazolam, by continuous infusion.
- *Propofol*: Propofol is best reserved for circumstances where agitation and sedation represent life-threatening emergencies.
- *Opiates*: Drugs such as morphine or fentanyl have calming effects in some patients.
- α_2 *agonists*: Clonidine has sedative, axiolytic analgesic effects in addition to attenuating the stress response.
- β *blockers*: Agents such as esmolol suppress noradrenergic hyperfunction.

Drug dependence and withdrawal

Tolerance to sedatives and analgesic drugs may develop in patients on long-term infusions leading to an increase in the amount of drug required [32, 33]. Sudden cessation or too rapid weaning of these drugs may precipitate withdrawal symptoms with a potential incidence in excess of 30% [34].

The diagnosis of drug dependence and withdrawal in critically ill patients is challenging because many of the signs of acute withdrawal are:

- non-specific (tachycardia, hypertension, fever, tachypnoea, mydriasis, agitation, delirium and seizures) [35];
- difficult to elicit in ventilated patients (opioid craving, cramps, aches and dysaethesia) [35].

Gradual reduction in sedative and opioid infusion rates and/or supplementation with drugs such as methadone may help decrease the incidence of withdrawal phenomena.

The establishment of balanced sedation and analgesia, and its subsequent smooth withdrawal, may be further complicated as a result of patients' existing habituation to alcohol and nicotine at the point of their admission to intensive care.

In addition, increasing numbers of patients are regular users of pharmacological substances for recreational purposes and, indeed, may be admitted to intensive care as a consequence.

Consideration of alcohol, nicotine and narcotic analgesic replacement therapy for habituated patients whilst in intensive care has been recommended by some authorities [36] though the related ethical questions remain a subject of debate.

Pharmacological muscle paralysis

- The use of muscle relaxants is usually necessary for safe intubation. Suxamethonium (1–1.5 mg/kg) is the muscle relaxant of choice provided the serum potassium level is in the normal range.
- Whilst most ventilated patients do not need continued neuromuscular blockade to facilitate ventilation, in certain circumstances neuromuscular blockade is indicated.

The following are examples of such circumstances:

- Minimisation of peak inflation pressures in ventilated patients with severe acute asthma.
- Control of surges in intra-cranial pressure associated with coughing in patients with severe head injury.
- Possible improvement of effective mechanical ventilation in patients with critical oxygenation and poor lung compliance undergoing inverse ratio or prone ventilation or high frequency oscillation.
- Assurance of safe transport of the critically ill ventilated patient.
- Assurance of full ventilatory control during airway procedures such as tracheostomy and bronchoscopy.
- Control of muscles spasms in tetanus and rabies.

Therapeutic agents

- *Atracurium*: In general the properties of atracurium (0.5–1 mg/kg/h) make it an ideal muscle relaxant for use by infusion. Significant haemodynamic instability is rare and the production of active metabolites does not pose a problem. Dose requirements are reduced in hypothermic patients and increased in pyrexial and hyperdynamic septic patients.
- *Cis-atracurium*: Whilst cis-atracurium is a costly alternative it does not generate the histamine release often observed with the mixed isomer.
- *Vecuronium and rocuronium*: Medium duration muscle relaxants such as vecuronium and rocuronium may also be used for continuous infusion in ICU though their duration of action may be unpredictable and prolonged against a background of hepatic or renal dysfunction.

Problems with neuromuscular blockade

Neuromuscular blockade can lead to the following problems for ICU patients:

- Awareness which cannot be communicated to critical care staff.
- A variant of critical care myo-neuropathy especially if concurrent use of steroids.
- Prolonged weaning as a result of loss of muscle bulk secondary to pharmacological-induced disuse atrophy.
- Inability to clear secretions through prevention of effective coughing.

Patients on infusions of muscle relaxants should have their level of neuromuscular blockade regularly checked with a peripheral nerve stimulator to avoid over dosage. One or two "twitches" in response to a supra-maximum stimulus of four twitches at 2 Hz is satisfactory in practice.

FURTHER READING

Jacobi J, Fraser GL, Coursin DB, Riker RR et al. Clinical practice guidelines for the sustained use of sedatives and analgesics in the critically ill adult. *Crit Care Med* 2002; 30(1): 119–41.

Murray MJ, Cowen J, DeBlock H, Erstad B et al. Clinical practice guidelines for sustained neuromuscular blockade in the adult critically ill patient. *Crit Care Med* 2002; 30(1): 142–56.

Ostermann ME, Keenan SP, Seiferling RA, Sibbald WJ. Sedation in the intensive care unit: a systematic review. *J Am Med Assoc* 2000; 283(11): 1451–9.

REFERENCES

1. Murdoch S, Cohen A. Intensive care sedation: a review of current British practice. *Intens Care Med* 2000; 26: 922–8.
2. Aurell J, Elmquist D. Sleep in the surgical intensive care unit: continuous polygraphic recording of nine patients receiving postoperative care. *Br Med J* 1985; 290: 1029–32.
3. Stickgold R. Sleep: off-line memory reprocessing. *Trend Cogn Sci* 1998; 2: 484–92.
4. Schacter DL. The hypnagogic state: a critical review of the literature. *Psychol Bull* 1976; 83: 452–81.
5. Jones C, Griffiths RD, Humphris G, Skirrow PM. Memory, delusions, and the development of acute posttraumatic stress disorder-related symptoms after intensive care. *Crit Care Med* 2001; 29: 573–80.
6. Kress JP, Pohlman AS, Hall JB. Sedation and analgesia in the intensive care unit. *Am J Respir Crit Care Med* 2002; 106: 1024–8.
7. Jones C, Griffiths RD, Humphries G. Disturbed memory and amnesia related to intensive care. *Memory* 2000; 8: 79–94.
8. Shelly MP, Mendel L, Park GR. Failure of critically ill patients to metabolise midazolam. *Anaesthesia* 1987; 42: 619–26.
9. Roekarts PMHJ, Huygen FJPM, DeLange S. Infusion of propofol versus midazolam for sedation in the intensive care unit following coronary artery bypass surgery. *J Cardiothorac Vasc Anesth* 1993; 7: 142–7.
10. Barrientos-Vega R, Mar-Sanchez-Soria M, Morales-Gracia C, Robas-Gomaz A et al. Prolonged sedation of critically ill patients with midazolam or propofol: impact on weaning and cost. *Crit Care Med* 1997; 25: 33–40.
11. Riker RR, Fraser GL, Cox PM. Continuous infusion of haloperidol controls agitation in critically ill patients. *Crit Care Med* 1994; 22: 433–40.
12. Kulkarni SK, Parale MP, Kulkarni GK. Clonidine in alcohol withdrawal: a clinical report. *Methods Find Exp Clin Pharmacol* 1987; 9: 697–8.
13. Cushman PJ, Sowers JR: Alcohol withdrawal syndrome: clinical and hormonal responses to α-2 adrenergic treatment. *Alcoholism* 1989; 13: 361–4.
14. Venn RM, Grounds RM. Comparison between dexmedetomidine and propofol for sedation in the intensive care unit: patient and clinician perceptions. *Br J Anaesth* 2001; 87: 684–90.
15. Novaes MA, Knobel E, Bork AM, Pavao OF, Nogueira-Martins LA, Ferraz MB. Stressors in the ICU: perception of the patient, relatives and health care team. *Intens Care Med* 1999; 25: 1421–6.
16. Turner JS, Briggs SJ, Springhorn HE, Potgieter PD. Patient's recollection of intensive care unit experience. *Crit Care Med* 1990; 18: 966–8.
17. Osborne RJ, Joel SP, Slevin MI. Morphine intoxication in renal failure: the role of morphine-6-glucuronide. *Br Med J* 1986; 292: 1548–9.

18. Breen D, Wilmer A, Bodenham A, Bach V et al. Offset of pharmacodynamic effects and safety of remifentanil in intensive care unit patients with various degrees of renal failure. *Crit Care* 2004; 8: R21–30.

19. Brook AD, Ahrens TS, Schaiff R, Prentice D et al. Effect of a nursing implemented sedation protocol on the duration of mechanical ventilation. *Crit Care Med* 1999; 27: 2609–15.

20. Hansen-Flaschen J, Cowen J, Polomano RC. Beyond the Ramsay scale: need for a validated measure of sedating drug efficacy in the intensive care unit. *Crit Care Med* 1994; 22: 732–3.

21. De Jonghe B, Cook D, Appere- De- Veecchi C, Guyatt G et al. Using and understanding sedation scoring systems: a systematic review. *Intens Care Med* 2000; 26: 275–85.

22. Sedation Guidelines. UK ICS 1999.

23. Carrasco G. Instruments for monitoring intensive care unit sedation. *Crit Care* 2000; 4: 217–25.

24. Edmonds HL, Paloheimo M. Computerised monitoring of EMG and EEG during anaesthesia: an evaluation of the anaesthesia and brain function monitor. *Intens Clin Monit Comput* 1985; 1: 201–10.

25. Simmons LE, Riker RR, Prato BS, Fraser GL. Assessing sedation during intensive care unit mechanical ventilation with the bispectral index and the sedation–agitation scale. *Crit Care Med* 1999; 27: 1499–504.

26. Barr G, Anderson RE, Samuelsson S, Owall A et al. Fentanyl and midazolam anaesthesia for coronary bypass surgery: a clinical study of bispectral electro-encephalogram analysis, drug concentrations and recall. *Br J Anaesth* 2000; 84: 749–52.

27. Frenzel D, Greim CA, Sommer C, Bauerle K et al. Is the bispectral index appropriate for monitoring the sedative level of mechanically ventilated surgical ICU patients? *Intens Care Med* 2002; 28: 178–83.

28. Kress JP, Pohlman A, O'Connor MF, Hall JB. Daily interruption of sedative infusions in critically ill patients undergoing mechanical ventilation. *New Engl J Med* 2000; 342: 1471–7.

29. Kress JP, Gehlbach B, Lacy M, Pliskin N, Pohlman AS et al. The long-term psychological effects of daily sedative interruption on critically ill patients. *Am J Respir Crit Care Med* 2003; 168: 1457–61.

30. Inouye SK. The dilemma of delirium: clinical and research controversies regarding diagnosis and evaluation of delirium in hospitalized elderly medical patients. *Am J Med* 1994; 97: 278–88.

31. Ayd FJ. Intravenous haloperidol–lorazepam therapy for delirium. *Int Drug Ther Newslett* 1984; 19: 33–5.

32. Shafer A, White P, Schuttler J, Rosenthal MH. Use of fentanyl infusion in the intensive care unit: tolerance to its anesthetic effects? *Anesthesiology* 1983; 59: 245–8.

33. Busto U, Sellers E. Pharmacologic aspects of benzodiazepine tolerance and dependence. *J Subst Abuse Treat* 1991; 8: 29–33.

34. Cammarano WB, Pittet JF, Weitz S, Schlobohm RM et al. Acute withdrawal syndrome related to the administration of analgesic and sedative medications in adult intensive care unit patients. *Crit Care Med* 1998; 26: 676–84.
35. Kress JP, Pohlman AS, Hall JB. Sedation and analgesia in the intensive care unit. *Am J Respir Crit Care Med* 2002; 166: 1024–8.
36. Shelly MP. Personal communication 2004.

15

Continuous renal replacement therapy

R. Brits

Renal replacement therapy (RRT) forms a very important part of the combined management of multiorgan failure along with mechanical ventilation and cardiovascular support:

- Severe acute renal failure (ARF) is a common complication in patients with multiorgan failure (10–20% of all critically ill patients) and 70% of these patients will require RRT [1, 2].
- In previous studies mortality rates have been reported to be as high as 33–93% [1, 2].
- In contrast, single organ ARF has a much lower-mortality rate – less than 10%.

RRTs

RRTs can be classified as continuous or intermittent. Units differ nationally as well as internationally regarding their preference of therapy. In Europe and Australia continuous renal replacement therapy (CRRT) predominates while in the USA intermittent replacement therapy (IRT) is preferred.

Haemofiltration (CRRT)

There are several methods of CRRT:

- Continuous veno-venous haemofiltration (CVVH) uses a double lumen venous cannula and a peristaltic pump which allows higher blood flows and increased membrane surface area, thus higher ultrafiltration rates and better uraemic control. CVVH produces an ultrafiltrate by maintaining a pressure difference over a highly permeable membrane (convection). Water is pushed across the membrane and carries dissolved solutes (known as solvent drag). A physiological substitution fluid is infused into the patient to maintain hydration status and chemical balance.

CVVH is the most commonly used CRRT in intensive care unit (ICU). Less common or historical methods of CRRT are as follows:

- Continuous arterio-venous haemofiltration (CAVH) uses the arterio-venous pressure difference across a membrane to continuously produce an ultrafiltrate. Disadvantages include cannulation of both artery and vein which is associated with a much higher morbidity and also limited solute clearance.
- *Slow continuous ultrafiltration* (SCUF): Fluid removal by ultrafiltration.
- *Continuous veno-venous haemodialysis* (CVVHD): Fluid and toxins are removed through a process of diffusion with the use of a dialysate.
- *Continuous veno-venous haemodiafiltration* (CVVHDF): Widely used in Australia but less so in other countries. Fluid and toxins are removed through a combination of diffusion, convection and ultrafiltration.

Haemodialysis IRT

- Haemodialysis produces dialysate by counter circulation of the patient's blood and dialysis solution while being separated by a semi-permeable membrane. Solutes move down a concentration gradient across the membrane – the process is known as diffusion.
- Treatments are intermittently 3–4 times per week, each treatment lasting approximately 4 h. However, if IRT is to be used in ICU there is evidence that daily dialysis decreases mortality in medical ICU patients [3].
- IRT is mainly used in the management of end stage renal failure or single organ ARF. IRT is still the preferred method of RRT in the USA. However, even in the USA, CRRT is gaining increasing acceptance in many units.

Advantages of CRRT

- CRRT is slow and "gentle" on the cardiovascular system of these unstable patients. However, despite this, large volumes of fluid can still be removed if required. The continuous removal of fluid creates room for the administration of nutrition and other fluids.
- Adequate uraemic control is achieved even in very severely catabolic patients.

- CRRT may have other advantages like removal of cytokines and proinflammatory materials (the "middle molecules") from the circulation of the critically ill (see below). This is, because of the bigger pore size of the filter membrane.
- Techniques of CRRT are easy to learn.
- IRT is associated with hypotension, which is more severe in those patients with cardiovascular instability.

Advantages and comparisons are further explored below when discussing controversies.

Indications for starting RRT

Most common indications are:

- anuria or oliguria (urine volumes less than 200 ml/12 h),
- hyperkalaemia (serum potassium persistently more than 6.5 mmol/l),
- severe acidaemia (pH <7.1),
- azotaemia (urea >30 mmol/l or creatinine >300 mmol/l),
- pulmonary oedema.

Other indications may include:

- diuretic resistant cardiac failure,
- anasarca,
- uraemic complications (encepholopathy, pericarditis, neuropathy or myopathy),
- dysnatraemia (sodium >160 mmol/l or <115 mmol/l),
- temperature control (hyper or hypothermia),
- drug overdose (salicylates, methanol, barbiturates, lithium, amino glycosides, cephalosporins),
- sepsis.

Timing of CRRT

Most clinicians would prefer to prevent complications arising from the development of uraemia and institute CRRT early. In addition, recent studies examining the role of early versus late intervention of renal support are of interest. For example:

- Early initiation of CVVH in a small study of patients with septic shock has been shown to improve haemodynamic and metabolic responses and improve survival [4].

- Early haemofiltration is associated with better than predicted survival in ARF after cardiac surgery [5].
- Despite similarities in injury severity and risk of developing renal failure, survival was increased in the early filtration group in a retrospective review of 100 trauma patients [6].

Thus, many ICUs institute support at an early stage before biochemical decompensation occurs.

Efficacy of CRRT

Size of molecules cleared by CRRTs

Type of molecule	Size	Example	Mode of removal
Small	<500 Da	Urea, creatinine, amino acids	Convection, diffusion
Middle	500–5000 Da	Vit B12, inulin, vancomycin	Convection > diffusion
Low-molecular weight proteins	5000–50,000 Da	B2 microglobulin, cytokines	Convection or absorption
Large proteins	>50,000 Da	Albumin	Only minimal removal by CRRT

As regards creatinine and urea clearances; high-volume CVVH may approach clearances associated with intermittent haemodialysis (IHD). Creatinine clearances of 30 ml/min are not unrealistic [7]. Clearance increases with increasing ultrafiltrate volumes and decreases with decreased filter life.

Practicalities

Initial settings

- An adequate pump speed is required, for example, approximately 200 ml/h blood flow through the machine.
- A fluid exchange/ultrafiltrate rate of 35 ml/kg/24 h is recommended (see below).
- Fluid deficits can be set as required (automatically on many modern machines).

Filters (membranes)

As blood comes into contact with the filter (membrane) surface, complement and leucocytes can be activated, therefore triggering the inflammatory and coagulation cascade. The degree of activation is variable, depending on the degree of the biocompatibility of the membrane. Greater triggering occurs with bioincompatible membranes and it has been suggested that biocompatible membranes are associated with better outcomes.

Membranes used during RRT can be divided into two groups:

(1) *Cellulose based membranes*:
   • cuprophan, hemophan, cellulose acetate,
   • generally considered low-flux membranes and are very thin,
   • strongly hydrophilic,
   • bioincompatible.
(2) *Synthetic membranes*:
   • polysulfone, plyamide, polyacrylonitrile,
   • high flux-membranes,
   • hydrophobic,
   • biocompatible,
   • better than cellulose membranes in removing "middle molecules" which include proinflammatory mediators.

Four randomised controlled trials have been published comparing the use of biocompatible versus bioincompatible membranes in the critical ill patient [8–11]. Two trials found a significant difference in survival and recovery of renal function in favour of biocompatible membranes. A third study did not show any difference, but it must be pointed out that the trial was sponsored by a bioincompatible membrane manufacturer and one of the most potent inducers of complement was used as the biocompatible membrane. The fourth study did not show any difference either, but compared a semi-synthetic membrane with a synthetic membrane.

Replacement fluid

During RRT a sterile replacement fluid is infused to replace the ultrafiltrate removed with haemofiltration or haemodiafiltration. There are two ways of infusing the replacement fluid:

(1) *Pre-dilution*:
   • Fluid is infused before the filter.

- Lowers haematocrit of blood passing through the filter and, therefore, reducing anticoagulant requirements.
- There are 10% less solute clearance compared to the post dilution method.

(2) *Post-dilution*:
- Fluid is infused into blood leaving the filter.

The concentration of sodium, potassium and glucose can be varied according to the patient's requirements, but the fluid does not contain phosphate and this may need to be supplemented.

Buffers

The main buffers in replacement fluid are lactate or bicarbonate. A study by Barenbrock et al [12] found bicarbonate buffer solutions to be superior in normalising acidosis and reduced the incidence of cardiovascular instability in patients with renal failure.

Acetate buffered solutions are also available, but studies have shown both lactate and bicarbonate buffer solutions to be superior.

Note: Lactate-free haemofiltration replacement fluid contains no buffer, so bicarbonate must be infused separately at an appropriate rate to supply this.

Vascular access

Extracorporeal treatments require vascular access and there are mainly two approaches:

(1) *Veno-venous mode*:
- Most commonly used method in critical ill patients.
- Requires cannulation of a large central vein with a double lumen catheter.
- A peristaltic pump, pumps blood through the filter, drawing blood through an "arterial" or outflow limb and returns via a "venous" or inflow limb.
- Blood flow is usually between 150 and 200 ml/min.

(2) *Arterio-venous mode*:
- Rarely used.
- Requires cannulation of artery and vein, hence higher-complication rates.
- The arterio-venous pressure gradient drives blood through the circuit.
- Blood flow is usually 50–150 ml/min.

Anticoagulation

All forms of RRT expose blood to contact with a non-biologic surface and therefore, activation of the clotting cascade. Despite coagulation abnormalities often seen in critical care patients, they still require anticoagulation to prevent filter and circuit clot formation during CRRT. No correlation has been found between routine coagulation variables and duration of filter survival.

Anticoagulation options include:

- anticoagulant free,
- continuous pre-filter unfractionated heparin infusion,
- low-molecular weight heparin,
- sodium citrate,
- regional heparisation,
- prostacyclin,
- recombinant hirudin.

Anticoagulant free

- Critical ill patients often have deranged clotting, thrombocytopenia or a combination of both. Anticoagulation-free CRRT is made easier with good venous access, good blood flow rates and pre-dilution.
- Tan et al have reported the safe use of CRRT with pre-dilution and no pharmacological anticoagulation in patients with coagulation abnormalities [13].

Continuous pre-filter unfractionated heparin infusion

- Infusion of doses (5–10 IU/kg/h) that does not alter activated partial thromboplastin time.
- It may have some unpredictable and undesirable effects on systemic clotting mechanisms.
- Infusion doses are adjusted, aiming for an activated clotting time (ACT) of 180–200 s.

Low-molecular weight heparin

- Reeves et al showed identical filter life, comparable safety but increased cost when they compared fixed dose low-molecular weight heparin (dalteparin) with unfractionated heparin [14].

Regional anticoagulation

- Heparin or sodium citrate.
  Heparin is infused pre-filter while protamine is infused post-filter as the neutraliser.
- Sodium citrate may be used as an alternative to heparin in order to avoid heparin induced thrombocytopenia.
- A technique that involves the pre-filter infusion of sodium citrate and post-filter infusion of calcium as a neutraliser.
- Although earlier techniques were associated with metabolic complications, two recent studies with simplified protocols have shown the safe use of citrate anticoagulation [14, 15].

Prostacyclin

- Prostacyclin inhibits the interaction between platelets and artificial membranes and, therefore, prevents extra corporeal thrombus formation. Heparin is relative ineffective towards platelets.
- It inhibits fibrin, leucocyte and platelet base micro-aggregates which might prevent renal, pulmonary and neurological dysfunction.
- A study by Kozek-Langenecker et al showed that prostaglandin's were most effective in prolonging filter life, when co-administered with heparin. Bleeding complications were also less in the group receiving both prostacyclin and heparin, than in the group receiving heparin alone [16].

Drug removal

Many of the drugs we administer to patients may be removed during CRRT including drugs which normally accumulate in renal failure. Some drugs may suffer increased removal. Thus, dosages may have to be increased or decreased or dosage intervals changed to achieve an adequate therapeutic effect.

A detailed description of the proportional removal of different drugs is beyond the cope of this text. Readers are advised to check the large reference texts available, consult the drug data sheet or take advice from their hospital pharmacy.

The controversy – CRRT or IRT?

No conclusive evidence exists to determine the best form of RRT for critically ill patients. There is, therefore, controversy over which type of RRT should be used in ICU, with practitioners in Europe and Australia increasingly adopting CRRT, while the American nephrologists choose to remain with IRT:

- After adjusting for poor quality and severity of illness, a meta-analysis of 13 studies by Kellum et al showed that mortality was lower in patients treated with CRRT [17]. The fact that trials have excluded patients with cardiovascular instability from intermittent renal replacement therapy (IRRT) probably supports the use of CRRT in critically ill patients [18].
- The French HEMODIAFE study is as yet unpublished but early presentations at scientific meetings suggest mortality of approximately 70% in patients in ICU given either CVVHDF or IHD. It is of interest that the IHD groups showed improved survival through the length of the study, that is intermittent dialysis got "better" in critically ill patients with more training, longer duration of treatment and increase in the dialysis "dose". Definitive studies comparing CVVH and IHD remain to be performed.

In addition to potential benefits in terms of survival, there may be other benefits associated with the use of CRRT compared to IRT:

- The rapid fluid shifts and haemodynamic upset associated with dialysis are associated with further ischaemic insults to the kidney in animals.
- Creatinine clearance falls after dialysis! (but does not after CVVH) – presumably because of these shifts [19].
- Computed tomographic (CT) studies of the brain demonstrate changes after dialysis consistent with increased brain water which are not present after CVVH [20].
- A randomised clinical trial (RCT) has shown that intrinsic renal function among survivors of ARF recovers to a predetermined level in over 90% of patients treated with CVVH but in only 59% of patients treated with dialysis (i.e. more patients will require chronic renal support when ARF is managed with intermittent dialysis) [21].

High-volume haemofiltration?

- The volume of ultrafiltrate may be important. Large volumes of ultrafiltrate (high volume or "aggressive" CVVH) increase creatinine clearance and may remove greater quantities of inflammatory mediators. The only large RCT of over 400 patients demonstrated improved survival with high volumes of ultrafiltrate compared to lower volumes [22]. The authors recommend ultrafiltrate volumes of at least 35 ml/kg/h.

- In addition a study of over 300 patients from Holland managed with high volume CVVH had a mortality of 33% compared with a predicted mortality of 67% given by the Madrid ARF score [23]. A subsequent smaller, randomised study from the same group has, however, failed to confirm these findings.

Fluid and electrolyte control

Another controversial area where CRRT may prove to be beneficial is the control of fluid and electrolyte balance:

- Patients with acute respiratory distress syndrome (ARDS) have increased extra vascular lung water and in an attempt to improve oxygenation a negative fluid balance can be introduced. Loop diuretics usually results in the loss of water but not in a salt diuresis, therefore hypernatremia develops and extra vascular lung water remains high. In such circumstances CRRT will normalise sodium levels and remove extra vascular water. This often leads to a substantial improvement in gas exchanges and lung compliance.
- Some patients in cardiogenic shock post-cardiac surgery might require extra corporeal membrane oxygenation and will usually also require large amounts of clotting factors. CRRT can be used to maintain an even fluid balance by removing fluid while clotting factors are transfused. The development of ARDS and pulmonary oedema can be prevented, while factors are infused.
- One study comparing CVVHDF with IRT showed that normalisation of sodium, potassium and bicarbonate levels was more frequently achieved with CRRT [24].
- It has been suggested that transfusion requirements may be associated with filter life – frequent clotted filters resulting in greater requirement for blood transfusion.

Septic shock, multiorgan failure, ARF and RRT

- Many patients with ARF have severe sepsis, multiorgan failure and a major systemic inflammatory response. The activation and amplification depends on the release of proinflammatory mediators into the circulation. Targeting the systemic effects of these mediators seems to be a logical goal in the treatment of patients with severe sepsis. Specific single mediators has been targeted, but with disappointing results. Therapies targeting the removal of several circulating inflammatory mediators may prove to be more effective. CRRT is one of these therapies.

- Standard CRRT (exchange rate 1–2 l/h) has shown clinical improvement with severe septic shock, independent of fluid balance, but has failed to reduce inflammatory mediator plasma concentrations. Recent animal and human studies have suggested that if haemofiltration is to have an additional role in the management of severe sepsis, the plasma exchange rate has to be increased [25–27].
- Blood purification using high-volume haemofiltration (6 l/min) or coupled plasma filtration with adsorption has been shown to decrease the need for vasopressor therapy in septic shock.
- In experimental studies results were more striking when the therapy used was high volume and convective. Cole et al found high volume haemofiltration to be associated with significant decrease in vasopressor requirements [25]. The decrease was greater than during standard CVVH. Secondly they also showed a significant decrease in plasma levels of C3a, C5a and IL-10. Changes were more striking during the early part of therapy, thus suggesting that the early decline in plasma concentration is due to membrane adsorption as the major removal modality. High volume haemofiltration (HVHF) increase adsorption because of an increase in transmembrane pressure and larger filtering membrane area. Convective clearance will mainly take place after membrane saturation has taken place through adsorption.
- Other possible explanations for improved haemodynamic parameters are the possibility that other unmeasured vasodilatory solutes are removed during CVVH causing vasoconstriction and decreased vasopressor requirements. Hypothermia induced by CVVH might also reduce requirements. It is also possible that sedative removal is greater during HVHF, therefore also reducing vasopressor requirements. Cole et al found during their study that more than half of the patients required more sedation [25].
- Protective molecules, such as vitamins and aminoacids, might also be removed during HVHF having a negative effect on an already critically ill patient. No studies have yet been done to look at this effect.

FURTHER READING

Acute Dialysis Quality Initiative. http://www.ADQI.net

Bellomo R, Baldwin I, Ronco C, Golper T. *Atlas of Haemofiltration*. Saunders, Philadelphia, 2002.

Molitoris BA (Ed.). *Critical Care Nephrology*. Remedica, London, 2004.

REFERENCES

1. Brivet FG, Kleinecht DJ, Loirat P, Landais PJM. French Study Group on Acute Renal Failure. Acute renal failure in intensive care units – causes, outcome, and prognosis factors of hospital mortality: a prospective, multicentre study. *Crit Care Med* 1996; 24: 192–8.

2. Guerin C, Girard R, Selli JM, Pedrix JP et al. Initial versus delayed acute renal failure in the intensive care unit. A multicentre prospective epidemiological study. *Am J Resp Crit Care Med* 2000; 161: 872–9.

3. Schiffl H, Lang SM, Fisher R. Daily hemodialysis and the outcome of acute renal failure. *New Engl J Med*; 346: 305–10.

4. Honore PM, Jamez J, Wauthier M et al. Prospective evaluation of short-term, high-volume isovolemic hemofiltration on the hemodynamic course and outcome in patients with intractable circulatory failure resulting from septic shock. *Crit Care Med* 2000; 28: 3581–7.

5. Bent P, Tan HK, Bellomo R et al. Early and intensive continuous hemofiltration for severe renal failure after cardiac surgery. *Ann Thorac Surg* 2001; 71: 832–7.

6. Gettings LG, Reynolds HN, Scalea T. Outcome in post-traumatic acute renal failure when continuous renal replacement therapy is applied early vs. late. *Int Care Med* 1999; 25: 805–13.

7. Brocklehurst IC, Thomas AN, Kishen R, Guy JM. Creatinine and urea clearance during continuous veno-venous haemofiltration in critically ill patients. *Anaesthesia* 1996; 51: 551–3.

8. Schiffl H, Lang SM, Konig A, Strasser T et al. Biocompatible membranes in acute renal failure: prospective case-controlled studies. *Lancet* 1994; 344: 570–2.

9. Hakim RM, Wingard RL, Parker RA. Effect of dialysis membrane in treatment of patients with acute renal failure. *New Engl J Med* 1994; 331: 1338–42.

10. Himmelfarb J, Tolkoff, Rubin N, Chandran P et al. A multicentre comparison of dialysis membranes in the treatment of acute renal failure requiring dialysis. *J Am Soc Nephrol* 1998; 9: 257–66.

11. Jorres A, Gahl GM, Dobis C, Polenakovic MH et al. Haemodialysis-membrane biocompatibility and mortality of patients with dialysis-dependent acute renal failure: a prospective randomised multicentre trial. *Lancet* 1999; 354: 1337–41.

12. Barenbrock M, Hausberg M, Matzkies F, De La Motte S et al. Effects of bicarbonate- and lactate-buffered replacement fluids on cardiovascular outcome in CVVH patients. *Kidney Int* 2000; 58: 1751–7.

13. Tan HK, Baldwin I, Bellomo R. Continuous veno-venous hemofiltration without anti-coagulation in high risk patients. *Int Care Med* 2000; 26: 1652–7.

14. Reeve JH, Cumming AR, Galagher L, O'Brien JL et al. A controlled trial of low-molecular-weight heparin (dalteparin) versus unfractionated heparin as anticoagulant during continuous venovenous hemodialysis with filtration. *Crit Care Med* 1999; 27: 2224–8.

15. Tolwani AJ, Cambell RC, Schenk MB, Allon M et al. Simplified citrate anticoagulation for continuous renal replacement therapy. *Kidney Int* 2001; 60: 370–4.

16. Kozek-Langenecker SA, Kettner SC, Oismueller C, Gonano C et al. Anticoagulation with prostaglandin E1 and unfractioned heparin during continuous venovenous hemofiltration. *Crit Care Med* 1998; 26: 1208–12.

17. Kellum JA, Angus DC, Johnson JP, Leblanc M et al. Continuous versus intermittent renal replacement therapy: a meta-analysis. *Int Care Med* 2002; 28: 29–37.

18. Kenningham J. Controversies in haemofiltration. *CPD Anaesthesia* 2002; 4: 115 –20.

19. Manns M, Sigler MH, Teehan BP. Intradialytic renal hemodynamics: potential consequences for the management of the patient with acute renal failure. *Nephrol Dial Transp* 1997; 12: 870–2.

20. Ronco C, Bellomo R, Brendolan A et al. Brain density changes during renal replacement in critically ill patients with acute renal failure. Continuous hemofiltration versus intermittent hemodialysis. *J Nephrol* 1999; 12: 173–8.

21. Mehta R, McDonald B, Gabbai F et al. Acute renal failure in the ICU: results from a randomised multicentre trial. *Am J Soc Nephrol* 1996; 5: 7.

22. Ronco C, Bellomo R, Homel P et al. Effects of different doses in continuous venovenous haemofiltration on outcomes of acute renal failure: a prospective randomised trial. *Lancet* 2000; 356: 26–30.

23. Oudemans-van Straaten HM, Bosman RJ, van der Spoel JL et al. Outcome of critically ill patients treated with intermittent high volume hemofiltration: a prospective cohort analysis. *Int Care Med* 1999; 25: 814–21.

24. Uchino S, Bellomo R, Ronco C. Intermittent versus continuous renal replacement therapy in ICU: impact on electrolyte and acid–base balance. *Int Care Med* 2001; 27: 1037–43.

25. Cole L, Bellomo R, Journois D, Davenport P et al. High-volume haemofiltration in human septic shock. *Int Care Med* 2001; 27: 978–86.

26. Van Deuren M, Van der Meer JWM. Hemofiltration in septic patients is not able to alter the plasma concentration of cytokines therapeutically. *Int Care Med* 2000; 26: 1176–8.

27. Bellomo R, Tipping P, Boyce N. Continuous veno-venous hemofiltration with dialysis removes cytokines from the circulation of septic patients. *Crit Care Med* 1993; 21: 522–6.

16

Withholding and withdrawing therapy in the ICU

I. McConachie

"To cure sometimes, to relieve often, to comfort always"

15th Century French quote

Many patients die in intensive care unit (ICU) either as a result of failed therapy or, increasingly, as a result of withheld or withdrawn therapy. It wasn't always so; in the early days patients were only seen as appropriate for ICU admission if they were clearly recoverable. Now ICU is sometimes seen as a place where patients go to die.

Indeed, it is estimated that:

- 20% of all Americans over the age of 65 die in or having recently been in ICU (half of all the deaths in hospital),
- 10–12% of *all* health care expenditure in America is spent in the last 6 months of patients' lives.

Almost certainly these percentages will be less in Europe and the UK (so far) but, even in the UK, dying is almost an everyday occurrence in ICU.

Thus it is increasingly important to address:

- end-of-life (EOL) care in the ICU,
- withholding and withdrawing of therapy,
- optimal care of the dying patient.

This chapter will discuss these three aspects of ICU therapy, although unlike other chapters, there may be as many questions raised as answered. Much is, and will probably remain, controversial.

EOL care in the ICU

Who makes decisions?

Ideally the patients would make these decisions in conjunction with their families and after discussions with their nursing and medical carers. Autonomy and other ethical matters will be discussed below. Decisions should be made *early* (before ICU admission) so that decisions do not need to be made during a time of crisis, or grief and so as to avoid families feeling under any form of duress.

ICU is just a place in the hospital in this context. There is sometimes a reluctance to engage in discussion of EOL issues on general wards but this is often the best place for such discussions.

In most instances the discussions are initiated by the team of carers with a small proportion of discussions initiated by the family or patient. Often there is little consultation – decisions are exclusively made by the carers with the results just communicated to the patient or family. Often discussions may be implicit, that is, prognosis or futility alone are talked about with the family with the result of withdrawing therapy glossed over. Direct, explicit agreements are to be preferred where it is made clear that withholding or withdrawal will lead to death.

Nurses should have a major role in influencing the decisions made by both physicians and families due to the unique and central nature of their relationship with all involved parties.

Sjokvist [1] asked lay people, nurses and doctors in Sweden who should make these decisions on EOL care. He outlined two scenarios for discussion – a mentally competent patient in ICU and an incompetent, comatose patient in ICU.

- For the competent patient: 48% of the public, 31% of nurses, and 8% of physicians thought that decisions about continuing ventilator treatment should be made by the patient and family; 87% of doctors would wish to make the decision themselves with the aid of the family and patient.
- For the incompetent patient: 73% of the public, and 70% of the nurses thought that a joint decision should be made by the doctors and the family; 61% of the physicians would wish to decide this on their own – a view supported by only 5% of the public and only 20% of the nurses.

Thus, in Sweden, the public favour more patient and family involvement than the doctors would wish.

In practice, there are geographical and cultural differences re-decision-making for EOL care.

- Family should decide – US Guidelines.
- Physician should decide – European Guidelines.

There are arguments in favour of both approaches, and indeed, some combination of the two would seem ideal. The American legal system places more emphasis on transfer of responsibility to the family – a substituted decision maker. In Europe, the families have less legal status and, in general, are not legally able to make consent type decisions on behalf of the patient. European arguments for physician based decision-making include the undoubted emotion and distress caused to families by being involved in these decisions (and in rare cases, genuine concern re personal or financial motivation).

When making these decisions one must never forget that one must take note of the views expressed by a *competent* adult. In the ICU, it is often too late – few of our patients can be considered competent and even fewer have some form of advance directive. Advance decisions or directives are increasingly accepted in the UK. Surrogates have recently been defined by law in Scotland.

Which patients?

Which ICU patients should be considered for discussions re-EOL care issues? Should we include:

- 77-year-old postoperative laparotomy admitted for overnight ventilation?
- 22-year-old hypotensive trauma patient?
- 55-year-old patient admitted with metastatic disease?
- Patients with predicted length of stay of more than 5 days?
- Predicted mortality of more than 25%?
- Certain groups, for example multiple organ failure?
- Certain chronic premorbid conditions, for example congestive cardiac failure (CCF) or chronic obstructive pulmonary disease (COPD)?

Individual ICUs may wish to develop their own policies.

Training in EOL care and communication

EOL care should be part of the core competencies of ICU doctors but formal training and assessment of this rarely occurs. Doctors in training, when asked often express dissatisfaction with their skills and training in this area. In one survey [2]:

- 96% of ICU residents thought EOL care was important,
- 42% felt their training in this area had been "fair to poor"(compared to only 7% giving a similar poor rating for their training on sepsis),
- Alarmingly 88% thought they had been asked to prolong the dying process inappropriately.

Communication and communication skills are the key. There is evidence of widespread dissatisfaction with communication in the ICU [3]. However, studies show that doctors can be taught:

- improved communication skills,
- to reduce emotional distress during discussions.

Language is important and it must be clear and unambiguous.

"Easy" words calculated not to upset the relatives often serve only to confuse and underplay the realities of the situation. Certain words, phrases and technical expressions, in particular, which are clear to us may not be clear to lay people. For example:

"Wrong" words?	"Better" words?
Arrest	Heart stopped
Stable	Drugs are still required to…
Ventilator	Breathing machine
Filter	Kidney machine
Asleep	Sedated
Paralysed	Drugs to relax the muscles
Critical	Might die
Passed on	Died
Gone to a better place	Died

Certain metaphors and cliches are also best avoided, for example:

Had a good innings (successful at cricket?)
At peace (previously at war?)
Expired (past sell by date?)

Doctors sometimes avoid difficult decisions and difficult discussions with patients and/or their relatives. Although perhaps understandable, this must be resisted. Families will have these EOL discussions once, twice or at most three times in their life whereas they are a regular part of life for ICU doctors! However, one implication of this is that the family *will* remember what you say to them and how you say it. Therefore, doctors have a duty and professional responsibility to prepare for these discussions and be prepared to have unpleasant discussions and potential disagreements with families.

Mixed messages and differing opinions within the team are unhelpful and cause considerable distress and confusion amongst the family. Any differences between members of the team should be sorted out in private so a "team message" can be presented to the family.

All communications should be witnessed, preferably by the nurse involved, and recorded in the form of a written summary including all the key points raised and the family's reaction.

Withholding and withdrawing therapy in ICU

Historical background

The evolution of the history of withholding and withdrawing ICU therapy is well documented in the USA. In the early ICUs in the 1960s therapy could not, in general, be withdrawn. (Prior to that ICUs did not exist as we know them so the ethical and legal dilemmas associated with life-support technology did not occur.)

The following is a summary of some of the landmark events and cases which illustrate the changes since the 1960s.

1968	Harvard	The original description of brainstem death was published partly because it was not believed that Intermittent positive pressure ventilation (IPPV) could be stopped unless the patient had already been declared dead.
1975	Quinlan	A case of persistent vegetative state. After 9 months coma, family petitioned the courts for the right to take patient off the ventilator (against the will of the attending doctors). Court ruled that family can speak for patient as surrogate decision-maker.
1983	Herbert	Patient was removed from the ventilator and feeding was stopped. After death, the District Attorney charged two Doctors with Homicide!
		They were acquitted but, understandably, this caused much disquiet amongst ICU doctors and led to a marked reluctance to withdraw ICU therapy.

| 1990 | Cruzan | Another patient with persistent vegetative state. The Supreme Court allowed the physicians as, surrogate decision makers, to make the decision and remove the patient from the ventilator. |
| 1990 | Wanglie | In this case the husband insisted on full treatment against the judgement of the doctors. The hospital went to court to ask for permission to remove the husband as decision-maker so as to enable them to withdraw therapy. |

In essence, the position had come full circle from a time when therapy could not be withdrawn (prior to Harvard) even though the family wished to do so (Quinlan) to a position where the hospital were prepared to withdraw care against the wishes of the family (Wanglie). In other words doctors in America have changed their attitudes and now are prepared to fight for the right to let patients die (Wanglie) even against family wishes whereas previously they were prepared to fight to keep the patient alive against family wishes (Quinlan).

There have been several recent landmark cases in the UK:

- A doctor was found guilty of attempted murder in 1992 after administering KCl to a terminally ill patient in severe pain in an attempt to relieve her suffering. (The charge was attempted murder rather than murder because it could not be proved conclusively that the injection killed her.) Thus, euthanasia or doctor assisted suicide is illegal in the UK.
- In 1993, the courts permitted the removal of nutritional support in the case of Anthony Bland who had been in a persistent vegetative state for over 3 years.
- In 1999, a general practitioner (GP) was acquitted of murder after admitting giving a large, lethal dose of diamorphine to a terminally ill patient with cancer. He claimed that it was his intent to relieve pain rather than to kill. This case ruling provides some legal backing and protection to the so-called "double effect" principle, that is, it is permissible to give potent analgesics to relieve suffering even though it is recognised that it could hasten the death of the patient. It is still illegal for the primary intent of the doctor to be to kill.
- In 2002, Diane Pretty died a natural death after she lost, in both the UK and European courts, her fight to allow her husband to assist her to commit suicide.
- Also in 2002, Miss B, who was quadriplegic, asked to be removed from her ventilator. The court granted her petitioned to be moved to another hospital where the doctors would permit her request (her doctors at the original hospital had refused). She subsequently was removed from the ventilator and died. This case

arguably is based more on the principle of the right of a competent adult to refuse treatment rather than a "right to die".

Definitions

Withholding is not offering or providing therapy. Not admitting a patient to ICU for organ support is the easiest example but not increasing vasopressors or not providing CPR are examples of withholding therapy while in the ICU.

Withdrawing is stopping or removing therapy with an intent to substitute other (palliative) therapies. Examples on ICU include:

- stopping vasoactive drugs,
- stopping ventilatory support,
- reducing inspired oxygen concentrations,
- removing the haemofilter,
- extubating the patient.

Both withholding and withdrawing are likely to lead to the patient's death from their disease and, as such, are ethically equivalent (no ethical difference between positive and negative acts).

Withdrawal may be seen as easier (for the doctor!) in some circumstances:

- *Easier*: Multiple organ failure on ventilator.
- *More difficult*: Poor neurological state, low oxygen requirements but ventilator dependent.
- *Most difficult*: Awake, ventilator dependent patient. This type of patient may be mentally competent to be involved in the decision.

Euthanasia (from the Greek words for "good death") is the administration of therapy, at the specific request of the patient with the *sole* aim of causing death (see below re-palliative care, the "double effect" principle and the ethics of intent). As such neither withholding nor withdrawal can be considered to be the same as euthanasia.

Withdrawal, for example of IPPV, at the request of the patient could be considered equivalent to passive euthanasia but, as we have seen, the competent patient has the right to refuse any or all treatments.

Palliative care is the care of terminally ill patients where the focus is on holistic support of the patient and relief of symptoms rather than seeking to cure the patient. Management is *active*, intends neither to hasten nor to postpone death and is not guided by hopelessness or fatalism. Good palliative care should reduce any requirement or need for euthanasia.

Differences between killing and letting die

Crippen [4] makes the point that if extraordinary support is withdrawn, and the patient dies, it is the disease that has killed them *not* the withdrawal of support, as these supports (e.g. IPPV, inotropes, etc.) are not required for life under normal circumstances.

Thus, withdrawal of IPPV does not cause death. IPPV, up to the point of withdrawal, has merely temporarily prevented the occurrence of death.

If one cannot accept this [5]:

- One would have to accept that withdrawal of *any* therapy may lead to death rather than the disease process.
- One would conclude that doctors *cause* the vast majority of deaths in terminally ill patients.
- All cases where cardiopulmonary resuscitation (CPR) is stopped would be doctors causing death as the CPR is supporting the circulation and maintaining life and could have been continued for longer!
- The law would have to examine thousands of medical cases as potentially manslaughter or murder. If withdrawing therapy is considered to cause death then the legal situation would only be manageable if the law was changed to permit causing death!
- Interestingly, in a trauma case, withdrawal of therapy has led to a plea that the assault did not cause the death. Fortunately, this has been rejected by the courts.

Reasons to withhold or withdraw therapy [5]

(1) Ineffective or futile treatment. Doctors do not have a duty to provide futile treatment and patients and families cannot expect such treatment. Futility is discussed further below. However, it is not acceptable to provide no treatment when some would be beneficial, for example analgesia or sedation.

(2) Treatment would impose excessive burdens in the opinion of the patient (assuming the patient is not motivated by suicidal intent). Excessive burdens may include:
    - pain (there are limits to everyone's courage),
    - emotional and psychological burdens,

- restrictions on liberty (e.g. balance between an extra year of life gained versus that year being spent in hospital),
- financial burdens (hopefully not in UK),
- in the ICU, burdens of tubes, ventilators, monitoring, etc.

(3) Treatments not considered to further the patient's medical good, for example nasogastric feeding in advanced cancer which may prolong survival only for the patients to die of other complications of the cancer.

(4) Treatments not considered to further the patient's total good, for example antibiotics to treat pneumonia in comatose patients who have had a massive stroke.

The first two reasons are most common especially in ICU and related areas. The latter two are most difficult and arouse considerable emotion amongst carers.

Factors in the decisions for withholding or withdrawing therapy

Firstly, the wishes of the competent or autonomous patient should be taken into account followed by an acknowledgment of the wishes of the family. Other members of the multidisciplinary team have a right to be included in the discussions and decision-making.

"Quality of life" is very subjective and what is an unacceptable quality to the carers may be acceptable to the patient and vice versa. Actual studies of quality of life following ICU admission show variable results:

- Konopad [6] found ICU survivors to have a decreased level of activity 1 year after ICU discharge.
- Niskanen [7] found that quality of life of ICU survivors was good but that recovery of physical function was slower than mental and social recovery.
- Danis [8] found that 70% of patients and families would want ICU care again if it granted them one extra year of life. There was no relationship between this and quality of life. However, 88% of patients and 41% of families would refuse ICU if no chance of recovery.

Factors in the decision to withhold or withdraw therapy throughout the world that have been identified in studies include:

- previous quality of life (but many pitfalls);
- previous health;
- futility of proposed therapy;
- age; again, many pitfalls but many studies show no survivors from prolonged IPPV in patients over the age of 85 [9];

- cost (unacceptable to many on an individual basis but condoned by society e.g. unavailability of chronic dialysis facilities).

The decision should be direct and explicit including discussions on withholding and withdrawal. If doubt arises (as is often the case) one solution is to admit the patient according to the following classification:

- Patient reasonable chance of recovery – admit – full treatment.
- Patient no chance of recovery – do not admit – withholding.
- Patient low probability – admit – full treatment 24/48 h – reevaluate with the possibility of withdrawing.

Although sometimes seen as problematic there no ethical differences or difficulties with admitting for a trial of ICU therapy which is withdrawn if it is ineffective. This is sometimes called the ICU test – "we will admit for IPPV for a few days to give the antibiotics time to work". This approach is valid if actively managed. If the few days are up, and there is clearly no improvement, then "we will see tomorrow" is inappropriate.

Incidence of withholding or withdrawing therapy

In the USA, where most studies have been done, the proportion and number of patients having withdrawal (withholding commoner in Europe) of therapy is rising with time as is the "do not resuscitate (DNR)" rate. There are major variations:

- Some hospitals issue no DNR orders in dying ICU patients and no withdrawal of therapy.
- In some hospitals, up to 90% of dying patients in ICU involve withdrawal of therapy [10].
- The rate of withdrawal of therapy in one study in the USA was highest when the patients were cared for by ICU specialists compared to when the decisions were made by their private physicians [11].

There is an expectation that patients in whom ICU therapy is withheld or withdrawn will die:

- withholding – associated with an 89% mortality,
- withdrawing – associated with a 99% mortality.

Both statistics are from Ethicus (the European study on ethics in ICU) as yet unpublished.

It is interesting to speculate on these results:

- Would admitting the refused patients produce more survivors without imposing an excessive burden on the majority?
- Would the 11% who were not admitted have still survived if exposed to the hazards, side effects and complications associated with ICU care?

Futility

Futility is increasingly debated and the concept "used" frequently in the USA.

A good definition is that a treatment is futile if it has no reasonable chance of producing benefit capable of being perceived by the patient not just some measurable improvement in some parameter or merely prolonging a period of support.

A treatment may be futile but care is never futile (so do not use the term "futile care"). Palliation is never futile (but may not include admission to ICU).

The definition of what therapy is futile in a certain circumstance is a matter of clinical judgement on an individual basis (as long as the decision is consistent with general medical opinion in that field).

There are grey areas and disagreement but to take one example: studies have shown no survivors amongst 400 patients who develop multiple organ failure after receiving a bone marrow transplant and require IPPV [12]. Is it not futile to offer IPPV to such patients on the grounds of reasonable certainty? If not, how many patients must be cruelly exposed to the burdens of this treatment in the hope of achieving one survivor? Is this moral?

The issue is whether the treatment can deliver its intended benefits not whether the patient is "worth" treating (otherwise we could stop all care and end what has been judged as a worthless life).

Sometimes treatment is suggested because it gives the patient or family hope – this provides false hope, is without counterbalancing benefit and, therefore, causes harm. Our duty is to do no harm.

Outcome prediction and futility

There are many scoring systems to assess severity of the patient's critical illness. Although these systems may enable a calculation to be done which predicts the probability of death during that admission (based on the databases from which the scoring system has been devised) these are not designed to be used to determine the outcome of an individual patient. Their main use is in prediction in populations and for audit. They may predict probability of death but care is necessary with this concept as the general public, and many doctors do not really understand probability.

In terms of predicting an individual patient's outcome, studies suggest that an experienced clinician is probably as accurate as the scoring systems [13]. Our judgement is able to take into account local experiences as well as large statistical databases. Referring physicians are less accurate at predicting patient survival [14].

Outcome prediction models:

- Are most accurate in very low risk and very high risk situations.
- Cannot predict side effects of treatments.
- Are probably more accurate as time passes (trends) in the ICU, that is, take into account the response to treatment.
- Do not fully allow for the detrimental effect on prognosis of delays in diagnosis and treatment or the problem of no clear underlying diagnosis (except for the effect these delays may have on physiological parameter scoring).
- Do not fully allow for the detrimental effect on prognosis of extreme age as few patients of extreme age in the databases!

The more recent development of early warning scores do not help guide our decisions re-prognosis, outcome and futility as they tell us who is sick enough to go to ICU but they do not tell us who is *too* sick to go to ICU.

Thus, severity scoring and formal models for outcome prediction only provide some general guidance in decisions regarding futility and withholding and withdrawing therapy.

What do ethical principles tell us about decision-making?

The four main principles of medical ethics are:

- *Beneficence*: The desire and aim to do good.
- *Non-maleficence*: The desire and aim not to do harm.
- *Autonomy*: Self awareness and the right to self determination. Linked to mental competence.
- *Justice*: Equal access for all.

Most ICU patients have lost their autonomy. Autonomy should always be respected but should not be the overriding principle. The goal of health care must be the promotion of health not the promotion of autonomy. If not, what would be the goals of treatment for non-autonomous patients?

Relatives may reflect patient wishes:

- Uhlmann [15] found that in given scenarios, families are better than doctors at predicting patient preferences.
- However, Emanuel [16] found that family were unreliable at following the patient's wishes.

Thus, doing what relatives want may not always be to the patients' overall good. Doctors, nurses and other carers should always act as the patient's advocate rather than doing what the relatives want. This may take some courage as doing what the family want may well be the easiest option!

The above is true also for autonomous patients. We should respect their wishes but should also do no harm. Indeed, it is our professional duty to act in the patient's best interests and to do no harm.

Problems with autonomy as overriding principle:

- Does a patient have the right to ask for bizarre, harmful treatment, for example beta blockers for asthma?
- If autonomy is the overriding principle, as some would suggest, then doing what the patient wants would be seen as "good" and anything else would be "bad". What would be the goals of treatment for non-autonomous patients?
- Harm and benefit would then be seen as totally subjective and doctors and nurses would be avoiding their professional responsibilities and accountabilities.
- There must, surely, be some objective assessment and understanding of the concepts of harm and benefit.
- If autonomy were the overriding principle, then we would have to legalise euthanasia and assisted suicide. Most would consider this undesirable.
- Autonomy would, in theory, override justice and lead to demands for treatment even if the result were unjust deprivation of others, for example, patients and their families cannot demand to stay in ICU if there is no clinical need thus denying critically ill patients the chance of life-saving treatment. The problems of scarce resources are also relevant to the principle of justice though preferably society should make these judgements. Health professionals arguably have an ethical duty to use resources appropriately.
- If autonomy were the overriding principle, then the next step is to see non-autonomous patients as having less worth and expendable in the interests of the autonomous.

Few ICU patients are autonomous. In one study [17], 62% of those that were competent still wanted a surrogate to act as decision maker in EOL decisions – mainly the family.

However, arguments based on the principle of justice favour the doctor as decision-maker – can't ask family to choose between their patient and another. The principle of non-maleficence extends to not desiring to impose the burden of decision-making to the family.

In America, Advance Directives such as:

- Living wills
- Durable power of Attorney orders

act to transfer autonomy and serve to free the family from the burdens of decision making.

The above promotion of the doctor as primary decision maker (in consultation with other carers and the family), reflecting the principles of beneficence and non-maleficence, is seen by some as paternalistic.

Paternalism (medical autonomy?) is an emotive term and seems somehow to be outdated and "bad" whereas autonomy is "good". However, both points of view are relative rather than absolute.

Doctors *do not* always know what is best but we do have a professional duty of care and it is unprofessional to pass the burden in its entirety to the family at a time when they are most vulnerable. Jacob interviewed 17 relatives involved in EOL decision making. The common theme reported was one of emotional burden [18]. Indeed, many relatives of ICU patients show symptoms of anxiety and depression [19].

We should also, where possible, protect them from the guilt of a "wrong decision". Such guilt may even interfere with the subsequent grieving process.

As has been stated before the ultimate decision and responsibility rests with the doctor after discussion with the other carers and the family. Ideally it is a shared decision and the answer to the conflict between autonomy and paternalism is that the correct approach lies somewhere along a spectrum as shown below:

$$\text{Autonomy} \longleftrightarrow \text{Paternalism}$$

Different families may be at different points along the spectrum.

Disagreements with family

If the family and the carers disagree, then a dilemma involving one "winner" and one "loser" can't be resolved ethically. The solution, however difficult, is to reach agreement.

- One solution is to defer to autonomy unless to continue is clearly futile. The concept of futility itself is not a solution; it merely helps structure, the discussion and may help in reaching agreement.

- Another solution is to avoid placing the burden on the family. Many families don't wish to be involved. It is reasonable to ask the family if they wish to be involved. If asked, and they want to be involved, they *still* may disagree!

Neither solution avoids disagreement but, nevertheless the principle is that agreement solves the problem.

Neither "I win because I am the doctor" or "You win because you are the family" are appropriate. Neither autonomy nor paternalism solve the problem. The "gold standard" is that long, difficult discussions must take place and agreement must, somehow, be reached. "Nobody wins" if the courts have to be involved (though rarely they may *have* to be involved).

Note: The longer the talks go on with treatment being continued, in a sense, the family win! If need to take a final decision suggest:

- Second opinion.
- Ethics consultation: Ethics consultations and ethics committees are an advisory and consultative service. They do not have decision-making powers for individual patients but have a valuable role in arbitration of difficult patients. Are ethics consultations "helpful" or merely "ethical" or are they only "helpful" when they agree with us?
- Multidisciplinary case conference.

Withdrawal of specific therapies

It may be appropriate to withdraw any or all therapies but when consideration is being given to withdrawal one should consider withdrawal of *all* therapies:

- Partial withdrawal strategies are confusing and difficult to carry out.
- Tapering of therapy, for example weaning of vasopressor infusions as opposed to cessation only serves to prolong needlessly the dying process.
- One should not give a timescale for death.
- Death is not to be hastened if withdrawal does not lead to death as quickly as anticipated.

IPPV is an intervention that is commonly withdrawn.

- Terminal weaning and rapid extubation are both acceptable techniques.
- Terminal weaning, for example no pressure support, "room air" and no positive end expiratory pressure (PEEP), may be preferable as it limits gasping and distressing obstruction.
- Extubation, however, has the advantage of being morally transparent [20] and cannot be confused with a normal weaning process.

- There were no differences in mental status, ventilatory status, age, or duration of survival between the patients who had support removed gradually and those from whom it was abruptly removed [21]. Interestingly, there seems to be no increase in pCO_2 but a decrease in pO_2 following removal of ventilatory support.
- If patient is to be abruptly separated from the ventilator some anticipatory analgesia and sedation may be required.

In those physicians who withdrew IPPV in one survey [22]:

> 13% preferred extubation,
> 33% preferred terminal weaning,
> 54% used both.

The differing groups both felt that family perceptions of care were improved by their method!

> An appropriate procedure is to:

- Decide to withdraw after discussion with colleagues and other carers.
- Discuss with family.
- Plan for performing procedure and dealing with complications.
- Ensure patient is in the right setting.
- Document in records *as for any other ICU procedure.* Full documentation reflects the conviction that palliative care is as important as restorative care.
- Evaluate outcomes to improve procedure and palliation techniques. EOL care is a highly appropriate topic for audit.
- Protocols and guidelines may be useful.

Reasons why therapy may not be withdrawn

There are several reasons why individual physicians may not consider withdrawal of therapy or why therapy may not be withdrawn in selected patients:

- Religious convictions on part of carers or physicians.
- Hope for a miracle (itself a religious concept) on part of family.
- Fear of failure.
- Pride (personal or professional).
- Fear of litigation/media involvement.
- Family aggression.
- Blind optimism.
- Pressure from physicians or surgeons (potential impact of development of league tables?).

- Compensating for or covering up of medical errors.
- Reverse ageism, that is, overtreatment of very elderly patients so as not to be accused of being ageist.

Problems with not withdrawing therapy

If treatment is not withdrawn when it perhaps should be there are potential problems:

- Danger of promoting false hope.
- Harmful effect on morale of nurses and other carers.
- May be against the ethical principle of justice especially if other patients are denied support.
- May impose an inappropriate burden on the patients or their families.
- Shamefully, there are instances reported where patients being maintained on a ventilator have developed rigor mortis of the limbs or putrefaction.

Optimal care of the dying patient

Patient and family experiences and wishes

Perhaps obviously, there are no reports in the scientific literature of patients reporting their satisfaction with their own dying process. Thus, there will probably always be certain unanswerable questions:

- Is it better to extubate?
- When is tachypnoea uncomfortable?
- Should comatose dying patients receive sedation?
- Should we sedate dying patients at all?

Surveys [20] suggest that patients fear a prolonged, painful (and in some countries), expensive death in an impersonal and technological environment surrounded by machines and prevented by incapacity from communicating with loved ones.

Does that not sound all too familiar?

Instead a "good death" is:

- free from avoidable pain and suffering,
- in accordance with the wishes of the family,

- consistent with clinical, legal, ethical, cultural and religious issues,
- at home or in a familiar environment.

Note: In surveys a high proportion of patients would wish spiritual issues to be addressed during their final illness. Physicians rarely consider this important.

Improving care of dying patients in the ICU

The key to optimal EOL care is relief of suffering including excellent palliative care (although relief of symptoms should be a goal for all ICU patients).

Is it appropriate for ICU to be a provider of palliative care? It may not be appropriate to admit patients to ICU for palliative care but it is entirely reasonable to provide palliative care for patients in ICU whose therapy has failed or been withdrawn, that is to switch to comfort measures and care of the dying process rather than trying to promote recovery of health. Palliative care includes such procedures as tracheal suction – which may not be adequately performed on a general ward.

EOL care in the ICU can include "keeping things going" until all the family is present. Dignity is improved by nursing the patient in a quiet, preferably side room with full visiting rights by all the family. Monitor alarms should be switched off.

The Society of Critical Care Medicine in America says that the goals of ICU care include assuring patients of a good death. They, and other societies strongly support a multidisciplinary approach with other professionals (including clergy) and the essential involvement of the family and close friends. Families should be encouraged to be involved in care and to touch patients – family are not just visitors.

The ICU societies also support a shared decision model in accord with the four ethical principles outlined earlier (without ranking them in priority or importance). They reject a narrow, medicalised approach to dying.

To improve quality of the dying process in ICU [20] one should:

- avoid inappropriate prolongation of the dying process,
- strengthen relationships with loved ones where possible,
- provide patients and families with a sense of control,
- provide good pain/symptom management,
- provide clear explanations to patients and families,
- provide privacy and comfort to patients and families,
- give opportunities for the family to voice concerns.

Studies show that patients and families wish the following from their doctors:

- emotional support,
- honesty,
- good communication,
- no contradictions,
- accessibility,
- continuity of care,
- information on diagnosis, treatment, prognosis and the dying process.

Another study [23] found that families were most satisfied with:

- nursing skills,
- caring attitudes of staff,
- sympathetic management,

and least satisfied with:

- the waiting room environment,
- physician communication.

A recent multicentre Canadian study [24] found that most of the patients' families perceived that the patients whose therapy was withdrawn died as follows:

- totally comfortably   37.2%
- very comfortably   24.5%
- mostly comfortably   29.6%

This is encouraging but still shows room for improvement.

Care of the dying patient in ICU may be improved by introducing checklists for aspects such as "do not resuscitate" and the process of Withdrawal of therapy [25].

Sedation, analgesia and paralysis

Pain and the distress from drips, drains, tubes, machines, etc. must be relieved by adequate doses of systemic analgesics. Occasionally regional analgesic techniques such as epidurals may play a part in providing sufficient analgesia. There may be distress from "fighting the ventilator" and a sensation of dyspnoea which may require analgesia and/or sedation. Opiods are often administered.

Strong opiod analgesics are associated with sedation and, in addition, specific sedatives are often administered to ensure lack of distress. Strong opiod analgesics also inhibit respiratory drive.

In one study [26], average dosages of sedative drugs before and after treatment withdrawal were examined:

Drug	24 h before withdrawal	24 h after withdrawal
Diazepam	2.2 mg/h	9.8 mg/h
Morphine	3.3 mg/h	11.2 mg/h

There were no differences in time from withdrawal to death between those patients who did and those who did not receive sedation (mainly comatose patients).

In the Canadian study already mentioned [24], the most frequently used drugs (though not all drugs were used in each patient) and the cumulative doses in the 4 h prior to death were:

Drug	Mean dosage (range)
Morphine	24 mg (2–450 mg)
Midazolam	24 mg (2–380 mg)
Lorazepam	4 mg (1– 80 mg)

There is a theoretical potential for conflict between

- a desire for the patient to be awake, surrounded by family to say "last good-byes" and
- the need to be sedated to relieve distress.

However, hypotension and low cardiac output itself lowers cerebral perfusion and impair conscious level. In practice, few families wish the patient to be unsedated during EOL care.

Paralysing agents should not be routinely given:

- not part of comfort care,
- not usually necessary if sufficient sedative and anlgesics are given,
- may mask patient's ability to show signs of distress.

All interested groups and societies support our professional obligation to relieve suffering even if the administration of the appropriate drugs may hasten death. This is the principle of double effect and is the ethical foundation for providing palliative care to the dying patient. Our intent is to relieve suffering and the "side effect" of hastening death by respiratory depression in an extubated patient is merely foreseen. It is considered better to administer an analgesic drug such as morphine by titrated infusion rather than by a large bolus.

- Titration to effect shows our intention to relieve suffering.
- There is no maximum dose and, indeed, high doses may be required.
- If a large bolus is given it may be less plausible that the intent is just to relieve pain.
- Since paralysing drugs have no analgesic effects, their use cannot be covered by the principle of double effect.

Despite the case of the GP in 1999 already mentioned many are uncomfortable that the double effect principle provides full protection from the courts. There are concerns that lack of intent may not be sufficient defence from a charge of manslaughter as, arguably, if the consequences of an action can be foreseen then that may be interpreted as intent.

Fortunately the judiciary seem unlikely to bring such cases from ICU to the courts as they recognise that an inability to provide palliative care in any form (which would be the clear consequence of negating the double effect principle) is clearly not in the interests of a civilised society.

However, we at all times must be certain of the purity of our intentions if only to satisfy our own moral and ethical conscience.

General aspects of care of the dying patient

- Good mouth care is essential and may reduce the prospect of distress due to lack of oral fluids.
- Pressure area care is important but turning patients for pressure area care has to be balanced against pain caused by the physical act of turning. Keeping the patient clean and dry is helpful for skin care.
- The benefits from nursing the patient in a side room have already been alluded to, where possible invasive lines, monitors and other technology should be removed.
- Chest suction may be appropriate but aggressive physiotherapy may not be.
- Non-palliative medications should be stopped. There are occasions where continuing anticonvulsants, non-steroidal anti-inflammatory drugs (NSAIDs), antipyretics and steroids may all be worthwhile. Blood products should no longer be given.
- Antibiotics are not appropriate in the dying patient unless, rarely, they may be given for painful conditions such as a painful otitis media.
- The patient should not be subjected to further laboratory tests or X-rays.

- If patients experience dyspnoea; symptomatic relief may occasionally be achieved by having air from a fan blowing air over the face (air may be as effective as oxygen at relieving dyspnoea [27]).

Thirst and hunger versus artificial feeding and hydration

The loss of body water is part of the normal dying process. If "near end of life" means the last few hours or days prior to death (as happens in ICU) then issues of hydration versus dehydration become irrelevant, superceded by issues of care, comfort and support for the patient. However, if "near end of life" is defined as last few days or weeks (as happens in Hospice care), then issues of hydration versus dehydration become more relevant – and controversial.

In ICU, some would argue that fluids and nutrition should be given to all patients, including those who are clearly dying, because:

- It is their "right".
- It is part of ordinary care.
- There may be distressing symptoms of either hunger or thirst/dehydration in the dying patient.

Here, it can be argued that discussions of "ordinary" versus "extraordinary" care only confuse in that one should do what is appropriate for the patient's needs. It is important to realise that dehydration at the end of life may not be associated with distress:

- Dehydration and loss of appetite are part of the dying process.
- Dehydration is associated with reduced conscious level.
- Dehydration may be associated with less gastric secretions.
- The discomfort from a dry mouth can be dealt with by local mouth care.

There may be additional problems and sources of additional distress arising from the process of hydration or nutrition:

- Discomfort or infection at the site of intravenous (IV) cannulae.
- Restriction of the patient's limb and restriction of family access and contact.
- Removal/reinsertion of nasogastric tube by the patient.
- Regurgitation of gastric contents following enteral feeding.

Occasionally a patient undergoing hospice care, who is mentally competent, feels strongly about being hydrated until the end. These wishes should, of course, be respected.

Care of the relatives

The family should be dealt with sympathetically. Many ICUs have access to short term accommodation for the use of the family of patients in the ICU. The family should have ready access to food, drink and pleasantly furnished areas to rest. Access to clergy is seen as important by many families. Providing a pager or mobile phone enables the family to be contactable even if not present on the ICU.

At the end the family should have some private time with their deceased relative prior to removal of the body from the ICU. Religious and cultural beliefs should, wherever possible be respected at this time.

FURTHER READING

Randall Curtis J, Rubenfeld GD. Managing death in the intensive care unit 2001. Oxford University Press, Oxford.

Withholding and Withdrawing Life-prolonging Treatments: Good Practice in Decision-Making. General Medical Council, London, 2002.

The Ethics Committee of the Society of Critical Care Medicine. Recommendations for end-of-life care in the intensive care unit. *Crit Care Med* 2001; 29: 2332–48.

Randall F, Downie RS. *Palliative Care Ethics*, 2nd edn. Oxford University Press, Oxford, 1999.

REFERENCES

1. Sjokvist P, Nilstun T, Svantesson M, Berggren L. Withdrawal of life support – who should decide? Differences in attitudes among the general public, nurses and physicians. *Intens Care Med* 1999; 25: 949–54.

2. Prendergast TJ. Fellowship education in end-of-life care (EOLC). *Am J Respir Crit Care Med* 2002; 165: B4 (Suppl).

3. Abbott KH, Sago JG, Breen CM et al. Families looking back: one year after discussion of withdrawal or withholding of life-sustaining support. *Crit Care Med* 2001; 29: 197–201.

4. Crippen D. Terminally weaning awake patients from life-sustaining mechanical ventilation: the critical care physician's role in comfort measures during the dying process. *Clin Intens Care* 1992; 3: 206–12.

5. Randall F, Downie RS. *Palliative Care Ethics* 2nd edn. Oxford University Press, Oxford, 1999.

6. Konopad E, Noseworthy TW, Johnston R, Shustack A, Grace M. Quality of life measures before and one year after admission to an intensive care unit. *Crit Care Med* 1995; 23: 1653–9.

7. Niskanen M, Ruokonen E, Takala J, Rissanen P et al. Quality of life after prolonged intensive care. *Crit Care Med* 1999; 27: 1132–9.

8. Danis M, Patrick DL, Southerland LI, Green ML. Patients' and families' preferences for medical intensive care. *J Am Med Assoc* 1988; 260(6): 797–802.
9. Meinders AJ, Van Der Hoeven JG, Meinders AE. The outcome of prolonged mechanical ventilation in elderly patients: are the results worthwhile? *Age And Ageing* 1996; **28**: 353–6.
10. Prendergast TJ, Luce JM. Increasing incidence of withholding and withdrawal of life support from the critically ill. *Am J Respir Crit Care Med* 1997; 155: 15–20.
11. Kollef MH, Ward S. The influence of access to a private attending physician on the withdrawal of life-sustaining therapies in the intensive care unit. *Crit Care Med* 1999; 27: 2125–32.
12. Rubenfeld GD, Crawford SW. Withdrawing life support from mechanically ventilated recipients of bone marrow transplants: a case for evidence based guidelines. *Ann Int Med* 1996; 125: 625–33.
13. Rocker G, Cook D, Sjokvist P, Weaver B et al. Clinician predictions of intensive care unit mortality. *Crit Care Med* 2004; 32: 1149–54.
14. Barrera R, Nygard S, Sogoloff H, Groeger J, Wilson R. Accuracy of predictions of survival at admission to the intensive care unit. *J Crit Care* 2001; 16: 32–5.
15. Uhlmann RF, Pearlman RA, Cain KC. Physicians' and spouses' predictions of elderly patients' resuscitation preferences. *J Gerontol* 1988; 43(5): M115–M121.
16. Emanuel EJ, Emanuel LL. Proxy decision making for incompetent patients. An ethical and empirical analysis. *J Am Med Assoc* 1992; 267: 2067–71.
17. Ferrand E, Bachoud-Levi AC, Rodrigues M, Maggiore S et al. Decision-making capacity and surrogate designation in French ICU patients. *Intens Care Med* 2001; 27: 1360–4.
18. Jacob DA. Family members' experiences with decision-making for incompetent patients in the ICU: a qualitative study. *Am J Crit Care* 1998; 7: 30–6.
19. Pochard F, Azoulay E, Chevret S, Lemaire F et al. Symptoms of anxiety and depression in family members of intensive care unit patients: ethical hypothesis regarding decision-making capacity. *Crit Care Med* 2001; 29: 1893–7.
20. Truog RD, Cist AF, Brackett SE, Burns JP et al. The Ethics Committee of the Society of Critical Care Medicine. Recommendations for end-of-life care in the intensive care unit. *Crit Care Med* 2001; 29: 2332–48.
21. Daly BJ, Thomas D, Dyer MA. Procedures used in withdrawal of mechanical ventilation. *Am J Crit Care* 1996; 5: 331–8.
22. Faber-Langendoen K. The clinical management of dying patients receiving mechanical ventilation. A survey of physician practice. *Chest* 1995; 108: 887.
23. Heyland DK, Rocker GM, Dodek PM, Kutsogiannis DJ et al. Family satisfaction with care in the intensive care unit: results of a multiple center study. *Crit Care Med* 2002; 30: 1413–18.
24. Rocker GM, Heyland DK, Cook DJ, Dodek PM et al. Most critically ill patients are perceived to die in comfort during withdrawal of life support: a Canadian multicentre study. *Can J Anaesth* 2004; 51: 623–30.

25. Hall RI, Rocker GM, Murray D. Simple changes can improve conduct of end-of-life care in the intensive care unit. *Can J Anaesth* 2004; 51: 631–6.

26. Wilson WC, Smedira NG, Fink C, McDowell JA, Luce JM. Ordering and administration of sedatives and analgesics during the withholding and withdrawal of life support from critically ill patients. *J Am Med Assoc* 1992; 267: 949–53.

27. Booth S, Kelly MJ, Cox NP, Adams L, Guz A. Does oxygen help dyspnea in patients with cancer? *Am J Respir Crit Care Med* 1996; 153: 1515–18.

ACKNOWLEDGMENT

Contributions to this chapter by Sister I. Frater, RN are gratefully acknowledged.

Part II

Specific problems

17

The surgical patient in the ICU

I. McConachie

This chapter brings together many aspects of relevance to "high-risk" surgical patients admitted to the intensive care unit (ICU).

For a full discussion of

- aspects of risk assessment,
- anaesthetic and surgical risk factors,
- cardiac risk, scoring systems and investigations,
- respiratory risk and the role of pulmonary function testing.

the reader is recommended to consult *Anaesthesia for the High Risk Patient* by the same author and publisher.

Preoperative assessment

The aim of preoperative assessment is to minimise morbidity and mortality.

Three questions should be asked when assessing surgical patients with the aim of minimising operative risk:

(1) Is the patient's medical and physiological status optimum?
(2) If not, can the patient's status be improved (time permitting)?
(3) If not, should the operation still proceed? In other words, do the risks of not operating outweigh the risks of operating? For example, medical status is almost irrelevant if the operation is clearly life saving. Thus, no patient is "not fit" for surgery – it just depends on the urgency of the situation. However, the patient should be considered salvageable by surgery. If not, palliative care may be more appropriate than heroic interventions.

Preoperative assessment should identify those patients who are at high risk of per- or postoperative organ failures. Such patients may need additional monitoring and may warrant admission to ICU or a high-dependency unit (HDU) postoperatively for organ function monitoring or support.

Patients are usually believed to be "high risk" because of the following:

- Respiratory disease predisposing to respiratory failure postoperatively.
- Cardiac disease predisposing to myocardial ischaemia or cardiac failure postoperatively.
- Less commonly, patients with renal insufficiency may develop renal failure postoperatively – vascular surgery patients are especially at risk.

One should not discount the effect of heroic surgery or increasing age (see below).

Respiratory disease

Presence of significant respiratory pathology will lead to an increased morbidity and, for major surgery, mortality. Anaesthesia may not pose much problem but respiratory failure may result in the postoperative period. This in part will be due to the inevitable changes in respiratory mechanics associated with anaesthesia and the surgery performed:

- Respiratory excursion will be impeded by pain which may result in atelectasis.
- Pain may also inhibit coughing resulting in sputum retention.
- The site of operation is important, for example, thoracic followed by abdominal sites being the worse – partly because these are the sites of incisions associated with most pain.

A review of preoperative respiratory function testing is beyond the scope of this text (readers are referred to standard anaesthetic texts) but certain risk factors are worth emphasising:

- Presence of hypoxia.
- Presence of hypercarbia.
- Breathlessness at rest.
- Smoking is a major risk factor [1].
- Increasing age is a risk factor due to, for example, increased closing volume and increased sensitivity to opioids.
- Site of surgery – highest for upper abdominal and thoracic surgery.

- Length of surgery.
- Obesity – increased closing volume and increased incidence of airway obstruction and sleep apnoea.

In order to attempt to reduce this risk the patient may be admitted preoperatively for

- abstinence from smoking,
- bed rest,
- physiotherapy,
- bronchodilator therapy if bronchospasm present,
- steroids may be beneficial in chronic obstructive pulmonary disease (COPD),
- antibiotics if infection present,
- nutritional assessment and supplementation if necessary,
- diuretics if cor pulmonale present.

Cardiovascular disease

Presence of pre-existing cardiac disease is undoubtedly a predictor of increased perioperative risk. More specifically many studies have identified cardiac risk factors which include:

• Previous myocardial infarction (MI)	• Left ventricular hypertrophy
• Hypertension	• Diabetes
• Renal failure	• Decompensated heart failure
• Old age	• Significant arrhythmias
• Emergency operation	• Severe valvular disease
• Unstable or severe angina or electro-cardiographic signs of ischemia	

The most important development in cardiac perioperative risk assessment and guidelines for perioperative investigations in recent years have been the joint guidelines from the American College of Cardiology and American Heart Association. These were first published in 1996 [2] and updated in 2002 [3]. These should be essential reading for all anaesthetists and critical care practitioners.

The overall message is that patients with severe heart disease and old and "sick" patients are at risk of increased adverse cardiac outcome. Although anaesthesia can be problematic, most problems occur in the postoperative period emphasising the importance of adequate monitoring and treatment of complications in the ICU in the postoperative ICU or HDU.

There are currently two main theories as to how cardiac disease might contribute to perioperative mortality in the surgical patient:

(1) Poor cardiopulmonary physiological reserve: The physiological reserve of the heart and lungs is insufficient to meet the increased demands of surgery. In physiological terms, oxygen delivery does not fulfil oxygen consumption (VO_2) requirements. End-organ ischaemia results in multi-organ dysfunction syndrome (MODS) and death. This is discussed further below in the section on perioperative optimisation.
(2) The development of myocardial ischaemia in patients with coronary artery disease (CAD).

A thought provoking review highlights the, at times, conflicting priorities in managing surgical patients at risk of myocardial ischaemia and those in whom the cardiac output and oxygen delivery need to be increased [4]. Both are at risk of an adverse outcome but the approach is different and identification of the group that patients belong to is important.

Prevention of myocardial ischaemia

- The majority of perioperative ischaemic episodes occur in the postoperative period.
- However, perioperative cardiac instability (especially tachycardia) is a major risk factor [5]. Thus, anaesthetic techniques and problems *are* important.
- Choice of anaesthetic drugs is, however, relatively unimportant providing myocardial oxygen balance is maintained, for example:
  - Factors increasing myocardial oxygen demand:
    (a) Tachycardia
    (b) Hypertension
    (c) Increases in contractility
    (d) Increases in wall tension (e.g. increased preload).
  - Factors reducing myocardial oxygen supply:
    (a) Tachycardia
    (b) Hypotension (especially low diastolic pressure)
    (c) Anaemia
    (d) Coronary artery spasm.
- Continuance of preoperative cardiac medications especially is vital.
- Perioperative Myocardial infarction (MI) (peak incidence on the second or third postoperative day) is commoner in patients with a recent MI but the incidence

can be reduced by invasive monitoring and careful control of haemodynamic parameters [6].

- Landmark studies have indicated that the prophylactic use of β-blockers in the perioperative period in patients with CAD, or risk factors for CAD reduces perioperative cardiac risk [7]. This is probably the most important intervention in order to reduce perioperative cardiac risk in these patients. However, chronic β-blockade does not seem to confer the same advantages as acute β-blockade.
- Smaller studies suggest a similar beneficial role from the sympatholytic effect of α2-agonists such as clonidine [8].
- Animal studies support the role of sympatholysis from thoracic epidural anaesthesia and analgesis in reducing cardiac ischaemia. Perhaps this may be valuable following coronary artery surgery but in vascular patients the evidence is conflicting – one study showing no difference in ischaemia between the use of thoracic epidurals and patient-controlled intravenous opioids [9]. A meta-analysis has claimed that the use of thoracic epidurals reduces the incidence of postoperative MI [10].

Ongoing ischaemia in the ICU may be a problem. This will be "silent" in the sedated, ventilated patient and may not be accompanied by overt ST changes on the electrocardiogram (ECG). A recent study [11] has suggested that mildly elevated Troponin I levels (below the threshold for MI) are not uncommon. This may reflect ongoing myocardial injury and may be associated with a worse outcome. The authors speculate that the administration of β-blockers and aspirin in the ICU may improve outcome.

Stress response to major surgery

- The intensity of the stress response is related to the degree of tissue trauma, that is, minor surgery stimulates a minor, transient response whereas major abdominal surgery may stimulate a stress response lasting days to even weeks. Other factors promoting the stress response after major abdominal surgery include gut stimuli via the sympathetic nervous system, local tissue factors and cytokines. Haemorrhage, hypothermia, sepsis and acidosis will all exacerbate the response.
- The response is multifactorial, thus neural blockade will not completely prevent this. Aspects of the cytokine response have been shown to be modified by the use of steroids, nonsteroidal anti-inflammatory drugs and the use of different catecholamines.

- The role of the stress response is to mobilise substrate and acute proteins for wound healing and the inflammatory response. Possible detrimental effects of a profound stress response following major surgery include increased demands on organs which may have reduced reserve, pulmonary complications, thromboembolism and pain and fatigue. The appropriateness of an unmodified response is, therefore, debatable.
- Intraoperative regional anaesthesia may only delay the development of the stress response. The optimum duration of blockade is not known.
- If the response is desired to be modified into the postoperative period a continuous regional technique is required – continuous epidural analgesia has been most studied.
- Epidural analgesia has significant modifying effects on the hormonal and catecholamine responses to lower abdominal surgery.
- The effects of epidural anaesthesia on the stress response following upper abdominal and thoracic surgery is less impressive. This could be due to failure to adequately block all afferent stimulation. For example, continuous spinal anaesthesia, with its denser block, is more effective at blocking the hormonal stress response compared with epidural anaesthesia.
- Central neural block may mitigate various aspects of postoperative morbidity but the evidence is really only convincing for decreased blood loss, reduction in deep vein thrombosis (DVT) and limiting gastrointestinal (GI) stasis after abdominal procedures.
- Spinal opioids have less effect on the stress response. Their effect on morbidity is unclear but is likely to be less due to lesser effects on stress response.
- The ability to influence changes in immune function after surgery is less well studied than the effects on metabolic responses. In general, any modification of the immune response to surgery by regional compared to general anaesthesia is probably of minor clinical importance.

The importance of adequate analgesia

In years past severe pain was accepted as an inevitable consequence of trauma and surgery, and little effort was made to provide adequate pain relief in the majority of unfortunate patients:

- Whilst adequate pain relief is a laudable objective from the humanitarian perspective, modern understanding of the pathophysiological effects of pain makes appropriate pain relief a primary objective in avoiding the common morbidities associated with surgery.

- There is little doubt that pain increases the stress response to surgery, promotes atelectasis and sputum retention and is a factor in myocardial ischaemia.
- The patient who is at "high risk" either because of the trauma of their surgery or their poor physiological reserve therefore requires effective pain relief to avoid these potentially lethal complications.
- If this is not achieved, then these are the patients most likely to slide down the slippery slope to critical illness.
- Early mobilisation can be facilitated by good pain relief and this in turn reduces the likelihood of deep venous thrombosis and pulmonary embolus and will reduce the likelihood of hypostatic pneumonia.

Modern approaches to the management of acute pain rely heavily on two analgesic techniques, patient-controlled analgesia (PCA) using an opioid self-administered in small doses by the patient, and epidural analgesic techniques. The provision of adequate analgesia may be more important than the method of analgesia employed.

Nevertheless, the use of PCA opiod techniques has not been shown to improve outcomes [12] (but provides good analgesia).

The problems of pain and analgesic regimens in high-risk surgical patients are fully discussed elsewhere by Duncan and Counsell [13].

Epidural anaesthesia and analgesia

A possible effect of epidural anaesthesia and analgesia on perioperative outcome is of major interest. This includes effects on coagulability and fibrinolysis with their impact on blood loss and thrombotic complications, which are part of the effect on the stress response. In addition, the role of regional anaesthesia and postoperative analgesia on overall morbidity and cardiac and respiratory complications has been increasingly investigated.

- There is no consensus on whether certain types of patient undergoing certain types of surgery benefit more from a regional, a general or a mixture of the two types of anaesthesia.
- In truth, there may not be a significant difference for all patients. Much will depend on how a technique is performed rather than which technique is performed, the skill of the practitioner, patient factors such as cardiac or respiratory disease and the occurrence of side effects or complications.

- Evidence obtained from systemic review of relevant randomised-controlled trials obtained by the Australian Working party group (National Health and Medical Research Council, NHMRC) demonstrates that postoperative epidural analgesia can significantly reduce the incidence of pulmonary morbidity [14].
- Several studies have examined whether epidural anaesthesia in association with general anaesthesia or, more, commonly, on its own results in less cardiac morbidity. This could be possibly related to a reduction in thrombotic tendency, reduction in catecholamine levels and avoidance of cardiac depression. Trials so far have found no significant reduction in cardiac morbidity from the use of epidural anaesthesia in vascular surgery patients [15].
- However, there are other benefits from the use of epidurals in aortic and peripheral vascular surgery such as improved graft patency due to reduced thrombotic tendency and improved graft blood flow [16].

The effect of epidurals on overall mortality

- In particular there is no clear consensus on whether the use of epidurals intra-operatively provides the same, lesser or even greater benefit than those epidurals carried on into the postoperative period. The role of epidurals on the ordinary ward versus those cared for in an ICU environment is unclear as is the desirability of continuing epidural infusions in the ventilated patient with haemodynamic instability.
- The original prospective randomised trial to address this issue reported beneficial effects from epidural anaesthesia in high-risk surgical ICU patients [17]. Unfortunately, this and other studies have shown conflicting results with interpretation of these studies hampered by their lack of statistical power and poor control of other management protocols.
- Subsequent studies of larger numbers of patients found no overall effect on mortality but one [18] showed important improvements in outcome in aortic surgery and the other showed a reduction in postoperative respiratory failure [19].
- Various meta-analyses have been performed including one [20] which claimed that epidurals reduce surgical mortality by one-third compared to general anaesthesia without an epidural.
- Reasons for the disparity between large trials and meta-analysis when looking at mortality may include the incorporation of older trials into the meta-analyses. In particular many of the older trials were performed at a time when DVT prophylaxis was not widespread – leading to a reduction in morbidity and

mortality in the epidural patients from the reduction in thrombotic complications. It is unlikely that there is as significant a benefit today from reduction in thrombotic complications in an era when DVT prophylaxis is standard practice.

Problems associated with the use of epidurals [13]

- The complications of epidural catheter insertion include epidural haematoma and abscess, intravenous injection of local anaesthetic and inadvertent dural tap. The risk of neurological complications either of a minor or major nature has yet to be clearly defined but must be considered when balancing the risks against the benefits of epidurals.
- Itching, nausea and vomiting are all recognised side effects of epidural opioids. Though respiratory depression is rare monitoring of sedation level is mandatory.
- Hypotension (systolic blood pressure <80 mmHg) is common. The fall in blood pressure results in loss of the often claimed benefit from epidurals (i.e. the potential increase in colonic blood flow).
- Care should be taken with the timing of prophylactic heparin injections in relation to insertion and removal of epidural catheters to reduce the likelihood of epidural haematoma.
- Epidural analgesia is associated with the development of pressure sores particularly on the heels. This can happen even in young healthy people and nursing vigilance is essential. Debilitated patients are at higher risk of developing this complication. Strong local anaesthetic solutions administered via the epidural in theatre may be a factor in the development of these sores. A sensible precaution is to switch off epidural infusions if patients' legs are still paralysed beyond 2 h after surgery. It can be recommenced when the block has regressed enough to allow leg movement. This precaution also facilitates early detection of epidural haematoma.

Aspects of surgical nutrition

- A large study demonstrated an increase in infectious complications in patients undergoing major surgery who received perioperative total parenteral nutrition (TPN) [21]. Guidelines suggest that preoperative TPN is not appropriate in patients with only mild to moderate degrees of preoperative malnutrition [22].

Postoperative TPN is only required if the patient cannot receive enteral nutrition within 7–10 days. The most important conclusion is that short-term TPN is probably to be avoided because the benefits do not warrant the complications.
• Early enteral nutrition (EN) feeding is clearly associated with improved outcome [23] (though a minority view would hold that EN is only better because TPN is worse, that is, EN avoids the metabolic and infectious complications of TPN). A recent meta-analysis of 11 studies has concluded that there are no benefits in keeping surgical patients "nil by mouth" after GI surgery [24]. However, some caution is required as most of these patients will not have been sick enough to require critical care support. Nevertheless, those patients receiving early enteral feeding had reduced septic complications and length of hospital stay. A further meta-analysis states that EN is to be preferred over TPN in patients with pancreatitis [25].

Oxygen transport in the high-risk surgical patient

Shoemaker in his original papers defined what he considered to be high-risk surgical patients [26]. Many studies have used these criteria:

Previous severe cardio respiratory illness (e.g. acute MI or chronic obstructive airways disease).
Extensive ablative surgery planned for malignancy (e.g. gastrectomy, oesophagectomy or surgery >6 h).
Multiple trauma (e.g. more than three organ injury, more than two systems or opening two body cavities).
Massive acute haemorrhage (e.g. more than eight units).
Age above 70 years and limited physiological reserve of one or more organs.
Septicaemia (positive blood cultures or septic focus) white cell count (WCC) >13, pyrexia to 38.3 for 48 h.
Respiratory failure (PaO_2 <8 Kpa on an FiO_2 >0.4 or mechanical ventilation >48 h).
Acute abdominal catastrophe with haemodynamic instability (e.g. pancreatitis, perforated viscus, peritonitis, GI bleed).
Acute renal failure (urea >20 mmol/l, creatinine >260 mmol/l).
Late stage vascular disease involving aortic disease.
Shock (e.g. mean arterial pressure (MAP) <60 mmHg, central venous pressure (CVP) <15 cmH$_2$O, urine output <20 ml/h).

Why might the surgical high-risk patient require increases in cardiac output and oxygen delivery? Reasons suggested are:

- Animal studies show that for an equivalent degree of blood loss, traumatic injury results in greater tissue hypoperfusion and a greater "injury" than simple haemorrhage.
- The wound is metabolically active with a resultant requirement for increased VO_2 and glucose oxidation – the concept of "the wound as an organ". In addition to the local reasons for increased metabolic demands, there are systemic inflammatory and catabolic causes of increased metabolic demand requiring an increased cardiac output compared to normal. This may imply a need for increased cardiac output and oxygen delivery in trauma and high-risk surgical patients – in line with Shoemaker's optimal goals as discussed in Chapter 1.
- There are studies demonstrating that high-risk surgical patients develop an intraoperative "oxygen debt", the magnitude and duration of which correlates with the development of lactic acidosis, organ failure and increased mortality [27]. This oxygen debt is postulated to potentially arise from anaesthetic cardiac depression, direct anaesthetic reductions in tissue oxygen uptake, failure to maintain adequate fluid levels during surgery and perhaps hypothermia.

Studies of high-risk surgical patients: Perioperative optimisation or perioperative optimism?

- The best evidence for a beneficial therapeutic effect of maximising oxygen transport is from studies where therapy was initiated very early in the presence of tissue hypoperfusion, that is, preoperatively in high-risk surgical patients [28]. Shoemaker's original prospective, randomised study demonstrating the virtues of optimising oxygen transport was performed in surgical patients [29].
- The crucial message is that high-risk surgical patients may have reduced cardiac reserves, especially in the elderly, suffer occult tissue hypoperfusion with a developing oxygen debt postoperatively, proceed to multiple organ failure if there is no intervention to reverse the tissue hypoperfusion and have a higher mortality than patients who *do* have sufficient reserves to reverse their oxygen debt and prevent serious tissue hypoxia.
- As stated in Chapter 1, a key issue may be timing – Shoemaker has suggested that there can be significant reductions in mortality in critical illness when patients are treated early to achieve optimal goals before the development of organ failure, when there were control group mortalities of >20% (otherwise

the patients are not sick enough) and when therapy produced differences in oxygen delivery between the control and protocol groups [30].

- In the most recent large study, the use of pulmonary artery flotation catheters (PAFCs) inserted preoperatively and used to guide the achievement of high oxygen delivery (see below) failed to show an improved outcome compared with "conventional" therapy [31].

The specific issue of dopexamine in high-risk surgical patients

- Boyd [28] in his study on perioperative optimisation showed improvements in survival in the high oxygen delivery group. It was later suggested that the improvement may have been related to the *choice* of inotrope – dopexamine – rather than the cardiac output achieved in the patients.
- Splanchnic blood flow may be increased with dopexamine, increased pHi may be normalised and indices of GI permeability reduced, but evidence comes mainly from animal studies. The significance of these with regard to outcome is currently unclear.
- The most interesting aspect of dopexamine and the most controversial is the suggestion that dopexamine may have specific anti-inflammatory properties [32]. (Catecholamines may have differing effects on inflammation, for example, β1-stimulation may be pro-inflammatory while α1- and β2-stimulation may be anti-inflammatory.) Most of the evidence for this to date is from animal studies but a few studies on surgical patients broadly support this hypothesis. Further evidence is eagerly awaited.
- Wilson's study [33] included three groups: a control group managed conventionally and two other groups who were admitted preoperatively to intensive care and given goal-directed therapy with either adrenaline or dopexamine. Both the treatment groups had significantly improved survival rate, however only the dopexamine group saw a significant reduction in morbidity. This is particularly interesting because the dopexamine treated group did not see an increase in cardiac index by as much as the adrenaline treated group. The reduced morbidity was due to a reduction in sepsis and acute respiratory distress syndrome (ARDS). An economic analysis on this trial data has shown that this approach to high-risk patients is cost-effective [34].
- However, a follow-up study from the same group found no apparent benefit from dopexamine in surgical patients [35] (though perhaps there was a benefit in both groups from volume loading).

- This echoed a multicentre European study which also failed to find any benefit from the routine perioperative use of dopexamine in elective surgery [36].
  However, the authors suggested, based on subgroup analysis and stratification
  according to the number of risk factors, that dopexamine should be further
  tested in patients at higher risk of complications or undergoing emergency
  surgery. This supports Shoemaker's contention that benefits will only be seen
  when the patients are sick enough and/or the control group have a high enough
  mortality to enable a benefit to be shown [30].

One conclusion from the above is clear, when the patients are not "high-risk" and
the expected mortality from surgery is low, there will be no benefit from perioperative optimisation.

GI surgery: the ultimate in high risk

The general public (and many practitioners) would no doubt consider such
surgery as open heart surgery as being amongst the most riskiest of surgical
operations in terms of immediate and early mortality. In fact, certain relatively
common GI operations are arguably amongst the highest risk procedures performed. For example, perusal of a recent standard surgical text [37] reveals the
expected operative mortality for the following operations and conditions:

Operation	Operative mortality (%)
Ca colon resection	5–10
Large-bowel obstruction	10
Small-bowel obstruction	30
Ca pancreas	20
Ca oesophagus	10

Predicted mortality may be expected to increase if the surgery is performed as an
emergency.

The lessons to be learnt are:

- GI surgery is high-risk surgery and warrants senior input and appropriate
  facilities.
- With the expected mortality, palliation may be better than attempting a cure in
  some patients.

Reasons for being high risk

- Coexisting medical diseases. Many of the patients are elderly with significant medical problems.
- Type of surgery. Often long procedures with significant blood loss, fluid shifts, electrolyte and nutritional problems, and significant postoperative pain.
- Abdominal surgery is associated with a profound physiological stress response.
- Emergency or elective. Many of these patients will present as urgent or emergent cases. This is well recognised to be associated with a worse outcome. Problems associated with emergency cases include less time to evaluate, investigate and treat patients.
- High incidence of fluid shifts and perioperative hypovolaemia.
- Abdominal surgery is associated with significant respiratory embarrassment – upper abdominal more than lower.
- Many patients will suffer from pre-, per- or postoperative sepsis. We all have a lethal dose of endotoxin contained within our gut!

Recovery of bowel function

- Epidural analgesia. Postoperative ileus involves sympathetic and parasympathetic pathways. These can be blocked by epidural analgesia leading to a reduction in the incidence of ileus following abdominal surgery [38]. The bowel is relatively contracted – which some surgeons dislike. Postoperative nitrogen balance after bowel surgery is improved by extradural anaesthesia [39]. Surgeons are often concerned that the increase in intestinal motility with epidurals may increase the incidence of anastomotic breakdown. However, a review of 12 trials has found no evidence of harmful effect [40] (but concluded that larger studies are needed for a definitive answer). Indeed, by increasing intestinal blood flow one might expect epidural anaesthesia to have a favourable effect on a bowel anastomosis.
- Opioids. Morphine has a major effect on bowel motility, significantly prolonging the time to recovery of bowel function after colonic surgery [41].
- Neostigmine increases intraluminal pressure (not prevented by atropine) and has been implicated in the past (mainly by surgeons) as a cause of anastomotic breakdown. Animal studies do not support this assumption. A large patient study found no difference in the rate of anastomotic leakage with or without neostigmine [42]. Surgical factors are undoubtedly more important than

anaesthetic factors in determining the fate of the anastomosis. Anaesthetists can help by maintaining good oxygenation (including into the postoperative period), prompt treatment of hypovolaemia and hypotension and avoiding hypocapnia.

Respiratory aspects of abdominal surgery

Respiratory function is significantly impaired after abdominal surgery, especially upper abdominal surgery. A combination of factors are involved:

- Reduced functional residual capacity (FRC).
- Pain leading to decreased cough and atelectasis. Pain is greater following upper abdominal incisions compared with lower abdominal incisions.
- Diaphragmatic dysfunction.

Several randomised trials have highlighted the role of physiotherapy in reducing respiratory complications following abdominal surgery. Physiotherapy is beneficial both prophylactically, that is, preoperatively and also postoperatively. One large study concluded that low-risk patients benefit from breathing exercises and high-risk patients benefit from incentive spirometry exercises [43].

Important factors

- Most studies have examined the effects of different analgesic regimens. Meta-analysis confirms that the excellent postoperative analgesia with continuous epidural analgesia leads to a reduction in respiratory complications [44]. The impairment in respiratory function following abdominal surgery is lessened – but respiratory function is still reduced compared to preoperative values.
- Large tidal volumes during anaesthesia are beneficial on respiratory function [45] but it is less certain if there are residual benefits postoperatively. Positive end-expiratory pressure (PEEP) has been shown to be beneficial in morbidly obese patients but not normal patients [46].
- Interestingly, pancuronium is associated with postoperative complications when given for patients undergoing lengthy operations compared with atracurium [47] – implying perhaps that repeated doses of pancuronium are associated with residual neuromuscular blockade.
- Surgical factors have been less well studied but it seems that length of surgery and blood loss are predictors of postoperative respiratory complications.

The elderly patient

Age should not be a discriminator to admission to a HDU or ICU. Indeed if it is felt that major surgery will be of benefit to the patient then it seems perverse to deny them appropriate postoperative care. A recent debate in the literature was provoked by a case report [48] that documented the pre- and postoperative care of a 113-year old on an ICU. The majority of aged patients will be adequately cared for on a general surgical ward but a few will require postoperative HDU or ICU care which, providing that surgery was appropriate, should be made available.

Nevertheless, it would be foolish to deny that surgical risk and ICU mortality is increased in the elderly patient [49]. Outcome is dramatically worse in the very old. Reasons for this include:

- Altered pharmacokinetics and pharmacodynamics.
- Altered physiology which can best be summarised as loss of homeostatic ability. There is a progressive loss of cardiorespiratory reserve (see monitoring strategies below) and a loss of tissue elasticity. This leads to:
    decreased myocardial and respiratory compliance,
    decreased maximum stroke volume (SV), heart rate (HR), vital capacity (VC),
    decreased lean muscle mass,
    increased work of breathing,
    increased closing volume (may be greater than FRC).
  Many of these changes are minimal at rest, but increased during stress, including surgical stress. Thus with surgery or trauma, cardiorespiratory reserve may not be sufficient and failure occur.
- In the kidney, nephron numbers fall leading, again, to loss of functional reserve and loss of problems with Na loading and depletion, problems with ability to concentrate or dilute urine and difficulty excreting an acid or alkali load.
- High incidence of comorbidities.
- High incidence of adverse drug interactions due to polypharmacy.
- High incidence of surgery for malignant disease.
- Malnutrition is common in the elderly and influences prognosis in many ways including decreases in immune function and decreases in wound healing.
- Sarcopenia [50]. Of these, sarcopenia is an under recognised problem in the anaesthetic, ICU and surgical literature as a cause of failure to thrive in ICU and increased perioperative morbidity and mortality. Its nature, implications and potential for improvement are subjects of much research in the geriatric literature.

Sarcopenia and the elderly patient

- Sarcopenia literally means lack of muscle. Skeletal muscle is approximately 40% of a young man's weight and 50% of his body protein. Total lean body mass (exclusive of bone) and total skeletal muscle mass both are greater in men than women and decrease progressively with age. Body composition, therefore, changes with ageing.
- It seems that there is a fall in muscle fibre number as well as atrophy. Thus, the sarcopenia seen in the elderly is not just muscle atrophy and differs from the atrophy seen after immobilisation following fracture – however it is accelerated by physical inactivity. It seems that the patient's body mass index (BMI) predicts the degree of sarcopenia [51].
- The muscle mass of the body is a major store of protein. This is a major physiological reserve called upon in critical illness. The "stress response" associated with surgery and critical illness promotes a catabolic state with mobilisation of muscle protein and muscle wasting. Thus the reduced muscle mass found in the elderly shortens and weakens the metabolic defence to illness leading to a worse impact of major surgery and critical illness. In addition the muscle loss in the elderly is from a reduced amount to start with!
- The loss of muscle mass obviously affects muscle strength. At the age of 80 years, muscle strength is approximately 50% what it was at the age of 20 years. One implication of this is that late in life, a large number of elderly people reach low levels of muscle strength that are associated with increasing physical disability. Less well recognised is the prognostic importance of the reduced muscle strength – reduced strength being associated with increased mortality [52] (probably more important prognostically than the loss of muscle mass). In addition, the reduced strength will result in the patient being easily fatigued, poor mobilisation and worsening chest problems associated with being immobile bed.
- With increasing age and muscle loss, an individual's maximal strength for a given everyday activity becomes the same as the minimum required to perform that same everyday activity. Thus, at that threshold, it only takes a small further decline to go from being "just able" to being "just unable" to perform that activity. Many elderly patients effectively are at that threshold.
- The small further decline may be caused by:
    major surgery,
    critical illness with catabolic loss of muscle protein, or
    disuse atrophy associated with immobilisation/bed rest.

- Indeed, a complication which slows progress is liable to have a considerable impact on outcome by prolonging the period of immobilisation, causing further muscle wasting which exacerbates their reduced reserve because of sarcopenia.

Interestingly, obesity does not seem as important a factor in predicting poor outcome as malnutrition and sarcopenia [53]. Whereas obesity leads to increased complications especially respiratory complications and longer length of stay in ICU, a low BMI is a definite predictor of increased risk of mortality.

Monitoring strategies in the elderly surgical patient

Invasive monitoring of elderly surgical patients has revealed a high incidence of "hidden" abnormalities reflecting their reduced physiological reserve even in patients "cleared" for surgery. Invasive monitoring during anaesthesia and in the postoperative period results in early recognition of problems, "fine tuning" of cardiovascular parameters and an improved outcome [54].

Postoperative hypothermia

Postoperative hypothermia has become recognised in recent years as a significant, and common, problem:

- Delayed awakening due to decreased clearance of anaesthetic agents.
- Most organ function is depressed by hypothermia.
- Haemodynamic instability during rewarming – increased fluids often needed as the patient vasodilates during rewarming. The hypotension thus produced can be confused with continued bleeding.
- The VO_2 is increased by about 140% by shivering during rewarming [55]. If oxygen delivery to the tissues is not able to match this increase, the oxygen debt is prolonged.
- Wound infection may be increased by reducing skin blood flow. In addition, cell mediated immune function may be reduced.
- Hypothermia causes coagulopathy and a decrease in platelet count. Intra- and postoperative blood loss is increased with hypothermia, for example, the typical decrease in core temperature during hip replacement increases blood loss by about 500 ml [56]. Normalisation of clotting problems will require normalisation

of temperature as well as giving clotting factors. *Note*: Laboratories perform coagulation studies at 37°C – regardless of the temperature of the patient at the time the sample was taken. Thus, these studies may underestimate the degree of impairment of coagulopathy in the hypothermic patient – what is after all a dynamic problem in vivo rather than in vitro.

- Adrenergic responses are increased postoperatively in hypothermic patients – responsible for increased cardiac morbidity. There is a 55% less relative risk of adverse cardiac events when normothermia is maintained [57].

The degree of hypothermia in many of the studies cited was not that severe – 35°C.

Thus, development of hypothermia after prolonged surgery *is* significant and warrants management in the ICU. Forced warm air rewarming systems seem most effective for rewarming such patients. However, prevention is better than cure!

Possum

This scoring system is of interest in that it was developed specifically to examine the overall perioperative risk of surgical patients.

Possum is an acronym for the *P*hysiological and *O*perative *S*everity *S*core for the *E*numeration of *M*ortality and *M*orbidity. Copeland et al [58] developed this scoring system in 1991 for audit purposes. It requires 12 physiological variables, a number of operative severity score factors and is reliant on outcome for final score and therefore is not suitable for preoperative risk prediction:

- It has mainly been utilised in the UK to date.
- Its main use is to compare hospitals for audit purposes and identify differences between individual surgeons.
- Possum is better than acute physiology and chronic health evaluation II (APACHE II) in predicting mortality in HDU patients [59].
- For colorectal surgery, predicted mortality with possum equals actual mortality but the score may overpredict mortality in low-risk patients and reports suggest it may not predict mortality accurately for ruptured aortic aneurysms or oesophagectomy patients. Modified forms have been developed, for example, for orthopaedic surgery and perhaps it is appropriate for different hospitals to modify its use for different types of surgery. This is exactly the opposite approach to, say, APACHE II scoring systems which are completely standardised with large databases.

FURTHER READING

Biccard BM. Peri-operative beta-blockade and haemodynamic optimisation in patients
    with coronary artery disease and decreasing exercise capacity presenting for major
    noncardiac surgery. *Anaesthesia* 2004; 59: 60–8.
Hanson GC. *Critical Care of the Surgical Patient.* Chapman and Hall, 1997; London.
McConachie I (Ed.). *Anaesthesia for the High Risk Patient.* Greenwich Medical Media, 2002;
    London.

All major textbooks of Anaesthesia will cover many of the topics included in this
chapter.

REFERENCES

1. Pearce AC, Jones RM. Smoking and anesthesia: preoperative abstinence and perioperative morbidity. *Anesthesiology* 1983; 61: 576–84.
2. Report of the American College of Cardiology/American Heart Association Task Force on Practice Guidelines (Committee on Perioperative Cardiovascular Evaluation for Noncardiac Surgery). *Anesth Analg* 1996; 83: 854–60.
3. A report of the American College of Cardiology/American Heart Association Task Force on Practice Guidelines. ACC/AHA Guideline Update for Perioperative Cardiovascular Evaluation for Noncardiac Surgery – Executive Summary. *Anesth Analg* 2002; 94: 1052–64.
4. Juste RN, Lawson AD, Soni N. Minimising cardiac anaesthetic risk: the tortoise or the hare? *Anaesthesia* 1996; 51: 255–62.
5. Slogoff S, Keats A. Does perioperative myocardial ischaemia lead to postoperative myocardial infarction. *Anesthesiology* 1985; 62: 107–14.
6. Rao TLK, Jacobs TH, El-Etr AA. Reinfarction following anesthesia in patients with myocardial infarction. *Anesthesiology* 1983; 59: 499–505.
7. Martinez EA, Pronovost P. Perioperative beta-blockers in high-risk patients. *J Crit Care* 2002; 17: 105–13.
8. Stuhmeier KD, Mainzer B, Cierpka J, Sandmann W et al. Small, oral dose of clonidine reduces the incidence of intraoperative myocardial ischemia in patients having vascular surgery. *Anesthesiology* 1996; 85: 706–12.
9. Bois S, Couture P, Boudreault D, Lacombe P et al. Epidural analgesia and intravenous patient-controlled analgesia result in similar rates of postoperative myocardial ischemia after aortic surgery. *Anesth Analg* 1997; 85: 1233–9.
10. Beattie WS, Badner NH, Choi P. Epidural analgesia reduces postoperative myocardial infarction: a meta-analysis. *Anesth Analg* 2001; 93: 853–8.

11. Relos RP, Hasinoff IK, Beilman GJ. Moderately elevated serum troponin concentrations are associated with increased morbidity and mortality rates in surgical intensive care unit patients. *Crit Care Med* 2003; 31: 2598–603.

12. Ballantyne JC, Carr DB, Chalmers TC, Dear KB et al. Postoperative patient-controlled analgesia: meta-analyses of initial randomized control trials. *J Clin Anesth* 1993; 5: 182–93.

13. Duncan F, Counsell DJ. Analgesia for the high risk patient. In McConachie I (Ed.), *Anaesthesia for the High Risk Patient.* Greenwich Medical Media, 2002; London.

14. *National Health and Medical Research Council Report.* Acute Pain Management: The Scientific Evidence Canberra. NHMRC 1999.

15. Bode Jr RH, Lewis KP, Zarich SW, Pierce ET, Roberts M, Kowalchuk GJ, Satwicz PR, Gibbons GW, Hunter JA, Espanola CC. Cardiac outcome after peripheral vascular surgery. Comparison of general and regional anesthesia. *Anesthesiology* 1996; 84: 3–13.

16. Christopherson R, Beattie C, Frank SM, Norris EJ, Meinert CL, Gottlieb SO, Yates H, Rock P, Parker SD, Perler BA. Perioperative morbidity in patients randomized to epidural or general anesthesia for lower extremity vascular surgery. Perioperative Ischemia Randomized Anesthesia Trial Study Group. *Anesthesiology* 1993; 79: 422–34.

17. Yeager MP, Glass DD, Neff RK, Brinck-Johnsen T. Epidural anesthesia and analgesia in high risk surgical patients. *Anesth Analg* 1987; 66: 729–36.

18. Park WY, Thompson JS, Lee KK. Effect of epidural anesthesia and analgesia on perioperative outcome: a randomized, controlled Veterans Affairs cooperative study. *Ann Surg* 2001; 234: 560–9.

19. Peyton PJ, Myles PS, Silbert BS et al. Perioperative epidural analgesia and outcome after major abdominal surgery in high risk patients. *Anesth Analg* 2003; 96: 548–54.

20. Rodgers A, Walker N, Schug S, McKee A et al. Reduction of postoperative mortality and morbidity with epidural or spinal anaesthesia: results from overview of randomised trials. *Br Med J* 2000; 321: 1493–7.

21. The Veterans Affairs Total Parenteral Nutrition Cooperative Study Group. Perioperative total parenteral nutrition in surgical patients. *New Engl J Med* 1991; 325: 525–32.

22. Buzby GP. Overview of randomized clinical trials of total parenteral nutrition for malnourished surgical patients. *World J Surg* 1993; 17: 173–7.

23. Moore FA, Feliciano DV, Andrassy RJ et al. Early enteral feeding, compared with parenteral, reduces postoperative septic complications. The results of a meta-analysis. *Ann Surg* 1992; 216: 172–83.

24. Lewis SJ, Egger M, Sylvester PA, Thomas S. Early enteral feeding versus "nil by mouth" after gastrointestinal surgery: systematic review and meta-analysis of controlled trials. *Br Med J* 2001; 323: 773–6.

25. Marik PE, Zaloga GP. Meta-analysis of parenteral nutrition versus enteral nutrition in patients with acute pancreatitis. *Br Med J* 2004; 328: 1407.

26. Shoemaker WC, Czer LS. Evaluation of the biologic importance of various hemodynamic and oxygen transport variables: which variables should be monitored in postoperative shock? *Crit Care Med* 1979; 7: 424.

27. Shoemaker WC, Appel PL, Kram HB. Role of oxygen debt in the development of organ failure sepsis, and death in high-risk surgical patients. *Chest* 1992; 102: 208–15.

28. Boyd O, Grounds RM, Bennett ED. A randomized clinical trial of the effect of deliberate perioperative increase of oxygen delivery on mortality in high-risk surgical patients. *J Am Med Assoc* 1993; 270: 2699–707.

29. Shoemaker WC, Appel PL, Kram HB, Waxman K, Lee TS. Prospective trial of supranormal values of survivors as therapeutic goals in high-risk surgical patients. *Chest* 1988; 94: 1176–86.

30. Kern JW, Shoemaker WC. Meta-analysis of hemodynamic optimization in high-risk patients. *Crit Care Med* 2002; 30: 1686–92.

31. Sandham JD, Hull RD, Grant RF et al. A randomised, controlled trial of the use of pulmonary artery catheters in high risk surgical patients. *New Engl J Med* 2003; 348: 5–14.

32. Uusaro A, Russell JA. Could anti-inflammatory actions of catecholamines explain the possible beneficial effects of supranormal oxygen delivery in critically ill surgical patients? *Intens Care Med* 2000; 26: 299–304.

33. Wilson J, Woods I, Fawcett J et al. Reducing the risk of major elective surgery: randomised controlled trial of preoperative optimisation of oxygen delivery. *Br Med J* 1999; 318: 1099.

34. Fenwick E, Wilson J, Sculpher M, Claxton K. Pre-operative optimisation employing dopexamine or adrenaline for patients undergoing major elective surgery: a cost-effectiveness analysis. *Intens Care Med* 2002; 28: 599–608.

35. Stone MD, Wilson RJ, Cross J, Williams BT. Effect of adding dopexamine to intraoperative volume expansion in patients undergoing major elective abdominal surgery. *Br J Anaesth* 2003; 91: 619–24.

36. Takala J, Meier-Hellmann A, Eddleston J, Hulstaert P et al. Effect of dopexamine on outcome after major abdominal surgery: a prospective, randomized, controlled multicenter study. European Multicenter Study Group on Dopexamine in Major Abdominal Surgery. *Crit Care Med* 2000; 28: 3417–23.

37. Burnand KG, Young AE (Eds). *The New Aird's Companion to Surgical Studies.* Churchill Livingstone, London, 1998.

38. Liu SS, Carpenter RL, Mackey DC, Thirlby RC et al. Effects of perioperative analgesic technique on rate of recovery after colon surgery. *Anesthesiology* 1995; 83: 757–65.

39. Vedrinne C, Vedrinne JM, Guiraud M, Patricot MC et al. Nitrogen-sparing effect of epidural administration of local anesthetics in colon surgery. *Anesth Analg* 1989; 69: 354–9.

40. Holte K, Kehlet H. Epidural analgesia and risk of anastomotic leakage. *Reg Anesth Pain Med* 2001; 26: 111–17.

41. Cali RL, Meade PG, Swanson MS et al. Effect of Morphine and incision length on bowel function after colectomy. *Dis Colon Rectum* 2000; 43: 163–8.

42. Morisot P, Loygue J, Guilmet C. Effects of postoperative decurarization with neostigmine on digestive anastomoses. *Can Anaesth Soc J* 1975; 22: 144–8.

43. Hall JC, Tarala RA, Tapper J et al. Prevention of respiratory complications after abdominal surgery: a randomised clinical trial. *Br Med J* 1996; 312: 148–52.

44. Ballantyne JC, Carr DB, de Ferranti S et al. The comparative effects of postoperative analgesic therapies on pulmonary outcome: cumulative meta-analyses of randomized, controlled trials. *Anesth Analg* 1998; 86: 598–612.

45. Tweed WA, Phua WT, Chong KY et al. Large tidal volume ventilation improves pulmonary gas exchange during lower abdominal surgery in Trendelenburg's position. *Can J Anaesth* 1991; 38: 989–95.

46. Pelosi P, Ravagnan I, Giurati G et al. Positive end-expiratory pressure improves respiratory function in obese but not in normal subjects during anesthesia and paralysis. *Anesthesiology* 1999; 91: 1221–31.

47. Pedersen T, Viby-Mogensen J, Ringsted C. Anaesthetic practice and postoperative pulmonary complications. *Acta Anaesthesiol Scand* 1992; 36: 812–18.

48. Oliver CD, White SA, Platt MW. Surgery for fractured femur and elective ICU admission at 113 yr of age. *Brit J Anaesth* 2000; 84(2): 260–2.

49. Djaiani G, Ridley S. Outcome of intensive care in the elderly. *Anaesthesia* 1997; 52: 1130–6.

50. McConachie I. Sarcopenia in the elderly. *CPD Anaesthesia* 2003; 5: 3–6.

51. Iannuzzi-Sucich M, Prestwood KM, Kenny AM. Prevalence of sarcopenia and predictors of skeletal muscle mass in healthy, older men and women. *J Gerontol A Biol Sci Med Sci* 2002; 57: M772–7.

52. Metter EJ, Talbot LA, Schrager M, Conwit R. Skeletal muscle strength as a predictor of all-cause mortality in healthy men. *J Gerontol A Biol Sci Med Sci* 2002; 57: B359–65.

53. Tremblay A, Bandi V. Impact of body mass index on outcomes following critical care. *Chest* 2003; 123: 1202–7.

54. Del Guercio LRN, Cohn JD. Monitoring operative risk in the elderly. *J Am Med Assoc* 1980; 297: 845–50.

55. Frank SM, Fleisher LA, Olson KF, Gorman RB, Higgins MS. Multivariate determinants of early postoperative oxygen consumption in elderly patients. Effects of shivering, body temperature, and gender. *Anesthesiology* 1995; 83: 241–9.

56. Schmied H, Kurz A, Sessler DI, Kozek S, Reiter A. Mild hypothermia increases blood loss and transfusion requirements during total hip arthroplasty. *Lancet* 1996; 347: 289–92.

57. Frank SM, Fleisher LA, Breslow MJ, Higgins MS, Olson KF et al. Perioperative maintenance of normothermia reduces the incidence of morbid cardiac events: a randomised clinical trial. *J Am Med Assoc* 1997; 227: 1127–43.

58. Copeland GP, Jones D, Waiters M. POSSUM: a scoring system for surgical audit. *Br J Surg* 1991; 78: 355–60.

59. Jones DR, Copeland GP, de Cossart L. Comparison of POSSUM with APACHE II for prediction of outcome from a surgical high-dependency unit. *Br J Surg* 1992; 79: 1293–6.

18

The trauma patient

J. Costello

Trauma related deaths typically demonstrate a tri-modal distribution:

- Initial mortality, within 30 min of the traumatic event, (e.g. great vessel rupture, gross cerebral disruption) constitutes 50–60% of all trauma-related deaths.
- 30% constitute deaths within 4 h – usually due to considerable volume loss compounded by ventilatory failure.
- The remainder constitute mortality in the days/weeks following the initial event and is typically due to a combination of multi-organ failure and sepsis.

The notion of "The Golden Hour" suggests active resuscitation within the first hour of trauma impacts positively on mortality.

Epidemiology of trauma

In the UK:

- Trauma cases occupy 850,000 bed nights (Average hospital stay 10–12 days).
- 0.5–1.0 major trauma cases/1000 population/year.
- 75% major trauma cases admitted between 5 p.m. and 8 a.m. (80% <45 years).
- Males constitute 72% of trauma related deaths and 56% of non-fatal injuries.
- Road traffic accidents (RTA) are a major cause of trauma mortality (in the USA, mortality from RTA accounts for 40% of total trauma mortality).
- UK has the highest paediatric RTA rate in the world.

Trauma death rates per million of population/per annum:

- UK 88/18,000.
- US 111/165,000.

Trauma is the third commonest cause of death in all age groups (UK and US) and the commonest cause of death in <45-year-old age group.

One quarter of survivors from trauma have a disability lasting 6 months or longer and in the USA, there are 80,000 new patients with major permanent disability per year.

RTA

- Most RTA involve one (or more) of: speed, alcohol, non-restraint.
- Restraints offer 75% efficiency rate in prevention of fatality and 50% fatal head injuries could be avoided by use of such restraints.
- Bicycle crashes and Motorcycle RTA account for 1200 and 5000 fatalities every year (respectively) in the USA (Head Injury accounts for 85% of these deaths).
- 60% of RTA involve alcohol excess.

Mechanism of injury in the multiple injured patient

Penetration injury

- Common in the USA.
- Usually an isolated injury requiring definitive surgery.
- Amount of tissue damage is proportional to the object velocity as the kinetic energy of the object is transferred to the surrounding tissues.
- $KE = M \times V(squared)/2$ (KE: Kinetic Energy; M: Mass; V: Velocity).
- Missile velocity has a greater impact than missile mass.
- Surface area and density of affected tissues are important determinants of degree of tissue "cavitation" caused.

High velocity objects demonstrate a biphasic mode of tissue damage.

- The initial "positive" shock wave ("temporary pulsating cavity").
- The secondary "negative" aftershock (negative pressure phase).

The former involves "stretch/shear" the latter involves "disruption/extravasation".

Blunt injuries

- Common in the UK.
- Usually associated with multiple injuries (surgery frequently not definitive).

- Kinetic energy is transferred into shock waves (or "force").
- $F = M \times V/T$ (F: Force; M: Mass; V: Velocity change; T: Time interval).
- Blunt trauma force may be external (fall, RTA, Assault) or internal (compression, deceleration).

Blast injuries

These involve rapid transformation of small volumes of media (gas, solid, liquid) into expanding gaseous products. Energy transfer occurs as pressure waves induce oscillation in the media through which it travels.

- *Primary Blast Injuries* due to direct effect of pressure waves and are most injurious to gas containing organs (ears, lung, eyes, bowel).
- *Secondary Blast Injuries* are due to flying debris (thus usually penetrating).
- *Tertiary Blast Injuries* result in victim as missile (thus usually blunt).

Pathophysiology of trauma

Neuroendocrine response

Brainstem sympathetic outflow results in

- Increased Chronotropy, Inotropy and systemic vascular resistance.
- Increased Glucagon production and Lipolysis.
- Reduced Insulin synthesis.

Respiratory response

Respiration is initially compromised in trauma by a combination of "Direct" (blunt, penetrating, inhalational injury) and "Indirect" (hypovolemia, sepsis, over zealous fluid administration) insults.

Renal response

Hypovolemia results in reduced organ perfusion (mediated by Aldosterone and ADH).

Immunomodulation

Cytokine mediated cascade of pro-inflammatory mediators result in ion-pump dysfunction (cellular oedema), cellular dys-motility (leucocyte responsiveness to stress hormones) and cell death. This ultimately leads to over-whelming sepsis, systemic inflammatory response syndrome (SIRS) and multi-organ dysfunction syndrome (MODS) (see Chapter 22) and subsequent acute respiratory distress syndrome (ARDS), disseminated intravascular coagulation (DIC), Hepato-renal failure.

Note: Sepsis still accounts for three quarters of late mortality in the multiple injured patient.

Severity of illness trauma "scoring systems"

Whenever possible, level of risk (and outcome) should be assessed on a continuous basis as this has implications for clinical management decisions, cost and resource utility.

Trauma scoring systems (see further reading for references)

- Glasgow Coma Scale (GCS) – primarily for neurological status in Head Injuries.
- Trauma Score.
- Trauma Index.
- CRAMS scale (*C*irculation, *R*espiratory, *A*bdominal, *M*otor, *S*peech).
- Abbreviated Injury Scale (AIS).
- Injury Severity Score (ISS).
- The trauma and injury severity score (TRISS) Methodology.
- Pediatric Trauma Score.

The Trauma Score combines GCS with cardio-respiratory indices (systolic blood pressure (BP) and respiratory rate). The Trauma Index is primarily a pre-hospital tool incorporating injury (type and location) and indices of function (cardio-respiratory and neurological).

CRAMS constitutes a simplified "trauma score" for pre-hospital use but carries poor overall sensitivity. The AIS is a crude anatomical-based scoring system applied to blunt trauma patients but also carries poor sensitivity. The ISS, also, is based on anatomical systems incorporating AIS but is complex in application.

TRISS Methodology combines the revised trauma score ("RTS") with the ISS to provide a standard approach for evaluating outcome of trauma care and is primarily used in quality assessment reviews (applicable to all trauma types). Mortality from trauma depends on the degree of physio-anatomical derangement, age fit and type of injury. TRISS Methodology combines these to provide a measure of the survival probability.

These scoring systems have little predictive purpose during the intensive care unit (ICU) episode and do not aid clinical decision-making. Accrued mortality estimates are reviewed retrospectively thus they have little practical application. However some authors suggest such scoring systems complement ongoing management and concurrent non-trauma score systems.

Trauma scoring systems have been recently reviewed [1].

The concept of traumatic shock

Advanced trauma life support (ATLS) teaching and the RTS [2] emphasise the importance of monitoring progressive changes in heart rate and BP in the injured patient. This does not always happen in the multiple injured patient.

Heart rate

- Heart rate is thought to be of poor value in the assessment of traumatic hypovolemia [3].
- Evidence suggests the biphasic response of heart rate [4] (i.e. bradycardia following tachycardia depends on the injury type). Concomitant direct tissue injury attenuates the magnitude of the bradycardic response to severe "simple" blood loss (variceal rupture, vessel penetration) thus concealing the true extent of hypovolemia [5].

BP

- BP is usually maintained until a deficit of approximately 30% blood volume (Class 3 Shock). Earlier progressive blood loss is suggested by a drop in pulse pressure (Class 2 Shock)[6].
- In trauma, such alterations are unpredictable and delayed due to injury-induced endogenous pressor response and reduced sensitivity to baro-receptor reflex involving "nociceptive" stimuli [7].

This attenuation of cardiovascular response may offer some degree of protection against the effects of hypovolemia. However, animal studies have shown that induced blood loss and concomitant electrical nerve stimulation (to simulate injury) resulted in lower Cardiac Index (CI), systemic oxygen delivery (DO_2) and higher mortality than that of simple blood loss alone.

Assessment of the trauma patient

ATLS teaching is one of many accepted systems enabling a stepwise approach to management of the trauma patient and is followed here; although other management tools exist, historically they have received little attention.

"Team Leaders" in trauma should be ATLS trained. Designation of responsibilities to "team members" (prior to arrival of the injured patient) enables coordinated and prioritised approach. Enlist additional/senior help in the case of multiple victims.

Immediate priority

Detect and treat immediately life-threatening injuries in the order of:

- Airway (and C-Spine) → Resuscitate.
- Breathing (and Ventilation) → Resuscitate.
- Circulation → Resuscitate.

Concurrent team management of these systems is usual and to be expected.

Airway (and C-Spine)

Airway must be immediately assessed. If not patent, definitive airway must be established by intubation (oral, nasal or fibreoptic) or surgical (cricothyroidotomy in the emergent setting) means.

*R*apid *S*equence *I*nduction (RSI) (and *I*ntubation) following preoxygenation is frequently employed in the emergency setting of trauma but has been associated with 1–2% failure rate especially if performed by inexperienced practitioners. Strategies to deal with failed intubation should be tailored towards use in the Emergency department [8].

Cricoid pressure to reduce the risk of aspiration of stomach contents should be performed.

Intubation during C-Spine precaution necessitates in-line manual immobilisation. Routine use of a gum elastic bougie is recommended as poor laryngeal views are frequent. It is difficult to find good evidence that this technique, properly performed, has resulted in *additional* neurological impairment in any trauma patient with cervical spine injury. Neurological signs should be documented before intubation, if possible.

Other options include nasal or fibreoptic intubation but there are pitfalls in the use of such techniques in the trauma patient.

Fibreoptic awake intubation	Nasal intubation
Unfamiliar technique for most	Increased failure rate
practitioners	Epistaxis
Uncooperative or obtunded	Bacteraemia
patient	Potentially greater C-Spine movement.

Surgical airway is indicated if the above fail and requires personnel trained in its application.

C-Spine injuries occur in 2–12% of blunt trauma cases [9], in up to 20% of serious head injuries [10] and 1 in 300 RTAs [11]. The reported incidence of missed (or delayed diagnosis) cervical C-Spine injuries is said to be 4.6% [12] – with potentially up to 30% incidence of secondary neurological deficit in those patients.

There are no controlled trials comparing methods of C-Spine handling with radiological evaluation thus current standards of care (guidelines) are based on level two or three evidence.

- High levels of radiographic misinterpretation still exist.
- Always assume C-Spine injury in the trauma victim. Application of hard collar (or) side support blocks is mandatory until clinical/radiological screening is complete.
- Always immobilise C-Spine if injury mechanism is suspicious, if history is inadequate or victim communication is poor. Loss of (or) deficit in consciousness is predictive of unstable C-Spine injury [9].
- Hard collar application may increase intracranial pressure (ICP) in the head injured patient and is thus not considered an absolute requirement in the adequately sedated head injury patient who has normal plain radiography. Hard collars provide incomplete immobilisation, may utilise excess staff resource and cause tissue ulceration and necrosis.
- Plain Radiography (at least) is required in patients with GCS <15 [13], sedative drug or alcohol co-ingestion or distracting pain [14].
- If victim is uncooperative/agitated (head injury, shock, hypoxia) forced restraint is ill advised. Abandonment of manual immobilisation, victim reassurance

and reversal of obvious causes (fluid, oxygen) should be initiated. Allow the collar to remain in-situ to prevent extremes of movement. If this fails, consideration should be given to RSI [14].

- In the vomiting victim, a head-down tilt is ideal (even in the head-injured patient). Other options would include coordinated log-roll or spinal board-board tilt [14].

Once definitive airway is established, C-Spine can only be fully cleared when the patient regains consciousness.

Current guidelines suggest awaiting successful weaning before formal C-Spine assessment, particularly if consciousness is anticipated within 48 h.

If intubation is expected for >48 h satisfactory clearance of C-Spine should be actively sought by:

- Additional plain radiography [13].
- Plain radiography with computerised tomography (CT) of C1–C3 (false negative rate <0.1%) [14].
- Plain radiography with dynamic fluoroscopy/stress views.
- Magnetic Resonance Imaging [15].
- National guidelines for CT of C-Spine exist [16] but compliance is questionable and reliability remains to be established [17].

Considerable variation still exists in relation to C-Spine management between individual ICUs [18].

A recent review in Anaesthesia gives a thoughtful review of cervical spine immobilisation in the ICU – especially with regard to its limitations and complications [19]. The reader is also strongly recommended to read the recent British medical association (BMA) review article by Morris on spinal immobilisation for unconscious patients with multiple injuries cited in the *Further Reading* section. The authors suggest that the risks of prolonged immobilisation beyond 48–72 h exceed the risks of a serious missed cervical spine injury after normal plain film and CT studies.

Breathing (and ventilation)

Immediate administration of high flow oxygen (with reservoir) to all trauma patients is essential.

Adequate ventilation is determined by patency of airway and lung/diaphragm/chest wall function.

Immediate life-threatening causes of inadequate ventilation include:

- tension pneumothorax,
- flail chest (with pulmonary contusion),
- open pneumothorax,
- massive haemothorax,
  - all should be immediately recognised and resuscitated during the primary survey.

If doubt exists, it is safer to opt for elective intubation and ventilation.

Circulation (and haemorrhage control)

Haemorrhage is the commonest cause of preventable trauma-related mortality

- Assume hypotension is due to blood loss.
- Control obvious external haemorrhage immediately.

Assessment of circulation is by:

- Non-invasive indices (pulse, BP, skin colour, temperature, level of consciousness).
- Invasive indices (Central venous and arterial cannulation, Urine output).
- Normal pulse and BP does not always suggest normovolemia (see earlier) – especially in the elderly, multi-medicated or young trauma victim.

Immediate resuscitation requires at least two large bore cannulae with large volume warmed infusion. Due consideration must be given to "concealed" blood loss (up to 4 units from femoral fractures).

ATLS guidelines suggest blood transfusion is indicated if bolus intravenous crystalloid (or colloid) is ineffective. Cross-matched, Type specific and Group O negative is administered (in order of emergent priority).

The crystalloid/colloid debate continues and is discussed further in Chapter 5. Two litres (Crystalloid) or one litre (Colloid) is the accepted initial bolus in adult trauma prior to consideration of blood transfusion. (APLS teaching suggests blood product administration subsequent to 2×20 ml/kg bolus' crystalloid/colloid in paediatric trauma patients).

The use of at least one manufacturer's rapid infusion device has been shown [20] to be beneficial compared to standard fluid administration – resulting in less fluid required and less coagulopathy (both thought to be due to efficient heating of the fluids and less patient hypothermia).

The role of hypertonic crystalloid in trauma has gained popularity owing to

- positive mortality outcome,
- improved cardiac efficiency and (DO_2),
- improved immunologic function.

Its incorporation into practice, however, is not widespread in the UK.

Massive administration of blood product/fluid (dilutional coagulopathy), hypothermia (disruption of clotting cascade and platelet disruption) and head injury (neural thromboplastin release) all add to "traumatic coagulopathy". Transfusion of platelets, cryoprecipitate or fresh frozen plasma (FFP) should be guided by baseline coagulation parameters taken initially.

It is currently not advised to empirically administer such blood products unless a known coagulation disorder (or history of anticoagulant medication) exists [21].

Note: Blood transfusion requirement is an independent predictor of mortality, ICU admission and length of stay (ICU and Total Hospital) [22].

Permissive hypovolemia/hypotension

Bickell [23] suggested a survival benefit associated with "delayed" fluid resuscitation in cases of penetrating trauma (with presentations suggestive of hypovolemia).

Theoretical benefits (as suggested by animal studies) include:

- reduced rupture of microvasculature clot tamponades,
- reduced dilutional coagulopathy,
- increased haemoviscosity,
- reduced "hydraulic acceleration" of haemorrhage.

Clinical parameters suggest limiting fluid resuscitation to achieve a Mean arterial pressure (MAP) of approximately 50 mmHg until definitive surgical control of haemorrhage; thereafter, resuscitation is suggested as outlined in ATLS.

This approach is not favoured for many patients owing to:

- The false assumption of prompt surgical resource deployment. The patients will need *prompt* definitive intervention to minimise the oxygen debt. Delays in surgery for example in rural area may be better with "normal" resuscitation.
- Isolated penetrating torso trauma comprising the minority of all trauma cases.
- Inapplicability in the context of coexistent head injury.
- Equivocal therapeutic utility [24].

The biggest problem is that this study was performed in penetrating injuries. Patients with blunt trauma (the majority) are not so likely to have definitive surgical interventions.

Differences between blunt and penetrating trauma

Penetrating	Blunt
Common in the USA	Commoner in Europe
Often sole injury	Not usually in isolation
Diagnosis often simple	Diagnosis often complex
Surgery often definitive treatment	Surgery rarely definitive

Therefore, this approach is not recommended in patients suffering blunt trauma.

It would be unfortunate if improvements in trauma management related to an understanding of the importance of rapid resuscitation (the "Golden hour" concept) with volume infusion as a cornerstone of that resuscitation were lost because fluid restriction was seen as appropriate in any but a few specific (and uncommon) circumstances.

Resuscitation indices

Non-invasive

- BP Trend (includes pulse pressure).
- Heart Rate.
- Temperature.
- Level of consciousness.
- Urine Output.

Invasive

- Central Venous Catheterisation.
- Pulmonary Artery Flotation Catheter.
- Arterial Catheter.

Invasive indices are usually required if there is no resolution with current management. A lower threshold for instituting invasive monitoring should be adopted in the case of trauma in the elderly, blunt chest trauma or haemorrhagic shock.

Scalea [25] showed a 40% mortality reduction in cases of elderly blunt trauma with early invasive monitoring. Similar trends are reported in the younger population [26]. The improvements are thought to arise from early identification of occult low cardiac outputs which, if not promptly reversed, result in the development of organ failures.

Adequacy of resuscitation

Non-invasive goals

Normalisation of non-invasive goals is ideal although these may not always reflect the true status (see earlier).

Increase	Decrease
BP	Heart rate
Urine output	
Consciousness	

Invasive goals

The therapeutic goal must be to optimise tissue oxygenation.

The magnitude of the oxygen deficit is a key factor in determining outcome in patients with haemorrhagic or cardiogenic shock – see also Chapter 1.

Indices of systemic oxygen transport (CI, DO_2, Oxygen Consumption (VO_2)) provide the most direct measurement of resuscitative progress. Maintenance of adequate oxygen transport is thought to reduce endothelial hypoxia-induced inflammatory cascade activation ("the oxygen debt").

- Most studies relate to mortality reduction in critically ill surgical or septic patients, but evidence does also suggest benefit in the multiply injured [27].
- "Goal-directed therapy" has received criticism but it is thought that in some situations failure of this approach may be due to delay in achieving the goals.
- Mixed Venous Saturation is becoming an important component of goal-directed therapy [28] and may have a role in the multiple injured patient.
- Blood Lactate increases in proportion to the systemic oxygen deficit and is indicative of supply dependency of systemic VO_2 and of prognostic value in severe trauma. Similarly, Base Deficit correlates well with injury severity and outcome [29].

- The measurement of gastric mucosal pH (pHi) may be of benefit but has received little attention in the context of trauma [30].

Thoracic trauma

Europe and the USA demonstrate a predominance of blunt and penetrating chest trauma respectively.

Chest trauma carries an overall 10% mortality (in-hospital mortality is 5% and rises to approximately 33% in severe multi-system trauma) and surgical intervention is required in 15%.

The severity of the injury predicts clinical course and outcome [31].

Thoracic trauma profile

Six life-threatening injuries must be immediately identified and treated in the primary survey.

- Airway Obstruction.
- Tension Pneumothorax.
- Open Haemothorax (Sucking chest wound).
- Massive Haemothorax.
- Cardiac Tamponade.
- Flail Chest.

Immediate management

- Ensure patent airway (definitive if required) and administer oxygen.
- Immediate needle decompression if suspecting tension pneumothorax.
- Obtain vascular access.
- Intercostal drain placement subsequent to needle decompression *or* for suspected or confirmed pneumothorax (apical placement) or haemothorax (basal placement).
- Tube placement may occasionally not initially be required owing to delayed presentation or small size traumatic pneumothorax.

Beck's Triad consists of elevated jugular venous pressure (JVP), hypotension, muffled heart sounds, Kussmaul's sign and pulsus paradoxus. Patients may have normal cardiac silhouettes on Chest X-rays (CXR). This may occur with Cardiac Tamponade, Tension Pneumothorax, Myocardial dysfunction or Systemic Air

Embolism. Pericardiocentesis of as little of 5 mls in Cardiac Tamponade may temporarily augment stroke volume by 25–50%.

Six "potentially" life-threatening injuries are usually identified in the secondary survey.

- Aortic Disruption.
- Myocardial Contusion.
- Pulmonary Contusion.
- Traumatic Diaphragmatic Rupture.
- Tracheobronchial Disruption.
- Oesophageal Disruption.

A detailed discussion on recognition and management of the above is out with the scope of this text.

Indications for emergency thoracotomy

Cardiac arrest

Emergency Thoracotomy may be appropriate for victims with penetrating chest trauma with witnessed signs of life during transport or in the emergency department and at least cardiac electrical activity on arrival [32]. However, there is no general consensus on what "signs of life" constitute. They may include any combination of palpable pulse, BP, reactive pupils, corneal reflex, gag reflex or respiratory effort.

ATLS Guidelines suggest thoracotomy is indicated for penetrating chest trauma with PEA (pulseless electrical activity).

Note: Animal studies show that external cardiac massage is ineffective at providing organ perfusion if preload is reduced that is external cardiopulmonary resuscitation (CPR) is unlikely to be successful in cases of exsanguinations [33].

For blunt trauma, some authors suggest thoracotomy is only indicated if signs of life are present at least on patient arrival. However, ATLS guidance recommends that thoracotomy is *not indicated* in cases of blunt trauma irrespective of the existence of PEA.

Massive haemothorax

This constitutes less than 5% of all haemothoraces. Thoracotomy is indicated if initial blood loss (per drain) is >200 mls/hr or >1.5 litres on immediate chest tube placement.

Cardiac tamponade

Emergency Thoracotomy is indicated only if haemodynamically unstable with suspected penetrating myocardial injury.

Contusional injuries

Blunt myocardial injury

This is usually suggested by:

- mechanism of injury (accelerative-decelerative or compressive);
- examination (arrhythmia, isolated tachycardia, cardiac failure, any part of Beck's Triad) radiography (increased cardiac silhouette, high rib fractures);
- electrocardiographic (ST anomalies, conduction abnormalities that may mimic Myocardial Infarction).

Adverse outcome is rare [34]. Conservative management is the norm.

Pulmonary contusion

- Occurs in 20% of blunt trauma cases with ISS of 15 or higher.
- 85% present within 6 h (95% within 1 day).
- Over half present with haemoptysis.
- Overzealous fluid administration may result in lung injury – judicious use is advised.
- Typically no ventilatory support is required if <10% lung volume involved.

Management should include:

- Humidified oxygen therapy.
- Chest physiotherapy.
- Incentive spirometry.
- Intercostal nerve block or Epidural analgesia.

The role of ventilatory support

- Ventilatory support is typically required if >30% lung volume is involved.
- 40–60% ultimately require ventilatory support [35].

- Prognosis is variable and mortality rates vary between 40–60% – largely dependent on the presence of other injuries and the degree of parenchymal injury as reflected by the impairment of oxygenation.

Chest wall injuries

Rib injuries

- 50% not seen on X-ray. 90% are associated with other injuries.
- High rib fractures are associated with poor outcome (usually associated with head injury or great vessel rupture).
- Low rib fracture is associated with viscus damage – in multi-trauma, CT abdomen should be considered.
- Elderly patients admitted after rib fractures have increased mortality even after taking comorbidities into account.

The management goal is:

- to detect significant complications such as haemopneumothorax, pulmonary contusion, vascular injury,
- to provide adequate analgesia.

Analgesic options include:

- Oral analgesia (non-steroidal anti-inflammatory drugs (NSAIDs), opiate-based analgesia).
- Intravenous patient-controlled analgesia.
- Regional anaesthesia (intercostal, intrapleural, epidural). Epidural analgesia is generally considered to be superior [36].

Flail chest

This is a clinical diagnosis. The pathophysiological insult includes parenchymal contusion, impaired compliance and intrapulmonary shunting resulting in reduced vital capacity.

There are three grades of severity:

- *Grade 1*: Can ventilate and cough/no associated injuries.
- *Grade 2*: Cannot cough/Has other injuries.

These are managed by combination of analgesia, physiotherapy and fluid restriction.

- *Grade 3*: Hypoxia, exhausted, multiple injuries, elderly.

These require ventilation.

Up to 50% are managed conservatively. The remainder require ventilation. Many will require an intercostal drain.

Progress is evaluated by:

- Repeated clinical assessment and examination.
- Arterial blood gas analysis.
- Serial vital capacity measurements.

Indications for early ventilation in flail chest

- Shock.
- Three associated injuries.
- Severe Head Injuries.
- Co-Morbid Lung disease.
- Eight Rib fractures.
- 65 years of age.

Ciraulo et al [37] suggests the degree of contusion as the best guide to estimating requirement for ventilatory support and emphasises that flail chest is a marker of high kinetic energy absorption.

Surgical fixation of flail segment remains controversial.

Operative intervention

- Many trauma patients will need surgery.
- In general, all the required surgical procedures should be performed acutely that is during one anaesthetic providing the patient has been appropriately resuscitated and is haemodynamically stable.
- The rationale is that, once the patient is resuscitated, the patient may be in the best condition that he will be in for some time that is before the development of sepsis, tissue oedema, malnutrition and metabolic complications.
- Delayed fixation of long bone fractures may increase the incidence of ARDS [38]. The mechanisms are uncertain but probably include ongoing bleeding, increased pain and physiological stress response and possible fat embolus.

- Conversely if the patient undergoing surgery *is* unstable, with developing hypothermia, coagulopathy and acidosis, prolonged surgery has a high mortality. Many surgeons now accept that the best way to manage these patients is to "bail out" for example pack the abdomen to stop bleeding, bring out bowel ends on to the abdominal wall etc. and take the patient to ICU for stabilisation and further resuscitation. Further surgical intervention is deferred to a later date. This has been described as "damage control surgery" [39].
- Blood clots, packing the abdomen, ileus and tissue oedema all, however, contribute to the development of an abdominal compartment syndrome where the increase in pressure literally squeezes the kidney. This causes a reduction in renal blood flow, glomerular filtration rate (GFR), direct compression of the renal parenchyma and increased release of ADH and Aldosterone from stimulation of abdominal wall stretch receptors. In general intra abdominal pressures of 15–20 mmHg are associated with oliguria while pressures greater than 30 mmHg may be associated with anuria.
- Interestingly, the use of large volumes of fluids in an attempt to achieve supranormal resuscitation goals has been shown to be associated with an increased incidence of abdominal compartment syndrome [40]. This variant of abdominal compartment syndrome has been called secondary compartment syndrome.

Injury associated organ failures and outcome

- Patients admitted to ICU following multiple injuries often have a protracted length of stay, duration of intermittent positive pressure ventilation (IPPV) and consume a lot of resources [41].
- Isolated pulmonary contusion in young trauma patients has a good prognosis [42].
- One study [43] found flail chest and pulmonary contusion to both be associated with approximately 16% mortality. The mortality was increased to approximately 42% if they were combined in the same patient.
- Length of stay and mortality are increased in the elderly trauma patient with a greater proportion requiring chronic care following discharge from ICU.
- Young trauma patients have a better prognosis and, those who survive, have a good prospect of rehabilitation and a fairly good ultimate outcome.
- Pelvic fractures in the elderly are of greater significance than in younger patients and are more likely to be associated with death [44].

- Delayed fixation of fractures has already been noted to be associated with the development of ARDS [38]. Later work has shown that early fixation of femur fractures (<24 hrs) is associated with better outcomes – even in patients with other head and chest injuries [45].

- Development of sepsis and multiple organ failure is responsible for much of the late mortality. Recently, it has been shown that single organ failure is associated with a good outcome – mortality being more related to the underlying injury [46]. It seems that the mortality for multiple organ failure may be less than what it was 15–20 years ago. However, mortality for patients with four or more organ failure remains almost 100% [46].

- The development of ARDS in trauma patients is associated with a prolonged ICU stay but, surprisingly is not a factor in a worse outcome – outcome being more closely linked to injury severity [47].

- Studies on tight glucose control and avoidance of hyperglycaemia (see Chapter 22) have been repeated in trauma patients [48]. Early hyperglycemia is associated with significantly higher infection and mortality rates independent of the injury.

- In many patients with multiple injury the single most crucial factor in predicting their outcome is the extent of their neurological injury.

FURTHER READING

Emergency Medicine – A Comprehensive Study Guide. 6th edn. American College of Emergency Physicians. McGraw Hill, 2004.

Morris CG, McCoy W, Lavery G. Spinal immobilisation for unconscious patients with multiple injuries. *Br Med J* 2004; 329: 495–9.

Scaletta TA, Schaider, JJ. *Emergent Management of Trauma.* 2nd edn. McGraw Hill, 2001.

TARN (The Trauma Audit and Research Network). www.tarn.ac.uk

REFERENCES

1. Chawda MN, Hildebrand F, Pape HC, Giannoudis PV. Predicting outcome after multiple trauma: which scoring system? *Injury* 2004; 35: 347–58.
2. Champion HR, Sacco WJ, Copes WS. A revision of the trauma score. *J Trauma* 1989; 29: 623–9.
3. Little RA, Kirkman E, Driscoll P. Preventable deaths after injury: why are the traditional "vital" signs poor indicators of blood loss? *J Acc Emerg Med* 1995; 12: 1–14.

4. Little RA. Heart rate changes after haemorrhage and injury – a reappraisal. *J Trauma* 1989; 29: 903–6.

5. Little RA, Marshall HW, Kirkman E. Attenuation of the acute cardiovascular responses to haemorrhage by tissue injury in the conscious rat. *Quart J Exp Physiol* 1989; 74: 825–33.

6. American College of Surgeons. Committee on Trauma 1997. *Advanced Life Support Course for Physicians,* (6th edn.) American college of Surgeons, Chicago.

7. Anderson ID, Little RA, Irving MH. An effect of trauma on human cardiovascular control: baroreflex suppression. *J Trauma* 1990; 30: 174–82.

8. Carley SD, Gwinnutt C, Butler J. Rapid sequence induction in the emergency department: a strategy for failure. *J Emerg Med* 2002; 19: 109–13.

9. Ross SE, O'Malley RF, de Long WG. Clinical predictors of unstable cervical spine injury in the multiply injured patient. *Injury* 1992; 23: 317–19.

10. Rockswold GL. Evaluation and resuscitation in head trauma. *Minn Med* 1981; 64: 81–4.

11. Heulke DF, O'Day J. Cervical injuries suffered in automobile crashes. *J Neurosurg* 1981; 54: 316–22.

12. Davis JW, Phreaner DC, Hoyt DB. The etiology of missed cervical spine injuries. *J Trauma* 1993; 34: 342–6.

13. MacDonald RL, Schwartz ML. Diagnosis of c-spine injury in motor vehicle crash victims: how many X-rays are enough? *J Trauma* 1990; 30: 392–7.

14. Kirshenbaum KJ, Nadimpalli SR. Unsuspected upper c-spine fractures associated with significant head trauma: role of CT. *J Emerg Med* 1990; 8: 183–98.

15. Benzel EC, Hart BL, Ball PA. Magnetic resonance imaging for the evaluation of patients with occult c-spine injury. *J Neurosurg* 1996; 85: 824–9.

16. NICE Guidelines. Head injury in infants, children and adults: triage, assessment, investigation and early management 2002. www.nice.org.uk

17. Dickenson G, Steill IG, Schull M. Retrospective application of the NEXUS low – risk criteria for cervical spine radiography in Canadian emergency departments. *Ann Emerg Med* 2004; 43: 507–14.

18. Gupta KJ, Clancy M. Discontinuation of cervical spine immobilisation in unconscious patients with trauma in intensive care units. Telephone survey of practice in the south and west region. *Br Med J* 1997; 314: 1652–5.

19. Morris CG, McCoy E. Cervical immobilisation collars in ICU: friend or foe? *Anaesthesia* 2003; 58:1051–3.

20. Dunham CM, Belzberg H, Lyles R, Weireter L et al. The rapid infusion system: a superior method for the resuscitation of hypovolemic trauma patients. *Resuscitation.* 1991; 21: 207–27.

21. DeLoughery TG. Coagulation defects in trauma patients: etiology, recognition and therapy. *Crit Care Clin* 2004; 20: 13–24.

22. Malone DL, Dunne J, Tracy JK. Blood transfusion, independent of shock severity, is associated with worse outcome in trauma. *J Trauma* 2003; 54: 898–905.

23. Bickell WH, Wall MJ, Pepe PE. Immediate versus delayed fluid resuscitation for hypotensive patients with penetrating torso injuries. *New Engl J Med* 1994; 331: 1105–9.

24. Dutton RP, MacKenzie CF, Scalea TM. Hypotensive resuscitation during active hemorrhage: impact on in-hospital mortality. *J Trauma* 2002; 52: 1141–6.

25. Scalea TM, Simon HM, Duncan AO. Geriatric blunt multiple trauma: improved survival with early invasive monitoring. *J Trauma* 1990; 30: 129–34.

26. Abou-Khalil B, Scalea TM, Trooskin SZ. Haemodynamic response to shock in young trauma patients: need for invasive monitoring. *Crit Care Med* 1994; 22: 633–9.

27. Bishop MH, Shoemaker WC, Appel PL. Prospective randomised trial of survivor values of cardiac index, oxygen delivery and oxygen consumption as resuscitation endpoints in severe trauma. *J Trauma* 1995; 38: 780–7.

28. Polenen P, Ruokenen E, Hippelainen M. A prospective randomised study of goal oriented hemodynamic therapy in cardiac surgical patients. *Anesth Analg* 2000; 90: 1052–9.

29. Rutherford EJ, Morris Jr JA, Reed GW, Hall KS. Base deficit stratifies mortality and determines therapy. *J Trauma* 1992; 33: 417–23.

30. Ivatury RR, Simon RJ, Havriliak D. Gastric mucosal pH and oxygen consumption indices in the assessment of adequacy of resuscitation after trauma: a prospective, randomised study. *J Trauma* 1995; 39: 128–34.

31. Richter M, Ketteck C, Otte D. Correlation between crash severity, injury severity and clinical course in car occupants with thoracic trauma: a technical and medical study. *J Trauma* 2001; 50: 10–16.

32. Branney SW, Moore EE, Feedhaus KM. Critical analysis of two decades of experience with post injury emergency department thoracotomy in a regional trauma center. *J Trauma* 1998; 45: 87–94.

33. Luna GK, Pavlin EG, Kirkman T, Copass MK et al. Hemodynamic effects of external cardiac massage in trauma shock. *J Trauma* 1989; 29: 1430–3.

34. Maenza RL, Scaberg D, D'Amico F. A meta-analysis of blunt cardiac trauma: Ending myocardial confusion. *Am J Emerg Med* 1996; 14: 237–41.

35. Miller PR, Croce MA, Bee TK. ARDS after pulmonary contusions: accurate measurement of contusion volume identifies high-risk patients. *J Trauma* 2001; 51: 223–8.

36. Luchette FA, Rudfshar MR, Kaiser R. Prospective evaluation of epidural versus intrapleural catheters for analgesia in chest wall trauma. *J Trauma* 1994; 36: 865–9.

37. Ciraulo DL, Elliott D, Mitchell KA. Flail chest as a marker for significant injuries. *J Am Coll Surg* 1994; 178: 466–70.

38. Johnson KD, Cadambi A, Seibert GB. Incidence of adult respiratory distress syndrome in patients with multiple musculoskeletal injuries: effect of early operative stabilization of fractures. *J Trauma* 1985; 25: 375–84.

39. Hirshberg A, Mattox KL. "Damage control" in trauma surgery. *Br J Surg* 1993; 80: 1501–2.

40. Balogh Z, McKinley BA, Cocanour CS, Kozar RA et al. Supranormal trauma resuscitation causes more cases of abdominal compartment syndrome. *Arch Surg* 2003; 138: 637–42.

41. Goins WA, Reynolds HN, Nyanjom D, Dunham CM. Outcome following prolonged intensive care unit stay in multiple trauma patients. *Crit Care Med* 1991; 19: 339–45.

42. Hoff SJ, Shotts SD, Eddy VA, Morris Jr JA. Outcome of isolated pulmonary contusion in blunt trauma patients. *Am Surg* 1994; 60: 138–42.

43. Clark GC, Schecter WP, Trunkey DD. Variables affecting outcome in blunt chest trauma: flail chest vs. pulmonary contusion. *J Trauma* 1988; 28: 298–304.

44. O'brien DP, Luchette FA, Pereira SJ, Lim E et al. Pelvic fracture in the elderly is associated with increased mortality. *Surgery* 2002; 132: 710–4.

45. Brundage SI, McGhan R, Jurkovich GJ, Mack CD et al. Timing of femur fracture fixation: effect on outcome in patients with thoracic and head injuries. *J Trauma* 2002; 52: 299–307.

46. Durham RM, Moran JJ, Mazuski JE, Shapiro MJ et al. Multiple organ failure in trauma patients. *J Trauma* 2003; 55: 608–16.

47. Treggiari MM, Hudson LD, Martin DP, Weiss NS et al. Effect of acute lung injury and acute respiratory distress syndrome on outcome in critically ill trauma patients. *Crit Care Med* 2004; 32: 327–31.

48. Laird AM, Miller PR, Kilgo PD, Meredith JW et al. Relationship of early hyperglycemia to mortality in trauma patients. *J Trauma* 2004; 56: 1058–62.

19

Acute coronary syndromes

R. Beynon and D.H. Roberts

Acute myocardial ischaemic events provide a large portion of the workload of hospitals in the developed world. Presentations may vary from an acute ST elevation myocardial infarction (STEMI) with chest pain to an asymptomatic perioperative event picked up on enzyme rise.

With the advent of new, more sensitive biochemical tests (troponins) many patients who would have previously been given a diagnosis of unstable angina have now been shown to have suffered small amounts of myocardial necrosis or "infarction". This has resulted in the need for a new definition for the term "myocardial infarction (MI)".

The current American College of Cardiology (ACC) and European Cardiac Society (ECS) consensus guidelines suggest the following definition [1].

Criteria for acute, evolving or recent MI

Either one of the following criteria satisfies the diagnosis for an acute, evolving or recent MI:

- Typical rise and gradual fall (troponin) or more rapid rise and fall (creatinine kinase MB, CK-MB) of biochemical markers of myocardial necrosis with at least one of the following:
  - ischemic symptoms;
  - development of pathological Q-waves on the electrocardiograph (ECG);
  - ECG changes indicative of ischaemia (ST segment elevation or depression);
  - coronary artery intervention (e.g. coronary angioplasty).
- Pathological findings of an acute MI.

Criteria for established MI

Either of the following criteria satisfies the diagnosis for established MI:

- Development of new pathological Q-waves on serial ECGs. The patient may or may not remember previous symptoms. Biochemical markers of myocardial necrosis may have normalized, depending on the length of time that has passed since the infarct developed.
- Pathological findings of a healed or healing MI.

The inevitable conclusion of this definition is an enormous expansion in the numbers of people being classified as having suffered an MI. As the definition encompasses such a heterogeneous population the ACC and ECS have stated the term MI should not be used without further qualifications such as size of infarct and timing [1]. In clinical practice this centres around the development of Q-waves, the presence or absence of ST elevation and the development of areas of poorly functioning myocardium on echocardiography.

Current management groups people into three categories. The first two are termed ACS and are discussed in this chapter:

(1) STEMI.
(2) ACS *without* ST elevation – encompassing all patients with ECG changes and/or troponin rises.
(3) Stable angina.

Acute STEMI

The pathogenesis of acute MI with ST elevation involves the rupture of an unstable atherosclerotic plaque and subsequent thrombus formation via platelet activation resulting in total coronary occlusion.

The natural history of acute MI treated in the community is poor with an overall fatality of between 30% and 50% in the first month of which about a half occur in the first 2 h [2]. Those patients that arrive in accident and emergency departments form a self-selected group. Studies on hospital groups have shown a reduction in 1-month mortality from 25% to 30% in the 1960s to 7–8% in the most recent trials [3].

Clinical presentation

- *Pain*: The most consistent feature of STEMI is pain. It is usually felt centrally or left sided in location and is described as tight or crushing in character. It often radiates to the neck and/or arm, and typically does not respond to sublingual glyceryl trinitrate (GTN). Diabetics can present silently without chest pain.
- *Breathlessness*: This often accompanies the pain and may be due to the myocardial ischaemia itself or be a manifestation of acute pulmonary oedema.
- Sympathetic and parasympathetic over activity. This often leads to vomiting, sweating, dizziness, palpitations and feeling clammy.
- Typically symptoms have no obvious precipitating factor but in a proportion of patients an MI occurs following anxiety or strenuous activity. There is also a well-documented circadian variation, with a peak occurring in the early morning (6–9 a.m.). This is probably related to increases in catecholamines and platelet aggregability.
- Regrettably one of the commonest presentations of acute MI is sudden death, where the MI has usually been associated with sudden fatal ventricular dysrhythmias. 50% of MIs may present this way.

Diagnosis

The clinical management of patients with ST elevation has progressed following clinical trials involving thrombolysis and percutaneous coronary intervention (PCI). The following criteria are required before considering thrombolysis or primary angioplasty:

- typical cardiac chest pain not responding to GTN spray;

  and ECG changes:

- 1 mm ST elevation in two or more adjacent limb leads *or*
- 2 mm ST elevation in two or more adjacent chest leads *or*
- new left bundle branch blockage (LBBB).

Clinical conditions which can look similar to acute STEMI include pericarditis and previous infarcts with an aneurysmal segment. The presence of an evolving ECG can be invaluable. If there is doubt then an opinion should be sought from a senior or specialist colleague. Those patients who do not fulfil current diagnostic criteria with less ECG changes should currently be managed as ACS without ST elevation.

Patients with STEMI classically exhibit a rise in biochemical markers including CK, CK-MB and troponin:

- *CK*: It is released following any kind of muscle damage. It can give information as to the size of infarct sustained but is relatively non-specific. CK-MB, which is almost exclusively found in myocardium is a more sensitive assay. These enzymes increase within 4–6 h of infarction and can remain elevated for 3–4 days.
- *Troponins*: Both the I and T isoenzymes are more specific and sensitive than CK-MB. They can be detectable within 4 h but for a acceptable sensitivity have to be sampled at 12 h. They may stay elevated for up to 3 weeks.

Clinical management

Basic immediate management includes cardiac monitoring for dysrhythmias, inhaled oxygen, analgesia (morphine or diamorphine) and an antiemetic (metoclopromide or cyclizine).

Routine bloods should be sent for:

- full blood count (FBC);
- urea and electrolytes (U&Es), glucose and lipids;
- cardiac enzymes should be sampled following admission. Many institutions measure troponin and CK at 12 h.

The urgent requirement in a patient with acute STEMI is the restoration of coronary flow and tissue perfusion. This is performed with antiplatelet therapy, thrombolysis or PCI.

Antiplatelet therapy

Aspirin

- Give 300 mg stat.
- 75–150 mg daily lifelong.

The only licensed antiplatelet therapy for acute STEMI is currently aspirin. It inactivates cyclooxygenase and so inhibits platelet aggregation.

Aspirin alone is beneficial for treatment of evolving acute MI with a 35-day number needed to treat (NNT) of 50 [4]. This confers almost as much benefit as modern thrombolytic regimes.

Other antiplatelet agents: clopidogrel

- Give 300 mg stat.
- 75 mg daily.

Clopidogrel selectively prevents the activation of the glycoprotein (GP) IIb/IIIa complex, thereby inhibiting platelet aggregation. There is currently no evidence that clopidogrel has a role in acute STEMI, but its use would appear sensible in the small group of patients who are aspirin intolerant.

The use of various forms of the GPIIb/IIIa blockers (eptifibatide and abciximab) in the management of acute STEMI continues to be studied but has yet to be shown to be more beneficial than thrombolysis.

Thrombolysis

More than 150,000 people have been enrolled into studies comparing the use of thrombolysis versus control. Approximately 30 deaths are prevented per 1000 patients treated who present within 6 h of symptom onset, with ST segment elevation or bundle branch block. Twenty deaths are prevented per 1000 patients treated for those presenting between 7 and 12 h [5]. Beyond 12 h there is no convincing evidence of benefit. As a result thrombolysis should be considered in those patients presenting within 12 h of onset of symptoms who fulfil ECG criteria.

ECG changes

Most benefit is seen in patients with new LBBB or anterior changes. Inferior infarctions also benefit but the NNT to save one life is four times the number for anterior changes or LBBB [5].

ECG changes compatible with posterior infarction warrant the use of thrombolysis but the diagnosis is more difficult and best left to experienced hands.

Age

Thrombolysis is beneficial whatever the age of the patients but the degree of benefit for patients over the age of 75 is less. Potential complications should be explored fully prior to commencement of treatment [5].

Patients with diabetes have been shown to derive more benefit from thrombolysis than those people with normal blood sugar.

Which thrombolytic agent?

Currently there are four agents in routine clinical use:

- Streptokinase, given as an infusion over 30–60 min.
- Accelerated tissue plasminogen activator (tPA), given as a bolus then infusion.
- Reteplase, two boluses 30 min apart.
- Tenecteplase (TNK-tPA), given as a single bolus.

Most institutions offer two options, streptokinase and one other:

- tPA and streptokinase have been compared, and a small additional benefit was seen with tPA but at the expense of an increase in intracerebral haemorrhage. Benefit was highest in patients presenting within 4 h of onset of symptoms with anterior infarcts [6].
- TNK and reteplase are similar to tPA, and are both easier to administer. They are becoming more widely used.
- tPA, reteplase and TNK all require the use of concomitant intravenous (IV) heparin for 24–48 h after thrombolysis. Streptokinase does not require the use of heparin.

Complications

Complications following thrombolysis centre on the risk of serious bleeding. The chance of intracerebral haemorrhage is on average <1% but increases with increasing age, uncontrolled hypertension, low body weight and the use of tPA. With no risk factors the risk is about 0.3% but with three risk factors can reach 2.5% [7].

Contraindications

Patients who have significant contraindications to thrombolysis should be discussed with a regional referral centre regarding the need for transfer and PCI.

Mechanical reperfusion/PCI

Current practice in the UK involves the use of thrombolysis to achieve vessel patency after occlusion from a thrombus. However, there is much interest in the use of coronary angioplasty and stenting as an alternative to thrombolysis. This is termed primary angioplasty.

Trials have compared:

- thrombolysis versus PCI in patients presenting to a regional referral hospital,
- thrombolysis versus transfer to a regional referral hospital for PCI in patients attending a district general hospital (DGH) [8].

Current trials are looking into:

- thrombolysis versus thrombolysis then transfer for PCI,
- ambulance thrombolysis and PCI.

Most trials have not shown a significant mortality benefit from PCI as opposed to thrombolysis. There was however a significant reduction in non-fatal strokes and the need for readmissions due to angina.

Failed thrombolysis/reinfarction

A number of patients fail to fully respond to thrombolysis with:

- failure to achieve resolution of ST segments,
- continuing cardiac pain,
- further chest pain and ECG changes after successful thrombolysis.

These groups should be discussed with the regional centre with a view to potential transfer for urgent angiography and revascularization.

Adjunctive medical therapy

Beta blockade

Since the advent of thrombolysis there has been no significant evidence of a prognostic benefit for immediate beta blockade [9]. However, short-acting beta blockers (e.g. metoprolol) should be considered where the patient is tachycardic or still in pain as long as there is no evidence for heart failure.

Placebo-controlled trials have shown that chronic beta blocker therapy improves prognosis post MI. Most of these studies were in the prethrombolytic era but it would now be unethical to repeat these studies with thrombolysis [10]. Beta blockers should be increased to aim for a target heart rate of 50–60 beats per minute. The development of acute heart failure, asthma or heart block should lead to a reduction in dose or cessation in treatment.

Intensive insulin therapy

The use of insulin following MI has become standard treatment since the publication of the Diabetes mellitus, Insulin Glucose infusion in Acute Myocardial Infarction (DIGAMI) trial that showed prognostic benefit for early intensive insulin treatment [11]. The DIGAMI regime should be commenced on:

- any known Type 1 or 2 diabetic, or
- any patient with random serum blood glucose >11 mmol/l.

Patients should then be referred to the diabetes specialist team for further management. These patients require an admission haemoglobin A1c (HbA1c) level checked.

Secondary prevention

Statins

The use of cholesterol lowering medication post-MI has been extensively studied [12]. Current UK guidelines (National Service Framework for Coronary Heart Disease, NSF for CHD) suggest that statins and dietary advice should be given to aim to lower serum cholesterol concentrations *either* to:

- <5 mmol/l (low-density lipoprotein cholesterol (LDL-C) to below 3 mmol) *or*
- by 30% (whichever is greater).

Recent European guidelines have lowered targets to total cholesterol 4.5 and LDL to 2.5 [13]. Cholesterol levels will drop within 12–24 h after MI so consequently it is best to measure levels directly on admission.

Angiotensin-converting enzyme inhibitors

The benefits of angiotensin-converting enzyme inhibitor (ACEI) in patients with cardiovascular disease are well proven. Initial trials looked at patients with left ventricular (LV) dysfunction; however, recent data has shown that they are of benefit to all patients with cardiovascular disease and should be started post-MI in all patients no matter what age or degree of LV function [14]. Blood pressure and renal function should be monitored.

Free fatty acids

There is recent evidence that dietary supplementation with polyunsaturated fatty acids can reduce cardiac events following MI [15]. Only one company currently has a product in the form of Omacor. Its use is now becoming more widespread.

Symptomatic treatment

Nitrates, calcium channel blockers and nicorandil are all used for the symptomatic treatment of angina, pre- or post-infarction. There is no conclusive evidence that they have any prognostic benefit either acutely or long term. It is important to recognize that if symptomatic treatment is required post-ST elevation MI then the patient has post-infarct angina and thus an indication for urgent angiography to prevent further myocardial loss.

Complications

Right ventricular infarction

Right ventricular (RV) infarction should be suspected in patients with:

- hypotension,
- clear lung fields,
- raised jugular venous pressure (JVP).

It can be confirmed by echocardiography.

Inferior MIs complicated by RV infarctions have a poor prognosis with a 31% in-hospital mortality rate. This is compared with a 6% mortality rate in those without RV involvement [16]. Treatment of RV infarction includes:

- Maintenance of RV preload with IV fluids.
- Avoidance of preload reducing medication such as nitrates and ACEI.
- Inotropic support of the dysfunctional right ventricle.
- Early thrombolysis or PCI.

Heart failure

Heart failure is common after MI. It should be treated with:

- fluid restriction,
- nitrates,

- IV diuretics,
- ACEI therapy,
- spironalactone/beta blockers.

A close eye should be kept on the patients' blood pressure looking for signs of cardiogenic shock. Regular blood samples should be sent for U&Es. The investigation and treatment of heart failure is covered in Chapter 20.

Cardiogenic shock

Cardiogenic shock is a clinical state of hypoperfusion characterized by:

- systolic pressure <90 mmHg;
- central filling pressure >20 mmHg;
- cardiac index $<1.8 \, l \, min^{-1} m^{-2}$.

Patients should be investigated with echocardiography to look for mechanical complications that are treatable along with the presence of RV infarction that can improve with fluids. The use of inotropes should be considered.

Treatment with intra-aortic balloon pump (IABP) and angiography followed by PCI or coronary artery bypass grafting (CABG) has been investigated as a possible treatment for cardiogenic shock in an attempt to revascularize ischaemic and hibernating myocardium. Overall this was found to have a non-significant benefit at 30 days but survival was significantly improved at 6 months [17].

Free wall rupture

Sudden ventricular free wall rupture is almost invariably fatal. Subacute rupture may occur resulting in rapid haemodynamic compromise and the presence of pericardial tamponade on echocardiography. The need for pericardialcentesis is urgent and if necessary definitive surgical treatment.

Ventricular septal rupture

A clinical deterioration in the patients' condition with the development of a systolic murmur should raise the possibility of a ventricular septal defect (VSD). It can be confirmed by echocardiography and most patients will require urgent surgical treatment.

Mitral regurgitation

Mitral regurgitation commonly develops after MI and may be caused by:

- Ventricular dilatation leading to valve annular dilatation and resulting poor coaptation of valve leaflets.
- Ischaemia driven mitral regurgitation.
- Papillae muscle rupture leading to pulmonary oedema and cardiogenic shock.

Echocardiography is mandatory and if rupture is confirmed the placing of an IABP followed by urgent surgery is required.

Aneurysm/pseudoaneurysm

Post-infarction a thinning of the LV free wall may result in a ventricular bulge or true aneurysm. Alternatively a ventricular rupture may be sealed off by overlying, adherent pericardium resulting in a pseudoaneurysm formation. Consideration should be given to surgical resection of the aneurysm especially in symptomatic patients with LV dysfunction.

Pericarditis

Inflammation of the pericardium can follow soon after MI. Alternatively 1–3 weeks post-MI patients may develop fever, pleuritis and pericarditis in the form of Dresslers syndrome. Patients usually complain of sharp pleuritic pain that may be relieved by sitting forward. A pericardial rub may be present and ECG changes may be seen with concave or saddle-shaped ST segment elevation. Patients should have an echocardiogram to look for pericardial fluid, and treatment involves non-steroidal anti-inflammatory drugs (NSAIDs) and rarely steroids.

Heart block

- First degree and Mobitz Type 1 (Wenekebach) requires no treatment post-MI. Patients should be monitored.
- Patients with anterior infarction and Mobitz Type 2 require temporary cardiac pacing as it often progresses to complete heart block (CHB). Otherwise Mobitz Type 2 requires no immediate treatment.
- Patients with CHB should be temporary paced. The risk of asystole is significant, and permanent pacing is usually required.

Temporary pacing

Temporary pacing can occur via:

- internal jugular,
- subclavian,
- femoral venous access.

Balloon flotation devices can be extremely useful in an intensive care unit (ICU) environment as fluoroscopic control is not required and the patient need not move from ICU. These devices are best inserted from the internal jugular or subclavian route. Immediately post-thrombolysis venous cannulation of the internal jugular or subclavian vein can result in bleeding complications so the femoral route is usually advocated. Insertion of a temporary pacing wire can be a difficult procedure unless in skilled hands and the use of femoral access is usually the easiest approach [18].

Dysrhythmias

Dysrhythmias are common post-MI and should be closely monitored. Electrolytes should be optimized and the introduction of a beta blocker is usually helpful. The use of IV magnesium has been shown to be beneficial and if the patient is haemodynamically compromised then they should be electrically cardioverted. The introduction of amiodarone can help to cardiovert patients and suppress paroxysmal dysrhythmias.

Ectopics and runs of bigeminy are common immediately post-MI, but if they become regular and more prolonged can be a poor prognostic sign. Ventricular dysrhythmias should be investigated if necessary with angiography and revascularization.

The National Institute for Clinical Evidence (NICE) has stated that the use of implantable cardioverter defibrillators (ICDs) should be routinely considered for patients with a history of previous MI and all of the following [19]:

- Non-sustained ventricular tachycardia (VT) on Holter (24-h ECG) monitoring.
- Inducible VT on electrophysiological testing.
- LV dysfunction with an ejection fraction (EF) <35% and no worse than Class III of the New York Heart Association functional classification of heart failure.

ACS without ST elevation

The pathogenesis of ACS without ST elevation is similar to that of ST elevation MI. An atherosclerotic plaque ruptures and causes reduced blood supply to a coronary artery. Unlike ST elevation MI this occlusion is temporary or the artery is subtotally occluded resulting in critical ischaemia and brief cell necrosis.

Clinical presentation

Clinical features are usually similar but less severe than ST elevation MI. Cardiac chest pain and breathlessness are common but silent ischaemia, especially perioperatively, may occur. Symptoms may be worse on exertion.

Diagnosis and investigations

In patients presenting with cardiac symptoms the diagnosis is confirmed by:

• Rise in biochemical enzymes above reference ranges.
• ECG changes with ST depression and/or T-wave changes.

Perioperatively symptoms may be lacking and diagnosis rests with enzymes and ECG changes.

Patients should be thoroughly investigated and treated for secondary causes of ischaemia including anaemia, fever, thyrotoxicosis, hypoxia, tachyarrhythmias, aortic stenosis or sympathomimetic drugs.

Clinical management

The optimal clinical management of ACS has over the last 10 years seen a progression from purely symptomatic treatments alone to interventions designed to alter prognosis.

Basic immediate management includes cardiac monitoring for dysrhythmias and inhaled high flow oxygen.

Routine bloods should be sent for:

• FBC;
• U&Es, glucose and lipids;
• most institutions measure troponin 12 h following the commencement of symptoms to optimize sensitivity.

Antiplatelet therapy

Aspirin

- 300 mg stat.
- 75–150 mg daily lifelong.

Aspirin is the cornerstone of antiplatelet therapy in ACS. Studies shows clear benefit [20] with treatment for 3 months resulting in one less death or acute ST elevation MI for 20 people treated:

Clopidogrel

- 300 mg stat.
- 75 mg daily for 9–12 months.

For those patients who are aspirin intolerant then clopidogrel is an alternative. The Clopidogrel versus Aspirin in Patients at Risk of Ischaemic Events (CAPRIE) study showed clopidogrel to be at least as effective in preventing events as aspirin with minimal extra side effects [21]. The additional benefit of clopidogrel on top of aspirin was studied in the Clopidogrel in Unstable angina to prevent Recurrent Events (CURE) trial [22]. There was a 2.2% reduction in MI, stroke or cardiovascular death but a 0.6% increase in major bleeding. There is only limited data regarding its safety with GPIIb/IIIa inhibitors. Current ECS guidelines are that it should be given acutely, continued for 9–12 months and then discontinued as long-term effects are not known.

GPIIb/IIIa inhibitors

Activated GPIIb/IIIa receptors connect with fibrinogen to form bridges between activated platelets, leading to formation of platelet thrombin. The use of various GPIIb/IIIa inhibitors has been investigated with randomized-controlled trails (RCTs) and studies show a small but consistent benefit [23]. Current NICE guidelines indicate that GPIIb/IIIa inhibitors should be used in high-risk patients [24].

Anticoagulation

There is convincing evidence that in aspirin treated patients anticoagulation with low-molecular-weight heparin (LMWH) reduces rates of death, MI or recurrent ischaemia [25]. Choice of LMWH is dependent on hospital protocols and should be continued for at least 2 days.

Symptomatic management

- *Beta blockers*: It can be given orally or IV and doses should be titrated to keep the patients heart rate between 50 and 60 bpm.
- *Calcium channel blockers*: A useful adjunct in angina and if the patient is intolerant to beta blockers, verapamil or diltiazem can help to control ventricular rate.
- *Nitrates*: Given sublingually, orally or IV. Extremely useful in controlling symptoms.
- *Nicorandil*: A potassium channel opener given orally and useful for symptomatic relief.

These agents lower blood pressure, slow heart rate or depress LV contractility, and hence reduce myocardial oxygen demand. Whilst all the drugs help to reduce symptoms none have shown convincing prognostic benefit.

Insulin treatment

There is currently no evidence that intensive insulin management alters prognosis in ACS without ST elevation. However, the DIGAMI study was published prior to the advent of troponins and many institutions are adopting DIGAMI protocols for patients with ACS without ST elevation.

Invasive versus conservative management

The benefit of managing patients with ACS without ST elevation with a strategy of early angiography and revascularization as opposed to symptomatic treatment, and non-invasive risk stratification has been fully investigated [26]. There was a clear prognostic benefit seen in patients in the invasive groups. Current international guidelines [27] advocate predischarge angiography in patients with chest pain and any of the following:

- raised troponin,
- ST depression,
- recurrent ischaemic pain.

Within the UK this policy has yet to be fully adopted. Predischarge exercise tolerance tests are sometimes used to further risk stratify patients and identify high-risk groups.

The recent National Service Framework and increased central funding for cardiac services are increasing resources and invasive management may soon be the norm for all suitable patients.

Secondary prevention

As with ST elevation, MI secondary prevention measures include the introduction of beta blockers, statins, ACEI and free fatty acids. For full details refer to the same section covered earlier in this chapter.

FURTHER READING

Task Force of the European Society of Cardiology. Management of acute coronary syndromes in patients presenting without persistent ST-segment elevation. *Eur Heart J* 2002; 23: 1809–40.

The Task Force on the Management of Acute Myocardial Infarction. The European Society of Cardiology. Management of acute myocardial infarction in patients presenting with ST-segment elevation. *Eur Heart J* 2003; 24: 28–66.

Unstable angina and non-ST-segment elevation myocardial infarction: American College of Cardiology/American Heart Association 2002 Guideline. *J Am Coll Cardiol* 2002; 40: 366–74.

The above guidelines are all available online free of charge at the ACC and European Society of Cardiology web sites.

REFERENCES

1. Myocardial Infarction Redefined – A Consensus Document of the Joint European Society of Cardiology/American College of Cardiology Committee for the Redefinition of Myocardial Infarction. *J Am Coll Cardiol* 2000; 36: 959–69.

2. Armstrong A, Duncan B, Oliver MF et al. Natural history of acute coronary heart attacks. A community study. *Br Heart J* 1972; 34: 67–80.

3. Norris RM, Caughey DE, Mercer CJ et al. Prognosis after myocardial infarction. Six-year follow-up. *Br Heart J* 1974; 36: 786–90.

4. ISIS-2 (Second International Study of Infarct Survival) Collaborative Group. Randomised trial of intravenous streptokinase, oral aspirin, both, or neither among 17,187 cases of suspected acute myocardial infarction: ISIS2. *Lancet* 1988; ii: 349–60.

5. Fibrinolytic Therapy Trialists' (FTT) Collaborative Group. Indications for thrombolytic therapy in suspected acute myocardial infarction: collaborative overview of early mortality and major morbidity results from all randomised trials of more than 1000 patients. *Lancet* 1994; 343: 311–22.

6. The GUSTO Investigators. An international randomized trial comparing four thrombolytic strategies for acute myocardial infarction. *New Engl J Med* 1993; 329: 673–82.

7. Simoons et al. Individual risk assessment for intracranial haemorrhage during thrombolytic therapy. *Lancet* 1993; 342: 1523–8.

8. Bednar et al. Interhospital transport for primary angioplasty improves the long-term outcome of acute myocardial infarction compared with immediate thrombolysis in the nearest hospital (one-year follow-up of the PRAGUE-1 study). *Can J Cardiol* 2003; 19(10): 1133–7.

9. Freemantle N, Cleland J, Young P et al. Beta blockade after myocardial infarction: systematic review and meta regression analysis. *Br Med J* 1999; 318: 1730–7.

10. Hjalmarson A, Elmfeldt D, Herlitz J et al. Effect on mortality of metoprolol in acute myocardial infarction: a double-blind randomised trial. *Lancet* 1981; 2: 823–7.

11. Prospective randomised study of intensive insulin treatment on long term survival after acute myocardial infarction in patients with diabetes mellitus. DIGAMI (Diabetes mellitus, Insulin Glucose infusion in Acute Myocardial Infarction) Study Group. *Br Med J* 1997; 314(7093): 1512–5.

12. Sacks FM, Pfeffer MA, Moye LA et al. The effect of pravastatin on coronary events after myocardial infarction in patients with average cholesterol levels. Cholesterol and Recurrent Events Trial Investigators. *New Engl J Med* 1996; 335: 1001–9.

13. European Guidelines on Cardiovascular Disease Prevention in Clinical Practice – EHJ Executive. *Eur Heart J* 2003; 24(17): 1601–10.

14. Fox et al. Efficacy of perindopril in reduction of cardiovascular events among patients with stable coronary artery disease: randomised, double blind, placebo-controlled, multicentre trial (the EUROPA study). *Lancet* 2003; 362(9386): 782–8.

15. Dietary supplementation with n-3 polyunsaturated fatty acids and vitamin E after myocardial infarction: results of the GISSI-Prevenzione trial. Gruppo Italiano per lo Studio della Sopravvivenza nell'Infarto miocardico. *Lancet* 1999; 354(9177): 447–55.

16. Zehender M, Kasper W, Kauder E et al. Right ventricular infarction as an independent predictor of prognosis after acute inferior myocardial infarction. *New Engl J Med* 1993; 328: 981–8.

17. Hochman JS, Sleeper LA, Webb JG et al. Early revascularization in acute myocardial infarction complicated by cardio-genic shock. SHOCK Investigators. Should we emergently revascularize occluded coronaries for cardiogenic shock. *New Engl J Med* 1999; 341: 625–34.

18. Clarke N. Novices can reliably and safely perform temporary pacing from femoral route. *Br Med J* 2002; 324: 112.

19. Guidance on the use of implantable cardioverter defibrillators for arrhythmias. The National Institute for Clinical Evidence (NICE). 4 November 2002.

20. Lewis HDJ, Davis JW, Archibald DG et al. Protective effects of aspirin against acute myocardial infarction and death in men with unstable angina: results of a Veterans Administration Cooperative Study. *New Engl J Med* 1983; 309: 396–403.

21. CAPRIE Steering Committee. A randomised, blinded, trial of Clopidogrel versus Aspirin in Patients at Risk of Ischaemic Events (CAPRIE). 1996; 348: 1329–39.

22. Yusuf S. Effects of clopidogrel in addition to aspirin in patients with acute coronary syndromes without ST-segment elevation. *New Engl J Med* 2001; 345(7): 494–502.

23. PURSUIT Investigators. Inhibition of platelet glycoprotein IIb/IIIa with eptifibatide in patients with acute coronary syndromes. The PURSUIT Trial Investigators. Platelet glyco-protein IIb/IIIa in unstable angina: receptor suppression using integrilin therapy. *New Engl J Med* 1998; 339: 436–43.

24. NICE Technology Appraisal. Guidance on the use of glycoprotein IIb/IIIa inhibitors in the treatment of acute coronary syndromes. September 2002.

25. FRISC Study Group. Low-molecular-weight heparin during instability in coronary artery disease, Fragmin during Instability in Coronary Artery Disease (FRISC) Study Group. *Lancet* 1996; 347: 561–8.

26. Cannon CP, Weintraub WS, Demopoulos LA et al. Comparison of early invasive and conservative strategies inpatients with unstable coronary syndromes treated with the glycoprotein IIb/IIIa inhibitor tirofiban. *New Engl J Med* 2001; 344: 1879–87.

27. ECS Task Force Report. Management of acute coronary syndromes in patients present-ing without persistent ST-segment elevation. *Eur Heart J* 2002; 23: 1809–40.

20

Heart failure

R. Beynon and D.H. Roberts

The prevalence of symptomatic heart failure in Europe is thought to be between 0.4% and 2.0% with the mean age being 74 years. Where the underlying problem cannot be rectified the prognosis is poor with 50% of people dead within 4 years. In patients with severe heart failure 50% will die within 1 year [1].

Acute versus chronic

Heart failure may be acute with a low cardiac output resulting in hypotension with poor organ perfusion and/or pulmonary oedema. It may also be chronic with output insufficient to provide the optimal needs of metabolizing tissues resulting in decreased tissue performance. The patient may complain of lethargy or reduced exercise tolerance.

Systolic versus diastolic

Severe heart failure is usually due to poor myocardial contractility. However the myocardium may inadequately relax resulting in reduced stretch of myocardial filaments and decreased cardiac output. This is termed diastolic heart failure and often occurs with systolic failure but may exist with the presence of a normal ejection fraction.

Aetiology

The commonest cause of heart failure in the Western world is myocardial ischaemia from coronary artery diseases. However potentially treatable and reversible aetiologies should be considered.

Cardiac

- Valvular dysfunction
- Arrhythmias
- Hypertension
- Pericardial disease.

Non-cardiac

- High-output states; anaemia, pregnancy and thyrotoxicosis
- Vitamin deficiencies
- Alcohol
- Autoimmune diseases
- Infections
- Drug toxicity (e.g. calcium channel blockers, beta blockers).

Acute heart failure

For some patients the presentation of acute heart failure may be an exacerbation of a long running medical complaint, for others it may be a new finding.

Signs and symptoms

Patients present with symptoms of breathlessness, decreasing exercise tolerance and orthopnoea. Signs include:

- Tachycardia
- Hypotension
- Peripheral oedema
- Raised jugular venous pressure (JVP)
- Displaced apex beat
- Third heart sound
- Crackles and cardiac wheeze.

Investigations

Routine blood should be requested in all patients with suspected heart failure including:

- full blood count (FBC),

- urea (U) and electrolytes (Es), liver function tests (LFTS),
- thyroid function tests (TFTs) glucose and lipids.

Unless there is a high index of suspicion of ischaemia then troponins should not be requested as they have been shown to rise in pulmonary oedema. Other investigations include:

- *Electrocardiograph (ECG)*: Is usually abnormal with Q-waves, bundle branch block or signs of new ischaemia (e.g. ST segment or T-wave changes).
- *Chest X-ray*: Cardiomegaly can be seen and in patients with acute pulmonary oedema dilation of the upper lobe pulmonary veins, kerley B-lines and the presence of interstitial oedema can be seen.
- *Echocardiography*: An echo is not usually required to make the diagnosis of acute heart failure but once the patient is stable it can give an idea of prognosis and reveal important valvular pathology. If a mechanical cause (e.g. papillary muscle rupture or new ventricular septal disease (VSD)) is suspected then an urgent echo is required.

Clinical management

- Patients should be sat up and given high-flow oxygen. If there is a suspicion of chronic obstructive airways disease (COAD) then arterial blood gases should be sent otherwise oxygen saturation provides adequate information to guide treatment.
- 2.5–5 mg of diamorphine should be given. Diamorphine eases patient distress and promotes venous vasodilatation so offloading the heart.
- 50–100 mg of intravenous furosemide or an equivalent dose of bumetanide should be administered. They promote vasodilatation in a matter of minutes and a later diuretic effect off-loads the heart.
- *Venous vasodilators*: Intravenous nitroglycerine may be given, starting with 0.25 µg/kg/min, and increasing every 5 min until a fall in blood pressure by 15 mmHg is observed or the systolic blood pressure falls to 90 mmHg.
- Correct any acute arrhythmia that may promote poor cardiac output.
- Most patients will improve quickly with aggressive diuretic and nitrate therapy but a few will remain in pulmonary oedema. As treatment increases some may become hypotensive precluding further drug increases. They should be considered for inotropes and mechanical ventilation.
- Patients with hypotension and pulmonary oedema have cardiogenic shock. Inotropes should be considered along with the need for ventilatory support.

- The use of non-invasive ventilation has been extensively studied in exacerbations of chronic lung disease whereas only a few studies have looked at benefits in patients with cardiogenic pulmonary oedema. Three randomized controlled trial (RCT) have compared continuous positive airway pressure (CPAP) with standard medical therapy and found a decrease in need for endotracheal intubation but no significant mortality benefit [2]. Bi-level non-invasive positive pressure ventilation (NPPV) has not been compared with standard treatment in a RCT. CPAP has been compared with bi-level NPPV in one RCT [3]. NPPV was found to improve vital signs and ventilation more rapidly than CPAP but this was at the expense of a significant increase in the number of myocardial infarctions. On this basis the trial was terminated early. Currently it would seem sensible to offer CPAP to patients with severe pulmonary oedema in an attempt to reduce the need for invasive ventilation.
- For some patients there is the need for invasive mechanical ventilation. Given the poor prognosis for severe heart failure consideration should be given for the potential for improved function prior to intubation.
- For some patients who are not deemed suitable for mechanical ventilation the presentation may represent a terminal event. The use of diamorphine, an anti-emetic and midazolam should be considered to aide distress.

Surgical treatment

A minority of patients present with acute heart failure secondary to a sudden mechanical complication usually post-myocardial infarction. Papillae muscle rupture or a new VSD is a potentially curable medical emergency requiring urgent surgery.

Ventricular assist devices are mechanical pumps that take over the function of the damaged ventricle. They are used in patients with myocardial infarction, acute myocarditis or end-stage heart disease who are not expected to recover adequate cardiac function and who require mechanical support as a bridge to transplantation.

Chronic heart failure

Chronic heart failure is common and often goes undiagnosed. Its prognosis is significant and the recent NICE guidelines go some way to raise the profile of a much neglected disease group [4].

Signs and symptoms

Patients present with a heterogeneous range of symptoms depending on the severity of disease and current medication use.

Breathlessness, fatigue and decreased exercise tolerance are common whilst some patients may have variable signs of acute left ventricular (LV) failure or in some cases minimal clinical signs.

Investigations

Routine blood including FBC, U and Es, LFTS, TFTs glucose and lipids should be requested in all patients with suspected heart failure.

- Consider a chest X-ray, serial peak flows and pulmonary function tests in patients with sign or symptoms compatible with asthma or COAD.
- *ECG*: A 12-lead ECG should be requested in all patients. A normal ECG has a high negative predictive value for heart failure.
- *B-type natriuretic peptide (BNP)*: Several clinical and epidemiological studies have related decreasing cardiac, usually LV function with increasing plasma natriuretic peptide concentrations raising the possibility of a diagnostic "blood test" for heart failure. BNP is the most sensitive test and has a strong negative predictive value [5].
- *Echocardiography*: For patients with a positive BNP or abnormal ECG, echocardiography is the diagnostic tool of choice to diagnose heart failure. A normal BNP and ECG should point the physician to an alternative diagnosis.

Clinical management

The therapeutic approach to chronic heart failure centres on improving symptom status in the short term, and introducing medication to promote cardiac remodelling and hence long-term sustained improvement. There are three approaches:

(1) Non-pharmacological measures.
(2) Pharmacological therapy.
(3) Devices and surgery.

Non-pharmacological management

Patients and their families require counselling and advice. Recent NICE guidelines suggest this should be in a specialist setting if the disease is severe. If overweight the patient should be actively encouraged to loose weight and in patients with advanced heart failure fluid and salt intake should be restricted. Exercise should be encouraged and exercise training programmes have been shown to improve symptoms and quality of life.

Pharmacology

Angiotensin converting enzyme inhibitors

The use of angiotensin converting enzyme (ACE) inhibitors in patients with both symptomatic and asymptomatic LV dysfunction has been standard practice in the UK and abroad since the publication of a numbers of RCT showing clear mortality and morbidity benefit [6]. However, the indications for ACE inhibitor therapy have widened dramatically over the last few years with the publication of recent trials, which showed long-term benefits in high-risk patients with normal LV function [7].

ACE inhibitors should be used with caution in patients with renal vascular disease, a creatinine greater than 250 and a systolic blood pressure <100 mmHg. Potassium should be monitored along with U&Es at regular intervals. The most common side effect is a dry irritating cough. If not tolerated an ACE inhibitor may be substituted with an angiotensin 2 blocker.

ACE inhibitors should be titrated up to the maximal amount tolerated by the patient.

Angiotensin 2 blockers

A small group of patients are unable to tolerate ACE inhibitors, usually because of a dry irritating cough. For these people the addition of an angiotensin 2 blocker in place of an ACE inhibitor has been shown to improve morbidity and mortality but not to the same extent as ACE inhibitors [8]. Current interest surrounds the addition of an angiotensin 2 blocker to established ACE inhibitor therapy. Results from RCTs have been mixed to date.

Diuretics

For patients who are fluid overloaded the immediate concern is for the addition of a diuretic and a fluid restricted diet. Patients are generally treated with a loop diuretic as they are stronger than thiazides but doses should be kept at a minimum.

Blood pressure and renal function should be regularly monitored. A potassium sparing diuretic can often be added to aid diuresis and keep electrolytes within acceptable limits. Diuretics were introduced prior to the use of RCT and as a result there are no large prospective trials showing benefit.

Beta blockers

There is good evidence from a number of RCTs that the use of beta blockers in patients with chronic heart failure increases life expectancy and reduces hospitalizations [9]. Not all beta blockers are licensed in the UK for heart failure and current evidence suggest that carvedilol or bisoprolol should be used. A low dose should be used at the start and the dose doubled not less than at 2 weekly intervals. Aim for highest dose tolerated keeping heart rate >50 bpm.

Aldosterone antagonists

The use of spironalactone in patients with moderate to severe heart failure (NYHA 3 or 4) was found to increase life expectancy and reduce hospitalizations in the RALES study [10]. Patients should be given 25 mg and potassium and creatinine should be monitored regularly. The mechanism of action is not thought to be diuretic induced but involves the inhibition of aldosterone and hence a reduction in vascular fibrosis, decreased sympathetic activation and increased parasympathetic tone.

Digoxin

Digoxin has been shown to have positive inotropic effects but this has not been consistently borne out in large-scale randomized trials [11]. There are no published data in patients in sinus rhythm to suggest it improves quality of life, symptoms or life expectancy. There has been some evidence to show reduced hospitalizations. Its use should be restricted to patients with severe heart failure of those in atrial fibrillation.

Anticoagulation

In patients with a dilated poorly functioning LV there is a theoretical risk of intracardiac thrombus formation and thromboembolism. There is however no convincing evidence of benefit with the use of oral, intravenous or subcutaneous anticoagulation unless the patient is in atrial fibrillation.

Devices and surgery

Revascularization

The major cause of heart failure in the Western world is occlusive coronary artery disease. For some patients the presence of a critically narrowed stenosis can result in impaired myocardial function that would improve if the blood supply is restored to normal. These areas of myocardium are "hibernating". Dobutamine stress echocardiography and nuclear perfusion scanning can both be used to look for areas of hibernation that may improve with revascularization.

Resynchronization therapy

Thirty percent of patients with severe heart failure have evidence of intraventricular conduction disturbances manifest by bundle branch block on a surface 12-lead ECG with QRS duration being longer than 120 ms. The result can often be asynchronous contraction of the LV free wall, right ventricle and intraventricular septum with resulting impaired cardiac output. The use of a biventricular pacemaker with leads pacing the right atrium, right ventricular and left ventricle via the coronary sinus has been shown to resynchronize contraction and improve cardiac output and exercise tolerance.

Heart transplantation

Cardiac transplantation offers hope to patients with severe end-stage heart failure and has been shown to increase survival, quality of life and exercise capacity. Five-year survival approaches 70% but morbidity can be significant with the intense immunosuppression needed.

FURTHER READING

Chronic Heart Failure in the Adult: American College of Cardiology/American Heart Association Practice Guidelines. *J Am Coll Cardiol* 2001; 38: 2101–13.

National Institute for Clinical Evidence (NICE). Chronic heart failure: management of chronic heart failure in adults in primary and secondary care. October 2003.

REFERENCES

1. Cleland JG, Gemmell I, Khand A, Boddy A. Is the prognosis of heart failure improving? *Eur J Heart Fail* 1999; 1: 229–41.

2. Pang D. The effect of positive pressure airway support on mortality and the need for intubation in cardiogenic pulmonary oedema. *Chest* 1998; 114: 1185–91.

3. Mehta S. Randomised prospective trial of bilevel versus continuous positive airway pressure in acute pulmonary oedema. *Crit Care Med* 1997; 25(4): 620–8.

4. National Institute for Clinical Evidence (NICE). Chronic heart failure: management of chronic heart failure in adults in primary and secondary care. October 2003.

5. Maisel AS, Krishnaswamy P, Nowak RM, McCord J, Hollander JE, Duc P et al. Rapid measurement of B-type natriuretic peptide in the emergency diagnosis of heart failure. *New Engl J Med* 2002; 347: 161–7.

6. Flather M, Yusuf S, Kober L et al. Long-term ACE inhibitor therapy in patients with heart failure or left ventricular dysfunction: a systematic overview of data from individual patients. ACE-Inhibitor Myocardial Infarction Collaborative Group. *Lancet* 2000; 355: 1575–81.

7. Yusuf S. Effects of an angiotensin-converting-enzyme inhibitor, ramipril, on cardiovascular events in high-risk patients. The Heart Outcomes Prevention Evaluation Study Investigators. *New Engl J Med* 2000; 342(3): 145–53.

8. Jong P, Demers C, McKelvie RS, Liu PP. Angiotensin receptor blockers in heart failure: meta-analysis of randomized controlled trials. *J Am College Cardiolo* 2002; 39: 463–70.

9. Shibata MC, Flather MD, Wang D. Systematic review of the impact of beta blockers on mortality and hospital admissions in heart failure. *Eur J Heart Fail* 2001; 3: 351–7.

10. Pitt B, Zannad F, Remme WJ, Cody R, Castaigne A, Perez A et al. The effect of spironolactone on morbidity and mortality in patients with severe heart failure. Randomized Aldactone Evaluation Study Investigators. *New Engl J Med* 1999; 341: 709–17.

11. The effect of digoxin on mortality and morbidity in patients with heart failure. The Digitalis Investigation Group. *New Engl J Med* 1997; 336: 525–33.

21

Arrhythmias

S. Vaughan

Cardiac arrhythmias are common in the critically ill. This chapter will give an overview of the prevalence, aetiology, therapy and impact of cardiac arrhythmias in the intensive care unit (ICU).

Amiodarone is a drug increasingly being used to treat arrhythmias within the ICU, but it is not without hazard. Amiodarone will be discussed but there is no scope in this chapter for in-depth discussion of the other anti-arrhythmic agents.

Prevalence of arrhythmias in ICU

Some of the early work on the prevalence of arrhythmias in ICU came from South America [1]. Artucio and co-workers looked at over 2800 patients admitted to their ICU over a 12-year period between 1971 and 1983. They found:

- An overall prevalence of cardiac arrhythmia of 78%.
- Atrial tachyarrhythmias were the commonest arrhythmia (28%) followed by ventricular tachyarrhythmias (22%).
- Atrial fibrillation (AF) and atrial flutter accounted for 52% and 27% of the atrial tachyarrhythmias, respectively.
- Ventricular tachycardia accounted for 43% of the ventricular tachyarrhythmia which was only exceeded by ventricular premature beats (VPB) (56%).

The surprisingly high prevalence of arrhythmias in this study can be explained by the patient population and study design. The data was collected from medical ICU (that included post-cardiac surgery patients); a very high proportion of patients had been admitted with cardiac (63%) and respiratory (12%) disease. Not surprisingly subgroup analysis revealed the highest prevalence of arrhythmias in these groups. Moreover, arrhythmia diagnosis was all inclusive; in that sinus bradycardia, sinus arrhythmia, atrial and VPB as well as bundle branch block were included, and increased the prevalence of recorded arrhythmias.

More recent studies from mixed ICU or surgical high dependency units (SHDU) are more representative of the patient case mix seen within the UK.

- Bender found that 14% of post-operative surgical patients developed a supraventricular tachyarrhythmia [2].
- Batra and colleagues also found that 13% of patients on a SHDU developed an arrhythmia of which AF was the commonest [3].
- Reinhelt and co-workers found that nearly 20% of their patients on a mixed ICU developed an arrhythmia of which the majority were ventricular in origin [4]. They also showed that the majority of arrhythmias occurred in those patients with cardiac disease or who had undergone cardiac surgery.

In summary, the prevalence of cardiac arrhythmia within the ICU population is between 0% and 20%.

Aetiology [5, 6]

Arrhythmias can be broadly classified into:

- Disorders of conduction: heart block.
- Disorders of impulse formation (rate or site): bradycardias and tachycardias.

There are three basic electrophysiological mechanisms for disordered conduction and abnormal impulse formation which themselves result from the "recognised" causes of arrhythmias.

The "recognised" causes of arrhythmias are:

Congenital (prolonged Q–T interval)

Jervall–Lange–Neilsen disease (autosomal recessive and associated with deafness) and Romano–Ward syndrome (autosomal dominant).

Myocardial ischaemia

This is probably the commonest cause of arrhythmia outside of the ICU. However, patients may be admitted to the ICU with acute coronary syndromes, have chronic myocardial ischaemia as a co-morbidity or even suffer a myocardial infarction whilst on the ICU. Moreover, it has been shown that cardiac troponin I (cTnI) is elevated in critically ill patients and that higher levels are seen in those who have ECG evidence of ischaemia, tachycardia, arrhythmia, hypotension and inotrope therapy. This suggests that critical illness and/or therapy on ICU causes myocardial damage [7].

Electrolyte imbalance

Changes in K^+, Mg^{2+} and Ca^{2+} are all linked to arrhythmia generation. Hypokalaemia and hypomagnesaemia frequently co-exist as they are both lost through the kidney and gut. Calcium deficiency rarely causes clinical problems whilst the main effect of hypokalaemia and hypomagnesaemia is to prolong the Q–T interval (see below). Conversely the effect of hyperkalemia and hypercalcaemia is to shorten the Q–T interval. Hypermagnesaemia is iatrogenic and aside from first degree heart block, will be asymptomatic.

Hypoxia and hypercarbia

Arrhythmia genesis is from associated myocardial ischaemia and pH-induced electrolyte disturbance.

Drugs

Drugs which prolong the Q–T interval are pro-arrhythmogenic. Drugs with such actions include:

- phenothiazine,
- tricyclic antidepressants,
- antihistamine,
- pentamidine,
- cisapride (now withdrawn from use in the UK),
- erythromycin the latter which has been implicated in fatal ventricular fibrillation if given by rapid intravenous infusion [8].

The other major class of drugs that can initiate cardiac arrhythmias are the anti-arrhythmic agents themselves [9].

- Class Ia (quinidine, procainamide and disopyramide) and Class III (amiodarone and sotalol) drugs in the Vaughan–Williams classification. Like the drugs listed above, these drugs pro-arrhythmic action seems to be due to prolongation of Q–T interval.

- Flecanide, a Class Ic drug which shortens the action potential, should not be used in those patients with acute coronary syndromes as they have been shown to increase mortality from arrhythmia [10].
- Digoxin, which inhibits the Na^+–K^+ ATPase pump results in a rise in intracellular calcium as Na^+ is exchanged for Ca^{2+}. Raised intracellular Ca^{2+} is the mechanism for arrhythmias generation (see below).

It should be noted that all anti-arrhythmic agents have the potential to generate arrhythmias by local changes in cardiac muscle physiology.

ICU specific conditions

There are a few conditions that may provoke arrhythmias that are almost exclusive to the ICU environment.

- Central venous cannulation has been shown to produce arrhythmias in nearly one-third of all insertions, a rate reduced to <5% when the guidewire was inserted to only 20 cm at the skin [11]. The incidence of arrhythmia during Hickman line insertion was reported to be 14% [12].
- High-frequency oscillation (HFO) is a technique well established in paediatric ICU and is now increasingly used in adult ICU. This may be associated with severe bradycardia, particularly in the recovery phase when the lung compliance improves. This is thought to be due to excessive stimulation of the pulmonary stretch receptors and responds well to conversion to conventional ventilation [13].
- Therapy with inotropes (β_1 agonists) and phosphodiesterase inhibitors (increase intracellular cAMP), acid–base disturbance and raised intracranial pressure can all lead to arrhythmias.

The electrophysiological aetiology of arrhythmias

To discuss the electrophysiological basis of arrhythmias, one first needs to re-consider the cardiac muscle action potential.

- Phase 0 is the rapid depolarisation of the myocardial cell membrane caused by opening of fast Na^+ channels and Na^+ influx into the cell.

- Phase 1 is the initial repolarisation of the membrane from the closure of the fast Na^+ channels and the action of the Na^+–K^+ ATPase pump removing Na^+ from the cell in exchange for K^+.
- Phase 2 is the plateau phase caused by the opening of slow Ca^{2+} and slow Na^+ channels resulting in influx of Na^+ and Ca^{2+} and hence delaying repolarisation.
- Phase 3 is the closure of the slow Ca^{2+} and Na^+ channels and restoration of the resting membrane potential by the action of the Na^+–K^+ ATPase pump.
- Phase 4 only occurs in conducting cardiac tissue and is spontaneous depolarisation of the myocyte cell membrane from opening of slow Ca^{2+} and Na^+ channels.

There are three electrophysiological mechanisms for arrhythmia generation:

(1) *Re-entry*

This is the commonest cause of arrhythmia formation. In essence a wave of excitability spreads down one pathway whilst being "blocked" in another then to return to the original pathway via the "blocked" pathway to set up a circle of activity. It requires three pre-conditions:
- two pathways separated by non-conducting tissue;
- differing conduction speeds in the pathways;
- differing refractory periods in the pathways.

It follows that the fastest pathway must have the longer refractory period to enable a circle of electrical activity!

Myocardial ischaemia is the main cause of re-entry arrhythmias as it will result in non-conducting tissue surrounded by conducting tissue of varying quality although electrolyte disturbances can generate the same pre-conditions. Some patients may not have all of the pre-conditions but develop an arrhythmia when a second insult provides the other pre-conditions for re-entry arrhythmias.

(2) *Abnormal automaticity*

This is when spontaneous phase 4 depolarisation occurs in non-conducting or pacemaker myocytes. This commonly results from ischaemia but can also result from metabolic derangement, hypokalaemia, drugs and sympathomimetic agents.

(3) *Triggered activity*

This refers to abnormal depolarisations that occur in the plateau phase of the cardiac action potential. There are two types; early after depolarisations (EAD) and delayed after depolarisations (DAD).
- EAD result from delayed closure of the slow Ca^{2+} and Na^+ channels and, if of sufficient amplitude, may trigger an abnormal impulse. The formation

of EAD is favoured by conditions, which prolong the Q–T interval such as bradycardia, drugs, hypokalaemia and congenital conditions (see above). The presence of EAD is strongly associated with genesis of torsade de pointes ventricular tachycardia.
- DAD result from raised intracellular Ca^{2+} levels of which the classic example is digoxin (see above), but they can also be generated by ischaemia, catecholamines and tachycardia.

Treatment of arrhythmias [9, 14, 15]

The basic treatment aims of arrhythmia management are:

- To restore sinus rhythm and hence optimise cardiac filling and cardiac output.
- To control rate improve the balance between myocardial oxygen consumption and myocardial oxygen delivery.
- To treat complications, namely thrombo-embolic phenomena.

On the ICU, restoration of sinus rhythm and rate control will have a greater significance than prevention of complications, but these should not be ignored.

A few simple rules are presented to help as an aide memoir for treating an arrhythmia developing in an ICU patient. In a perverse way, although the critical illness and its treatment predispose to cardiac arrhythmias, the ICU actually provides an ideal environment in which to treat arrhythmias as one will have a (usually) sedated, ventilated and fully monitored patient!

(1) Treat the patient and *not* the monitor!
    The degree of haemodynamic disturbance will determine the urgency of therapy. It is obvious that hypotension, evidence of ischaemia on the ECG or cardiac monitor and signs of cardiac failure require urgent intervention and treatment of the rhythm disturbance.
(2) Rapid identification and treatment of as many potential contributing factors as possible.
    - Make sure the K^+ is at least 4.5 mmol/l or higher as a higher K^+ concentration will shorten the action potential and lessen the risk of triggered arrhythmias.
    - Correct magnesium deficiency, particularly if there is co-existing hypokalaemia. The plasma level of Mg^{2+} should be at least 1.0 mmol/l and perhaps be between 1.4 and 2.0 mmol/l as levels within this range have been

shown to be superior to direct current (DC) cardioversion in the termination of atrial tachyarrhythmias [16].

– Correct hypoxia, hypercarbia and acidosis as the patient's clinical condition allows.

(3) If the patient is *pulseless* treat according to current ACLS guidelines [15]. See also Chapter 30.

(4) If the patient has a palpable pulse, then treatment should be based upon the UK Resuscitation Council peri-arrest algorithms [15].

The reader is strongly advised to acquaint themselves with the algorithms.
The algorithms are extensive and cover the management of bradycardia, broad and narrow complex tachycardia and AF. However there are some important points to note from the algorithms:

- Magnesium is only included in the broad complex tachycardia algorithm. There is evidence that magnesium will convert atrial tachycardia to sinus rhythm [16] and so the author believes that magnesium should be administered for all types of arrhythmia. A suitable initial dose would be 8 mmols over 10–15 min.
- Except for the broad complex arrhythmia, Class Ia drugs (quinidine, procainamide and disopyramide) are *not* used because they have been shown to increase the mortality in the treatment of AF [9].
- Class Ib (lidocaine and mexilitine) drugs are only recommended in broad complex tachycardia. Class Ib agents are only effective for ventricular arrhythmias [9] and hence are included should the broad complex rhythm be ventricular in origin.
- Class Ic (flecainide) agents should only be used in the absence of coronary artery disease [10].
- Class II drugs (β-blocking agents) should *not* be used in conjunction with Class IV agents (calcium antagonists) as this may precipitate complete heart block.
- There is no algorithm or mention made of extrasystoles and whether these should be treated despite the fact that both atrial premature beats (APB) and VPB may herald a more sustained arrhythmia. The CAST trial showed that VPB should not be treated after a myocardial infarction as mortality was increased [10] and so it is difficult to recommend therapy for VPB beyond correcting electrolyte abnormalities, acidosis and hypoxia. Digoxin may be considered for APB occurring in a background of ischaemic or valvular heart disease.
- Amiodarone appears in the ACLS and all the peri-arrest algorithms (except bradycardia). Amiodarone is a drug that is being increasingly used in the critical care setting and is discussed in more depth below.

- *DC Cardioversion is safe*: The ICU patient is the "ideal" patient for cardioversion. Although the peri-arrest algorithms state that electrical therapy is for the unstable/ symptomatic patient, the author believes that if medical cardioversion of the arrhythmia is considered then D.C. cardioversion should be considered too.

Amiodarone [17]

Amiodarone is rapidly achieving the status of first line anti-arrhythmic agent in the ICU. Its use, though, is not without significant risk to the patient.

Pharmacokinetics

Amiodarone is a lipid-soluble drug and therefore has:

- high degree of plasma protein binding (96%),
- a large volume of distribution (1–65 l/kg),
- a mean half-life of 52 days (16–180 days),
- a single dose intravenous dose has a half-life of 18–36 h.

Amiodarone undergoes hepatic metabolism with production of a weak active metabolite, desethylamiodarone. Metabolites are excreted via the biliary system rather than the kidneys and so amiodarone is safe in renal failure. There is very little accumulation of active metabolite even after days of infusion. Extensive hepatic metabolism means that the oral bioavailability is low (30–50%).

The usual dosing regimen is:

- a loading dose of 5 mg/kg over 1 h but can be given over 3 min in an emergency, followed by
  - 15 mg/kg in the first 24 h reducing to
  - 11 mg/kg on day 2 reducing to
  - 7.5 mg/kg on day 3 until a total of 15 g is given and then
  - a maintenance dose of 200 mg/day.

Pharmacodynamics

- Although appearing as a Class III agent in the Vaughan–Williams classification, amiodarone is unique as it possesses Class I–IV actions. It is therefore useful in the termination of AF, supraventricular and ventricular tachycardias. However, when given intravenously it main effect is β blockade (Class II) with decreased conduction across the atrio-ventricular (A-V) node and an increased A-V node refractory period.

- Although negatively inotropic it is the least cardiac depressant of the anti-arrhythmic agents. A reduction in cardiac afterload compensates for the negative inotropicity such that cardiac output is unchanged or even increased.
- Heart rate and mean arterial blood pressure are unchanged or minimally reduced.
- A most important and under recognised effect of amiodarone is direct coronary vasodilatation.

Drug interactions

Amiodarone will:

- Prolong the Q–T interval if given with other drugs that prolong the Q–T interval.
- Result in a bradycardia or heart block if given with Class II or IV drugs.
- Increase plasma levels of digoxin.
- Reduce warfarin metabolism.

Side effects

- *Cardiovascular*: Amiodarone will prolong the Q–T interval predisposing to arrhythmias. It may give rise to heart block, bradycardias and hypotension.
- *Pulmonary*: It is well known that amiodarone causes chronic pulmonary fibrosis. More recently a more serious acute pulmonary toxicity has been described [18, 19]. The incidence is between 5% and 10% of all those treated and it usually occurs within the first few day or weeks of treatment. Signs and symptoms are fairly non-specific with a fever, cough, pleuritic chest pain with a pleural rub and crackles on chest auscultation. There may be a raised white cell count, erythrocyte sedimentation rate (ESR) and lactate dehydrogenase (LDH) and a chest radiograph may reveal diffuse fine reticulo-nodular shadowing. Diagnosis may well be very difficult on the ICU as most of the signs and findings can be found from other commoner causes, such as a ventilator associated pneumonia, so a high index of suspicion is needed for the diagnosis. Broncho-alveolar lavage will reveal foamy macrophages. Another interesting finding is that acute pulmonary toxicity may be related to high-inspired oxygen concentrations (<50%) [20]. Treatment is supportive with cessation of amiodarone whilst some have suggested the use of corticosteroids. Acute pulmonary toxicity may be fatal.

- *Other organ systems*: Amiodarone can cause damage in the eyes, liver, thyroid gland, skin and peripheral nerves.

Impact of arrhythmias in ICU

It is easy to focus on the immediate problems that arrhythmias can cause, such as hypotension, but to lose sight of the overall impact that the development of a new arrhythmia will have on an ICU patient. Two studies [2, 21] have shown that the onset of new atrial arrhythmias in the critically ill is associated with:

- a greatly increased mortality rate,
- an increase ICU length of stay,
- an increased hospital length of stay.

In both these studies the excess mortality was not directly related to the cardiac rhythm disturbance. The excess mortality seen in those with arrhythmias is also borne out in subgroup analysis of Artucio's work [1]. In all the patient groups, those with an arrhythmia had a higher mortality, for example although septic patients made up only 7% of the total admissions, those with an arrhythmia had a mortality rate of 70% compared to 50% without an arrhythmia (relative risk reduction, RRD >1.5).

Another very important finding is that the onset of a new arrhythmia can herald or be co-incident with the onset of new sepsis [2]. Therefore amongst the investigations of a new arrhythmia, one must consider a new focus of infection, particularly of central venous catheters or of pulmonary or intra-abdominal sites.

Summary

- Arrhythmias are common (up to 20%) and the commonest type are atrial tachyarrhythmias.
- Arrhythmias are caused by myocardial ischaemia, electrolyte imbalance, drugs, acid–base disturbance, inotropic therapy and hypoxia. Always think of new sepsis with the onset of an arrhythmia.
- Hypokalaemia and hypomagnesaemia frequently co-exist.
- Correct any identified contributing factors.
- Magnesium should be given even if levels are "normal" and the K^+ should be at least 4.5 mmol/l.
- Electricity is safe; anti-arrhythmics agents cause arrhythmias!

- Use amiodarone cautiously particularly if the patient is receiving high-oxygen concentrations (>50%) and limit it use to 24–48 h as most arrhythmias will not be sustained, particularly if contributing factors have been corrected.

FURTHER READING

Chung MK. Cardiac surgery: postoperative arrhythmias. *Crit Care Med* 2000; 28: N136–44.

Hollenberg SM, Dellinger RP. Noncardiac surgery: postoperative arrhythmias. *Crit Care Med* 2000; 28: N145–50.

Montgomery H. Managing arrhythmias. In Helen Galley (Ed.), *Critical Care Focus (6)*. BMJ Books, London, 2002, pp. 33–8.

Saxonhouse SJ, Curtis AB. Risks and benefits of rate control versus maintenance of sinus rhythm. *Am J Cardiol* 2003; 91: 27D–32.

REFERENCES

1. Artucio H, Pereira M. Cardiac arrhythmias in critically ill patients: epidemiological study. *Crit Care Med* 1990; 18: 1383–8.
2. Bender JS. Supraventricular tachyarrhythmias in the surgical intensive care unit: an under-recognized event. *Am Surg* 1996; 62: 73–5.
3. Batra GS, Molyneux J, Scott NA. Colorectal patients and cardiac arrhythmias detected on the surgical high dependency unit. *Ann R Coll Surg Engl* 2001; 83: 174–6.
4. Reinelt P, Karth GD, Geppert A, Heinz G. Incidence and type of cardiac arrhythmias in critically ill patients: a single center experience in a medical-cardiological ICU. *Intens Care Med* 2001; 27: 1466–73.
5. Ramaswamy K, Hamdan MH. Ischemia, metabolic disturbances, and arrhythmogenesis: mechanisms and management. *Crit Care Med* 2000; 28(Suppl 10): N151–7.
6. Francis GS. Cardiac complications in the intensive care unit. *Clinics Chest Med* 1999; 20: 269–85.
7. Noble JS, Reid AM, Jordan LVM, Glen ACA, Davidson JAH. Troponin I and myocardial injury in the ICU. *Brit J Anaesth* 1999; 82: 41–6.
8. Haefeli WE, Schoenenberger RA, Weiss P, Ritz R. Possible risk for cardiac arrhythmia related to intravenous erythromycin. *Intens Care Med* 1992; 18: 469–73.
9. Chaudhry GM, Haffajee CI. Antiarrhythmic agents and proarrhythmia. *Crit Care Med* 2000; 28(Suppl 10): N158–64.
10. The Cardiac Arrhythmia Suppression Trial (CAST) Investigators. Preliminary report: effect of ecainide and flecainide on mortality in a randomized trial of arrhythmia suppression after myocardial infarction. *New Engl J Med* 1989; 321: 406–12.

11. Lee TY, Sung CS, Chu YC, Liou JT, Lui PW. Incidence and risk factors of guidewire induced arrhythmia during internal jugular venous catheterisation: comparison of marked and plain wires. *J Clin Anesth* 1996; 8: 348–51.

12. Ray S, Stacey R, Imrie M, Filshie J. A review of 560 Hickman catheter insertions. *Anaesthesia* 1996; 51: 981–5.

13. Mellema JD, Baden HP, Martin LD, Bratton SL. Severe paroxysmal sinus bradycardia associated with high frequency oscillatory ventilation. *Chest* 1997; 112: 181–5.

14. Hollenberg SM, Dellinger RP. Noncardiac surgery: postoperative arrhythmias. *Crit Care Med* 2000; 28(Suppl 10): N145–50.

15. Resuscitation Council (UK). Advanced Life Support Provider Manual, 4th Ed. London: Resuscitation Council (UK), 2001 [also found at www.resus.org.uk].

16. Moran JL, Gallagher J, Peake SL, Cunningham DL et al. Parenteral magnesium sulphate versus amiodarone in the therapy of atrial tachyarrhythmias: a prospective, randomised trial. *Crit Care Med* 1995; 23: 1816–24.

17. Hughes M, Binning A. Intravenous amiodarone in intensive care. Time for reappraisal? *Intens Care Med* 2000; 26: 1730–9.

18. Van Meighem W, Coolen L, Malysse I, Lacquet LM et al. Amiodarone and the development of ARDS after lung surgery. *Chest* 1994; 105: 1642–5.

19. Leonard A, Corris P, Parums D. Amiodarone pulmonary toxicity: Authors did not emphasise typical radiological and histological features sufficiently. *Br Med J* 1997; 314: 1831–2.

20. Donaldson L, Grant IS, Naysmith MR, Thomas JS. Amiodarone should be used with caution in patients in intensive care. *Br Med J* 1997; 314: 1832.

21. Braithwaite D, Weissman C. The new onset of atrial arrhythmias following major non-cardiothoracic surgery is associated with increased mortality. *Chest* 1998; 114: 462–8.

22

The patient with sepsis

R. Markham

Sepsis is the leading cause of multiple organ failure and the most common cause of mortality in the intensive care unit (ICU): in the first 24 h of intensive care admission, 21.7% of patients in England, Wales and Northern Ireland fulfil the criteria for severe sepsis [1]. Of these, 35% die on ICU and a further 12% die before discharge from hospital. In the USA, sepsis is responsible for as many deaths as acute myocardial infarction [2].

The mortality of septic shock varies from 40% to 80%.

Definitions

In 1992, the American College of Chest Physicians (ACCP) and the Society of Critical Care Medicine (SCCM) proposed definitions of sepsis which were re-validated at a 2001 consensus conference [3]:

- *Sepsis*: A clinical syndrome defined by the presence of infection and a systemic inflammatory response.
- *Infection*: A pathological process caused by the invasion of normally sterile tissue, fluid or body cavity by pathogenic microorganisms.
- *Systemic Inflammatory Response Syndrome (SIRS)*: Two or more of the following:
  - temperature $>38°C$ or $<36°C$,
  - heart rate >90 beats/min,
  - respiratory rate >20 breaths/min or $PaCO_2$ <4.3 kPa,
  - white cell count (WCC) $>12,000$ or <4000 or $>10\%$ immature band forms.
- *Severe sepsis*: Sepsis associated with organ dysfunction, hypoperfusion or hypotension (but not requiring inotropes or vasopressors).

- *Septic shock*: Acute circulatory failure in the presence of sepsis. This is defined as sepsis with hypotension despite adequate fluid resuscitation.

SIRS may be triggered by localised or generalised infection, trauma, burns or sterile inflammatory processes (e.g. acute pancreatitis).

SIRS emphasises that the host response to infection and non-infectious stimuli is the same and that the severity of the response determines the outcome. However, the SIRS criteria are non-specific and are widely considered to be over-sensitive (more than two-thirds of ICU patients meet SIRS criteria) [4]; but until further immunologic and biochemical markers of sepsis have been identified, and more appropriate definitions introduced, it remains an important concept [5].

PIRO: a staging system for sepsis

A staging system was proposed by the consensus conference to stratify patients by baseline risk and potential to respond to therapy. It is based on the concept of the tumour, necrosis and metastasis (TNM) system for classifying malignant tumours:

- P: Predisposition. Premorbid factors such as illness or genetic predisposition may influence both incidence and outcome of sepsis.
- I: Insult. Site, type and extent of infection.
- R: Response. Nature and magnitude of the host response.
- O: Organ dysfunction. The number or severity of failing organs.

At present, the PIRO system has not been validated and remains an experimental concept.

Pathophysiology

Bacterial infection [6, 7]

- Previously, Gram-negative infections (especially *Escherichia coli, Klebsiella* species and *Pseudomonas aeruginosa*) were the most common cause of severe sepsis, however Gram-positive infections (particularly staphylococci and streptococci) have increased and now account for about half of all cases. Fungi, mainly Candida are responsible for about 5% of cases of severe sepsis.
- Invading microorganisms are detected by pattern recognition receptors on the surface of innate immune cells called toll-like receptors (TLRs), which activate intracellular signalling pathways to initiate the inflammatory response.

Gram-negative and Gram-positive infections are mediated via different receptors: endotoxin (lipopolysaccharide) requires TLR4 to activate the immune response, whilst TLR2 is involved in the recognition of cell wall components of Gram-positive bacteria such as peptidoglycan and lipoproteins.

- Clinical manifestations of different bacterial infections vary due to differential expression and release of inflammatory mediators. Hence streptococcal toxic shock syndrome produces a very different clinical picture to meningococcaemia. This suggests specific host responses for each pathogen.

Inflammatory and procoagulant response [8]

- Infection results in monocyte and macrophage activation with consequent platelet activation and aggregation, and the release of inflammatory cytokines; particularly interleukin (IL)-1β, IL-6 and tumour necrosis factor α (TNF-α).
- Cytokines are newly synthesised and released in response to inflammatory stimuli, and have synergistic, overlapping and antagonistic effects.
- Inflammatory cytokines stimulate the release of tissue factor from the endothelium, which activates the coagulation cascade resulting in the formation of thrombin and a fibrin clot.
- Thrombin is itself pro-inflammatory via multiple pathways including platelet activation and mast cell degranulation. It also impairs fibrinolysis by release of plasminogen-activator inhibitor-1 (PAI-1) from platelets and endothelium. PAI-1 inhibits the endogenous fibrinolytic pathway, tissue plasminogen activator.
- Activated protein C levels are reduced. The conversion of protein C to serine activated protein C occurs on the endothelium and requires thrombin bound to thrombomodulin. Endothelial injury results in reduced thrombomodulin levels. Activated protein C is an endogenous protein that promotes fibrinolysis by inhibiting PAI-1; it is anti-thrombogenic by inhibiting factors Va and VIIIa and hence thrombin production; and it is anti-inflammatory, possibly by inhibiting cytokine production.
- The end result is diffuse endothelial injury and microvascular thrombosis leading to organ ischaemia, multi-organ dysfunction and, eventually, death. Cell apoptosis may contribute to this effect.

Myocardial depression [9]

- Myocardial depression occurs due to a circulating myocardial depressant factor, with reduced left and right ventricular contractility.

- Initially, tachycardia and increased left ventricular (LV) compliance (by ventricular dilatation and increased preload), together with reduced systemic vascular resistance, attempt to compensate for this impaired contractility. However, cardiac output remains low to normal.
- Eventually, aggressive fluid resuscitation may compensate for these changes and adequate left ventricular preload is re-established, producing a high cardiac output, low systemic vascular resistance state.
- However, up to a third of patients with septic shock remain with a low cardiac output shock [10]. Such patients typically have bacterial peritonitis and this may reflect overwhelming myocardial depression especially in patients with pre-existing cardiac disease.
- A recent important study demonstrated significant increase in cardiac Troponin I levels in patients with septic shock [11] implying significant myocardial cell damage. (This is despite, in general, evidence of well-maintained coronary blood flow in septic shock.) Serum troponin levels tended to be lower in survivors than in non-survivors and tended to be higher in patients on large doses of inotropes and vasopressors. This study raises serious questions, at present unresolved:
  - Is the reduction in cardiac function and cardiac dilatation in septic shock related to myocardial depression or myocardial injury, or both?
  - Is the use of inotropes and vasopressors necessary because of the myocardial injury or a cause of myocardial injury by increasing myocardial oxygen requirements?

Vasodilatation

- Nitric oxide (NO) is released from the endothelium in response to cytokine stimulation and results in profound vasodilatation. NO is synthesised from the amino acid arginine by the action of NO synthase.
- In severe cases the vasculature can lose its responsiveness to vasopressors.

Capillary leak (relative hypovolaemia)

- The endothelial damage leads to neutrophil adhesion, activation and degranulation with release of oxygen-free radicals and proteases causing further injury.
- The endothelial damage results in increased vascular wall permeability and peripheral oedema.

- This hypovolaemia is in addition to surgical "third space losses": fluid and blood loss in surgical sepsis and peritonitis.

Distributive shock [9]

- Hypoperfusion occurs despite a normal or increased cardiac output due to maldistribution of blood flow. Splanchnic blood flow is reduced and micro-vascular shunting occurs.

Reduction in oxygen utilisation

- Oxygen consumption, VO_2 is reduced with evidence of tissue hypoxia such as elevated serum lactate, often despite well-maintained cardiac output and oxygen delivery, DO_2. This may be due to changes at the cellular level by cytokine or NO induced mitochondrial inhibition, as well as maldistribution of flow.

Metabolic changes

- Endotoxin and cytokines stimulate metabolic changes including protein catabolism and pancreatic secretion of glucagon and insulin. This induces a sequential progressive inability to use glucose, fat, then amino acids and energy sources.
- Mitochondrial dysfunction may be present. This is expressed initially peripherally in the muscles and results in an increase in anaerobic metabolism and gluconeogenesis.
- If prolonged this peripheral defect may result in central organ changes ultimately culminating in multi-organ failure.

Diagnosis of sepsis

The diagnosis of sepsis is made on clinical or laboratory findings in the setting of confirmed or suspected infection. At least two blood cultures should be obtained; both peripherally and from each vascular access device. Cultures of other sites such as urine, cerebrospinal fluid and respiratory secretions should be obtained if clinically indicated. Imaging is important to determine the source of infection, for example ultrasound in suspected intra-abdominal collection. Other occult sources of sepsis must be considered including otitis media and sinusitis, as well as intravascular catheters.

The consensus conference in 2001 [3] agreed the following list of symptoms and signs of sepsis, however it must be noted that none are specific to sepsis:

Generalised symptoms:

- Fever
- Hypothermia
- Tachycardia
- Tachypnoea
- Altered mental status
- Hypotension
- High cardiac output
- Raised mixed venous oxygen saturation (SvO_2 >70%) reduced in shock
- Slow capillary refill/mottling.

Signs of organ dysfunction:

- Hypoxia
- Oliguria
- Coagulopathy
- Thrombocytopenia
- Hyperbilirubinaemia
- Ileus
- Hyperglycaemia.

Laboratory signs:

- Leucocytosis or leucopenia
- Plasma C-reactive protein >2 standard deviations above normal range
- Plasma procalcitonin >2 standard deviations above normal range
- Hyperlactatemia.

Therapy of sepsis and septic shock

Prevention

- Follow guidelines in Chapter 13.
- Prophylactic antibiotics for certain surgical procedures are appropriate.

Eradicate the infection

- Prompt administration of antibiotic therapy should commence after appropriate cultures have been obtained. In severe sepsis or septic shock, broad spectrum antibiotic therapy is warranted until the causative organism and its sensitivities have been identified.

- Surgical collections and foci of infection should be identified and drained promptly. These include intra-abdominal abscesses, gastrointestinal perforation, cholangitis and pyelonephritis.
- Intravenous catheters suspected of being colonised or infected must be removed and cultured.
- Antibiotic therapy or cardiovascular support alone will provide disappointing results in the therapy of septic shock. Outcome is, perhaps obviously, improved when both are combined.

Initial resuscitation

Resuscitation should begin as soon as a diagnosis of severe sepsis is made, and not be delayed until ICU admission. In patients who are not hypotensive an elevated serum lactate indicates tissue hypoperfusion.

- A randomised-controlled trial into early goal-directed therapy [12] found a significant improvement in the 28-day mortality of severe sepsis or septic shock when resuscitation in the first 6 h of therapy was directed towards the following parameters:
  - central venous pressure (CVP) is 8–12 mmHg by infusion of crystalloid (500 ml every 30 min),
  - mean arterial pressure (MAP) >65 mmHg by administration of vasopressors,
  - Central venous (superior vena cava, SVC) oxygen saturation >70%,
  - if <70%, red blood cells were transfused to achieve a haematocrit of at least 30%; following this if the target was not attained dobutamine infusion was commenced (up to 20 μg/kg/min).
- There appears to be no benefit in attaining supranormal cardiovascular parameter in patients with sepsis.

Fluid loading

Fluids must be given to optimise preload as an initial step:

- However, it has been shown that some patients with septic shock show a diminished cardiovascular response to fluid loading – further evidence for the depressed cardiac function seen from sepsis.

- For example, a study has shown that similar increases in preload, as assessed with a pulmonary artery catheter, result in lesser increases in LV stroke work compared to "control" critically ill patients without sepsis [13].

Fluid loading alone is unlikely to restore haemodynamic stability. Thus, almost all patients will require cardiovascular support.

Inotropes and vasopressor (see also Chapter 12)

- Dobutamine is the inotrope of choice for optimising cardiac output in the presence of adequate fluid resuscitation and MAP.
- In the presence of hypotension, autoregulation in vascular beds may be lost and perfusion can become linearly dependent on pressure. Vasopressor therapy may be required to achieve a satisfactory perfusion pressure to maintain adequate flow.
- Noradrenaline increases MAP by vasoconstriction with minimal increase in heart rate, and is commonly used as a first-line vasopressor in sepsis. It may be associated in with an improvement in outcome in septic shock [14]. Dopamine is also used (especially in the USA), but its primary effects are via an increase in heart rate and stroke volume. Both are probably superior to epinephrine, which may impair splanchnic perfusion.
- Vasopressin may be useful in low dose in refractory shock, but it should be used in caution in patients with cardiac dysfunction and may result in decreased cardiac output and splanchnic flow. No outcome data are available as yet.
- The combination of fluid resuscitation, dobutamine and noradrenaline has much to commend it and it is the standard approach in many centres.

Renal replacement therapy

- There is no evidence currently to support the use of continuous venovenous haemofiltration for the treatment of sepsis; however, in acute renal failure renal replacement therapy may be indicated.

Corticosteroid therapy

- Corticosteroids inhibit exogenous NO synthase and the release of inflammatory cytokines including IL-1 and TNF from monocytes. They prevent leucocyte adhesion and complement activation, and also prevent prostaglandin synthesis by induction of phospholipase A_2 inhibitor. Such anti-inflammatory properties suggest therapeutic benefit, however high-dose short-course steroid therapy has previously been shown to be ineffective if not harmful in severe sepsis [15]. However, the hypothalamic–pituitary–adrenal axis is often suppressed in sepsis and there is new evidence that low-dose replacement therapy with steroids improves outcome in septic shock.

- Initial studies suggested an improvement in haemodynamic parameters with reduced vasopressor requirement following low-dose hydrocortisone (about 300 mg/day) [16].
- A subsequent multi-centre study demonstrated improved 28-day survival in patients with septic shock and relative adrenal insufficiency treated with intravenous hydrocortisone 50 mg every 6 h and fludrocortisone 50 μg enterally daily for 7 days [17]. Relative adrenal insufficiency was defined as non-responders to the short corticotrophin (adrenocorticotrophic hormone, ACTH) test: 250 μg of synacthen was administered and blood samples are taken 30 and 60 min later. Non-responders had a cortisol response of 9 μg/dl or less. There were no significant adverse effects and the number needed to treat (NNT) to save one additional life was seven.
- From this evidence it is recommended that low-dose steroids are commenced in vasopressor-dependent septic shock. A short synacthen test should be performed prior to commencing treatment and when the result is available, if there is, an adequate response therapy may be discontinued.

Activated protein C

- Activated protein C levels are reduced in sepsis, probably due to down-regulation of thrombomodulin by circulating cytokines. A large multi-centre randomised-controlled trial was carried out to assess the efficacy of recombinant human activated protein C in severe sepsis: the Protein C Worldwide Evaluation in Severe Sepsis (PROWESS) [18]. The 1690 patients were randomised before the trial was stopped because of a significant mortality benefit in the treatment group. Patients received either activated protein C (drotrecogin alfa activated) 24 μg/kg/h for 96 h, or a placebo infusion for the same period; and were eligible for inclusion if they fulfilled the consensus criteria for severe sepsis with organ dysfunction of <24 h duration. Those with increased risk of bleeding; either congenital or acquired (e.g. recent surgery, active gastrointestinal bleed or severe head injury) were excluded. The two groups were well matched for demographic characteristics and disease severity and at 28-day mortality in the treatment group was 24.7% compared with 30.8% in the placebo group; an absolute risk reduction of 6.1% (NNT = 16). The incidence of serious bleeding was higher in the treatment group (3.5% versus 2.0%), but this mainly occurred in patients with an identifiable predisposition to bleeding. The anticoagulant effect was only apparent during the period of infusion.

- Post hoc subgroup analysis has suggested that the greatest benefit is to patients with more severe disease [19]. Owing to this and cost implications the US Food and Drug Administration have restricted the use of activated protein C to patients with an Acute Physiology and Chronic Health Evaluation II (APACHE II) score of 25 or more, and at least two organ failures.
- A larger follow-up trial (ADDRESS trial) looking at long-term outcome in severe sepsis patients is as yet unpublished but early presentations at scientific meetings has stated that there is no mortality difference between the therapy and control groups irrespective of APACHE II scores greater or less than 25. The main difference between this and the PROWESS trial is that the therapy window was increased to 48 h, emphasising the importance of early interventions in septic shock.

Control of blood glucose

- Hyperglycaemia associated with relative insulin resistance is common in critically ill patients with or without diabetes, and may increase the risk of severe infections, polyneuropathy, multiple organ failure and death. A large single-centre randomised-control trial of mainly post-operative surgical patients found a significant improvement in intensive care mortality when intensive insulin therapy was used to maintain blood glucose between 4.4 and 6.1 mmol/l [20]. Hypoglycaemia was more common in the treatment group but there were no serious sequelae. The greatest reduction in mortality involved deaths due to multiple organ failure with a proven septic focus.
- A subsequent prospective observational study of mostly cardiothoracic surgery patients suggested that a target blood glucose of <8 mmol/l may be adequate and reduce the risk of hypoglycaemia; whilst infusing high doses of insulin may be harmful [21].
- The control of blood glucose level appears to be more important than the insulin dose administered [22], and a recent observational study found hyperglycaemia on admission to the ICU to be associated with increased serum concentrations of IL-6 [23].

- When a glycaemic control strategy is employed it is important to provide a continuous supply of glucose substrate, preferably by enteral feeding.

Sedation, analgesia and neuromuscular blockade

- The use of sedation protocols, along with either intermittent bolus sedation or continuous infusions with daily interruptions or lightening may reduce the duration of mechanical ventilation as well as length of ICU stay. Neuromuscular blocking drugs should be avoided if at all possible due to the risk of prolonged muscle weakness.

Less commonly used therapies

- Attempts to block the excess effects of NO with analogues of arginine showed initial promise in case series but later phase II trials were stopped due to unexpected adverse events.
- Methylene blue is a potent inhibitor of guanylate cyclase (the target enzyme in the endothelium-dependent relaxation mediated by NO). Several studies show improvement in haemodynamics but no improvement in survival. In addition there may be problems in terms of pulmonary vasoconstriction and adverse effect on oxygenation.

Experimental therapies

- Antithrombin III has been evaluated in severe sepsis and septic shock. Unfortunately no beneficial effect on 28-day mortality has been demonstrated and there may be an increased risk of bleeding when high doses are administered in combination with heparin.
- Recombinant tissue factor pathway inhibitor, a physiological inhibitor of coagulation and thrombin generation has been investigated. A large phase III trial failed to show any improvement in mortality or morbidity.
- Clinical trials of monoclonal antibodies against TNF-α have so far proved disappointing.

Outcome and consideration for limitation of support

- Managing the patient with septic shock in an ICU run by trained ICU specialists has been shown to improve survival [24].

- Lundberg in 1998 [25] showed that early interventions for septic shock were associated with reduced mortality. The data suggests that for patients with septic shock on wards, there are clinically important delays in transfer of patients to the ICU, receipt of intravenous fluid boluses, and receipt of inotropic agents.
- Poor outcome is associated with excessive vasodilatation and resistance to catecholamines [26], increased age, immunosuppression (including prior therapy with steroids) and the development of multiple organ failure.
- Early and frequent discussions of likely outcome and realistic goals of treatment should take place with patients and their families, to allow timely withdrawal of life-sustaining therapy if it is considered futile or inappropriate.
- The use of noradrenaline may be life saving in many patients with septic shock but giving it to patients who have already developed multiple organ failure during their stay in the ICU is associated with a poor outcome (and may even be considered futile by some authors [27]).

Future strategies [6]

Agents that neutralise microbial products or block their interaction with immune cell receptors are potential therapeutic targets and monoclonal antibody therapy against CD14, a plasma and membrane protein that binds to lipopolysaccharide is being evaluated. However there is inherent risk in inactivating cells that are pivotal to innate immunity. Inhibition of macrophage migration inhibitory factor, a cytokine that modulates the expression of TLR4, may be of benefit in sepsis; and targeted immunomodulatory therapies may be indicated in patients with genetic polymorphisms that increase susceptibility to sepsis.

FURTHER READING

Dellinger RP, Carlet JM, Masur H et al. Surviving sepsis campaign guidelines for management of severe sepsis and septic shock. *Crit Care Med* 2004; 32: 858–73.

Dellinger RP. Cardiovascular management of septic shock. *Crit Care Med* 2003; 31: 946–55.

Annane D, Bellissant E, Edouard PE, Briegel J et al. Corticosteroids for severe sepsis and septic shock: a systematic review and meta-analysis. *Br Med J* 2004; 329: 480–4.

Hollenberg SM, Ahrens TS, Annane D, Astiz ME et al. Practice parameters for hemodynamic support of sepsis in adult patients: 2004 update. *Crit Care Med* 2004; 32: 1928–48.

REFERENCES

1. Padkin A, Goldfrad C, Brady A et al. Epidemiology of severe sepsis occurring in the first 24 hours in intensive care units in England, Wales and Northern Ireland. *Crit Care Med* 2003; 31: 2332–8.

2. Angus DC, Linde-Zwirbe WT, Lidicker J et al. Epidemiology of severe sepsis in the United States: analysis of incidence, outcome, and associated costs of care. *Crit Care Med* 2001; 29: 1303–10.

3. Levy MM, Fink MP, Marshall JC et al. 2001 SCCM/ESICM/ACCP/ATS/SIS International Sepsis Definitions Conference. *Crit Care Med* 2003; 31: 1250–6.

4. Vincent J-L. Dear SIRS, I'm sorry to say that I don't like you. *Crit Care Med* 1997; 25: 372–4.

5. Dellinger RP. To SIRS with love. *Crit Care Med* 1998; 26: 178–9.

6. Bochud P-Y, Calandra T. Pathogenesis of sepsis: new concepts and implications for future treatment. *Br Med J* 2003; 326: 262–6.

7. Hotchkiss RS, Karl IE. The pathophysiology and treatment of sepsis. *New Engl J Med* 2003; 348: 138–50.

8. Blackwell TS, Christman JW. Sepsis and cytokines: current status. *Br J Anaesth* 1996; 77: 110–17.

9. Dellinger RP. Cardiovascular management of septic shock. *Crit Care Med* 2003; 31: 946–55.

10. Jardin F, Brun-Ney D, Auvert B, Beauchet A, Bourdarias JP. Sepsis-related cardiogenic shock. *Crit Care Med* 1990; 18: 1055–60.

11. Turner A, Tsamitros M, Bellomo R. Myocardial cell injury in septic shock. *Crit Care Med* 1999; 27: 1775–80.

12. Rivers E, Nguyen B, Havstad S et al. Early goal-directed therapy in the treatment of severe sepsis and septic shock. *New Engl J Med* 2001; 345: 1368–77.

13. Ognibene FP, Parker MM, Natanson CC, Shelhamer JH, Parrillo JE. Depressed left ventricular performance. Response to volume infusion in patients with sepsis and septic shock. *Chest* 1988; 93: 903–10.

14. Martin C, Viviand X, Leone M et al. Effect of norepinephrine on the outcome of septic shock. *Crit Care Med* 2000; 28: 2758–65.

15. Cronin L, Cook D, Carlet J et al. Corticosteroid treatment for sepsis: critical appraisal and meta-analysis of the literature. *Crit Care Med* 1995; 23: 1430–9.

16. Briegel J, Forst H, Haller M et al. Stress doses of hydrocortisone reverse hyperdynamic septic shock. A prospective, randomized, double-blind, single-center study. *Crit Care Med* 1999; 27: 723–32.

17. Annane D, Sébille V, Charpentier C. Effect of treatment with low doses of hydrocortisone and fludrocortisone on mortality in patients with septic shock. *J Am Med Assoc* 2002; 288: 862–71.

18. Bernard GR, Vincent J-L, Laterre PF et al. Efficacy and safety of recombinant human activated protein C for severe sepsis. *New Engl J Med* 2001; 344: 699–709.

19. Dhainaut J-F, Yan B, Claessens Y-E. Protein C/activated protein C pathway: overview of clinical trial results in severe sepsis. *Crit Care Med* 2004; 32(Suppl): S194–201.

20. Van den Berge G, Wouters P, Weekers F et al. Intensive insulin therapy in critically ill patients. *New Engl J Med* 2001; 345: 1359–67.

21. Finney SJ, Zekveld C, Elia A et al. Glucose control and mortality in critically ill patients. *J Am Med Assoc* 2003; 290: 2041–7.

22. Van den Berge G, Wouters P, Bouillon R et al. Outcome benefit of intensive insulin therapy in the critically ill: insulin dose versus glycemic control. *Crit Care Med* 2003; 31: 359–66.

23. Wasmuth H, Kunz D, Graf J et al. Hyperglycaemia at admission to the intensive care unit is associated with elevated serum concentrations of interleukin-6 and reduced ex vivo secretion of tumour necrosis factor α. *Crit Care Med* 2004; 32: 1109–14.

24. Reynolds HN, Haupt MT, Thill-Baharozian MC, Carlson RW. Impact of critical care physician staffing on patients with septic shock in a university hospital medical intensive care unit. *J Am Med Assoc* 1988; 260: 3446–50.

25. Lundberg JS, Perl TM, Wiblin T, Costigan MD et al. Septic shock: an analysis of outcomes for patients with onset on hospital wards versus intensive care units. *Crit Care Med* 1998; 26: 1020–4.

26. Groeneveld AB, Nauta JJ, Thijs LG. Peripheral vascular resistance in septic shock: its relation to outcome. *Intens Care Med* 1988; 14: 141–7.

27. Abid O, Akca S, Haji-Michael P, Vincent JL. Strong vasopressor support may be futile in the intensive care unit patient with multiple organ failure. *Crit Care Med* 2000; 28: 947–9.

23

Acute renal failure in the critically ill

R. Kishen

Introduction

- Acute renal failure (ARF) in the critically ill, almost always, develops as part of multiple organ dysfunction (or failure) syndrome.
- ARF in the critically ill has high mortality.
- Understanding renal physiology and pathophysiology of ARF in the critically ill (especially those with sepsis-associated ARF or SAARF) provides logical guidelines for prevention and/or management of patients at risk.
- To date there are no proven pharmacological therapies that "prevent" ARF.
- Our understanding of ARF in the critically ill is far from complete.
- ARF in the critically ill is distinctly different from "medical" ARF; and management of these patients is often challenging.
- Critically ill patients with ARF have higher mortality than a similar cohort of patients without ARF.

Incidence and definition

- ARF in the critically ill is not properly defined.
- In the literature, definitions for ARF, populations studied and timing of interventions seem to be different in different studies.
- This creates problems in interpreting the available literature.
- Besides that, defining points at which interventions like renal replacement therapy (RRT) should begin or stop also becomes difficult.
- Lack of definition also means that it is difficult to estimate accurate incidence of this disease in our intensive care unit (ICU) patients.

- In the literature, the incidence of ARF is quoted as 0.14% (community acquired or "medical" ARF) to 33% in the critically ill. In some recent studies, ARF complicating critical illness has been estimated to be of the order of 4–8%. Based on unpublished data (1997–2001), the incidence of ARF in author's ICU is about 15–20% (a tertiary referral unit).
- A recent survey of 53 centres in 23 countries gave an incidence of ARF of about 6.0% in ICU patients. However, another survey reported in 2003 showed an incidence of about 36% in European ICUs. This only confirms that the definition of ARF is still a matter of debate.
- There is no universally accepted definition of ARF. I use the following working definition:
  - a precipitating factor (e.g., sepsis, major trauma),
  - a reduction in urine volume to <0.25 ml/kg/h (<480 ml in 24 h in 80 kg adult),
  - a rise in plasma creatinine of >50% from the "usual" baseline creatinine,
  - development of metabolic acidosis that cannot be explained by hypoperfusion, untreated severe sepsis or other causes.
- This definition applies to patients with previously "normal" renal function and who have been fully volume resuscitated and have had their perfusion restored.
- Defining renal failure in the critically ill with pre-existing renal failure (sepsis-induced ARF in a patient with chronic non-dialysis dependent renal dysfunction) can be difficult despite this definition.
- Recent attempts at defining ARF as a "graded injury", much like acute lung injury (ALI) and acute respiratory distress syndrome (ARDS) may well be the way forward. However, defining a point at which RRT should be instituted in ARF may still not be easy.
- Renal recovery may be defined as the point when RRT is no longer required to maintain normal or near normal biochemistry along with the return of urine output of more than 500 ml/day. This, again, is an arbitrary definition of an end point and will vary in different patients and progress of the on ongoing critical illness.
- Notwithstanding the problems in defining ARF in the critically ill, it has been found that ARF is an independent factor for increased mortality in the critically ill and despite advances in supportive treatment (e.g., better resuscitation, technologically advanced equipment for supportive therapy), mortality remains high in the region of 50–80%.
- Thus, it is important to understand mechanisms that cause ARF and the strategies that may prevent it.

Physiology in relation to ARF of critical illness

A brief account of some of the physiological principals that are important for present discussion are given below:

- Kidneys receive about 20–25% of cardiac output (about 400 ml/gm tissue – highest blood flow for any single organ in adult). This high-blood flow is primarily for producing large quantities of glomerular filtrate (which is modified along the length of the nephron to ultimately be excreted as urine).
- Kidney's metabolic (oxygen) demand is not a determinant of renal blood flow (RBF).
- Renal vasculature is complex. There are also regional variations in blood flow in that the cortex is relatively well supplied whereas the medulla, especially regions of outer medulla have sparse blood flow.
- Afferent arteriole supplies blood to the glomerulus. Blood from glomerulus drains via efferent arteriole, which then breaks up to become peritubular tuft of capillaries (supplying blood to the cortical nephrons) or into vas recta (supplying blood to juxta-medullary nephrons).
- RBF is autoregulated under normal physiological conditions (i.e., RBF stays relatively constant over a wide range of blood pressure).
- Although the precise mechanisms for this autoregulation are still a matter of debate, it is thought that local myogenic factors (affecting smooth muscle of renal vessels) and tubulo-glomerular feedback (TGF) are important mechanism responsible.
- TGF is a protective mechanism for the nephron. It operates under various physio-pathological conditions. For example in low-perfusion state, TGF will cause afferent arteriolar constriction to reduce glomerular filtrate coming down the tubule in order to lessen oxygen demand of the later till perfusion improves. Thus TGF protects the nephron during metabolic stress. Substances like low-dose dopamine abolish TGF and are thus potentially harmful to "metabolically stressed" tubules.
- Systemic blood pressure is not a good indicator of RBF (or renal perfusion) especially under pathological conditions. For example, during hypovolaemia or other shock states, kidneys act as "guardians" of blood pressure via the angiotensin–renin mechanism. Thus RBF may severely be compromised despite the blood pressure being well within the "normal" range.
- Blood flowing through the medulla (especially in the vasa recta) has a low haematocrit (important for countercurrent mechanism and maintenance of

high osmolality of the medullary interstitium) and therefore, reduced oxygen carrying capacity. The reduced oxygen delivery, high osmolality and counter-current mechanisms (including that for oxygen) make the outer medullary interstitium very hostile for the structures within it (e.g., loop of Henlé).

- Nephron is the functional unit of the kidney but the proximal tubule (PcT) and the thick portion of the ascending limb of the loop of Henlé (mTAL) are the metabolically very active parts of the tubule.
- PcT and mTAL are sites of active sodium reabsorption (60% sodium being absorbed by PcT and 30% by mTAL); this sodium reabsorption accounts for about 80–90% of renal oxygen consumption by the kidney.
- As the outer medulla does not have good oxygen delivery, parts of nephron in or close to outer medulla (e.g., mTAL, part of PcT) are in a finely balanced envir-onment, often at verge of hypoxia. Even a small upset in this balance can cause hypoxic damage to these metabolically active parts of the tubule.
- This state of virtual hypoxia is the price that has to be paid for efficient con-centration of glomerular filtrate and conservation of fluid.

Important factors that ensure integrity of renal excretory function under differ-ent physiological (and some pathological) conditions are:

- *Integrity of RBF*: adequate cardiac output and adequate circulating volume.
- *Afferent and efferent arteriolar smooth muscle tone*, and their control.
- *Afferent arteriolar dilatation*: to maintain flow into the glomerulus.
- *Efferent arteriolar constriction*: to maintain glomerular filtration pressure.
- *Interplay and balance between dilatory (local prostacyclin) and constricting (thromboxanes, especially TXA$_2$) prostanoids.*
- *Interplay and balance between nitric oxide (NO) and endothelin* (especially endothelin 1, the most potent naturally occurring vasoconstrictor) under dif-ferent conditions.

Pathophysiology of ARF (more specifically sepsis-associated ARF or SAARF)

- Most of our present knowledge about ARF is derived from animal models of ARF using rat kidneys.
- In most of these models, ARF is produced by either clamping of the renal artery or by infusion of norepinephrine. Either technique stops the blood flow to the kidney almost completely.

- However, this model does not accurately reflect the clinical situation where blood flow is never zero.
- Traditionally, it is common to describe ARF as acute tubular necrosis (ATN).
- Little human material has been studied as the biopsies in these patients are lacking, thus making our knowledge of this condition far from complete.
- However, the sparsely available material that has been studied has shown little necrosis in the renal tubular cells.
- Rather, there is evidence that renal tubular cells mostly show sub-lethal injury and the process of damage is apoptosis (programmed cell death) rather than necrosis. Apoptosis requires energy (requiring oxygen and blood flow; *cf.* necrosis where there is cell death due to lack of perfusion).
- In sepsis, RBF may be normal or even enhanced in some; quite the reverse of what has hitherto been believed.
- Clinically, there is a disproportionately greater functional derangement than the pathological findings warrant. These findings distinguish this condition from ARF in patients on nephrology wards (in whom ARF exists as a "single" organ disease) where distinct and widespread pathological changes in renal parenchyma are usually found.
- Thus ATN is a misnomer and does not reflect the pathology of ARF in the critically ill.
- A triggering factor is required to initiate the cell damage, for example, hypoxia, hypotension (as may be seen in severe hypovolaemic shock), cytokines (in sepsis or trauma), etc.
- In morphological terms, the tubular cells show cellular and mitochondrial swelling, lose their luminal brush boarder and show apical blebbing.
- In advanced injury, cells detach from the basement membrane, protrude into the tubular lumen causing tubular obstruction.
- There is disruption of basolateral membrane (the part of tubular cell where, after having been absorbed from the tubular lumen, sodium is actively extruded into the medullary extra-cellular fluid) and loss of cell function.
- Tight junctions (between the lateral walls of the tubular cells) are disrupted causing back leak of tubular fluid into the medullary interstitium.
- These changes cause cell dysfunction and tubular obstruction with generalised oedema of the kidney.
- The important point to remember is that these apoptotic changes are reversible (in time) with complete regeneration of functioning tubular cells and thus nephrons, if appropriate resuscitation, treatment of the precipitating cause is undertaken without delay, further insults like furosemide and or

"renal dose" dopamine are avoided and appropriate renal supportive therapy is provided.

It is therefore clear that our traditional view of renal failure in the critically ill as a mostly "haemodynamic problem" needs challenging and revising. Haemodynamic upsets (especially shock and hypoperfusion) are important causes of ARF in these patients but do not explain the mechanisms of this disease fully especially as ARF may develop despite adequate resuscitation and support. It is therefore important to remember that SAARF has other aetiology. There is evidence to suggest that endotoxin lipo polysaccharide (LPS) and tumour necrosis factor (TNFα) (that macrophages release under its influence) have distinct damaging effects on kidney (e.g., they are stimulators of Apoptosis). Moreover, in an episode of severe sepsis, kidneys excrete LPS, TNFα and many other cytokines (as waste products), when these substances are found in concentrated amounts in renal tubules, increasing their tubulotoxicity and therefore the risk of ARF.

Causes of ARF in the critically ill

Basic principles

- Single insults of short duration (e.g., a single short period of hypotension) rarely cause ARF in patients with previously normally functioning kidneys.
- This may not hold true in patients with associated risk factors (see below).
- Absolute anuria (i.e., absolutely no urine in the drainage bag) is a blocked urinary catheter unless proven otherwise. Occasionally this may require a change of catheter.
- Truly obstructive causes, for example, ureteric obstructions (e.g., a stone causing hydropnephrosis in a single functioning kidney) are rare in ICU. However, they must be sought for/ruled out as management is simple (e.g., a percutaneous nephrostomy) and very rewarding in terms of renal function recovery.
- Majority of critically ill patients admitted to ICU are dehydrated rather than "overloaded".

Aetiology in the critically ill

- The commonest cause of "oliguria" is hypovolaemia and must be vigorously looked for and treated as the first clinically relevant and preventable cause of ARF.

- Relative or actual hypovolaemia is commonly present in patients presenting with severe sepsis and may well be the initial or contributing factor for renal dysfunction.
- Low-cardiac output syndromes (either primary cardiac failure or secondary cardiac dysfunction due to sepsis) also contribute to development of ARF.
- As indicated above, sepsis is a major cause of ARF in the critically ill.
- In ICU patients, nephrotoxins (e.g., nephrotoxic antibiotics, NSAID's) are also a common cause.
- ARF also occurs in major or severe inflammation without infection (e.g., severe acute pancreatitis).
- Major trauma can also cause ARF usually due to:
  - *crush injuries*: because of severe hypovolaemia, rhabdomyolysis;
  - *rhabdomyolysis*: due to myoglobinurea; hypovolaemia;
  - *delayed extrication*: due to hypovolaemia;
  - *massive inflammatory response*: from multiple trauma
  - *sepsis*: late cause.
- Another important cause of ARF in trauma victims is abdominal compartment syndrome and is now being increasingly recognised. Releasing abdominal pressure by a laparostomy incision may help in this situation. Abdominal compartment syndrome can also occur in non-trauma situations like postoperative patients and leaking aortic aneurysms (postoperative).
- Contrast nephropathy as a consequence of radiological contrast materials used for angiography is also an aetiological factor for ARF.
- Look out for unusual causes in semiconscious/unconscious patients (e.g., dehydration and rhabdomyolysis) due to chemical intake like ecstasy.

Risk factors for ARF are:

advanced age;
pre-existing renal dysfunction;
hypertension, pre-existing peripheral vascular disease;
pre-existing cardiac failure (even when cardiac failure is well compensated);
diabetes;
atherosclerosis;
sickle cell anaemia, malaria.
excessive endothelin production (hypoxia, endotoxaemia, cyclosporin, etc.).

ARF in the critically ill is multifactorial in aetiology and often develops as part of multiple organ dysfunction syndrome. Development of ARF in the critically ill not only denotes a severely ill patient but also adds to their mortality.

Prevention of ARF

- It is better to prevent ARF than to treat it.
- There are no "magic" bullets that prevent ARF in the critically ill.
- Attention to volume resuscitation is of paramount importance.
- This is especially true in crush injuries and rhabdomyolysis. Large quantities of fluids (6 l or more) may be required in such patients.
- As inadequate perfusion is one of the basic problems in the critically ill, it must be vigorously treated. This may involve merely adequate intravenous access and appropriate fluid prescription to advanced invasive/non-invasive monitoring of flow (i.e., cardiac output).
- Sepsis is perhaps the most important cause of ARF in ICU patients. Look for and treat sepsis adequately. There is little advantage in prescribing antibiotics (often nephrotoxic ones) for surgically drainable pus. Treatment of sepsis is as important as adequate and vigorous resuscitation.
- Appropriate antibiotics should be prescribed in adequate doses. Monitoring of toxic antibiotic levels is mandatory. Single daily doses of aminoglycosides (e.g., 4–5 mg/kg of gentamicin once daily) are more efficacious (as higher peak levels are obtained) and less nephrotoxic. "Prophylactic" antibiotics are often not necessary, are given in inadequate doses and if given should be limited to one or two large doses. Inappropriate use of antibiotics creates more problems than it solves.
- Aggressive fluid resuscitation of crush injury victims and those with rhabdomyolysis may be supplemented with bicarbonate infusion. Bicarbonate reduces tubulo-toxic effect of muscle breakdown products. Alkaline urine dissolves myoglobin and may help prevent tubular blockage.
- *N*-acetylcysteine has been suggested as a useful agent in preventing radiological contrast media induced renal failure along with aggressive fluid infusions. However, a recent meta-analysis has not substantiated these findings and more research is needed in this regard.
- Vasopressin has found some favour in hepato-renal syndrome. This is one of the few drugs that increase RBF by inducing splanchnic vasoconstriction and thus diverting blood to kidneys. However, it reduces cardiac output and has deleterious effects on intestinal mucosa. Vasopressin (or its synthetic derivative ornipressin) is, therefore, not recommended for prevention of ARF.
- There is no such thing as "renal dose" dopamine. Dopamine may improve renal function by augmenting cardiac output but its effect by so called "renal vasodilatation", although demonstrated in well-hydrated rats is not observed

clinically. Besides, low-dose dopamine can be potentially nephrotoxic in hypo-volaemic states as it abolishes TGF.

- Loop diuretics like furosemide reduce sodium reabsorption at the level of loop of Hénle and thus reduce oxygen consumption of the tubular cells. This sub-stance is therefore, theoretically attractive in preventing ARF. However, studies in this regard have been disappointing.
- It has been suggested that furosemide converts oliguric ARF into polyuric ARF, which has a better prognosis. This "assertion" is without any scientific founda-tion and not borne out by prospective studies.
- Mannitol has been tried but in many studies its place in prevention of ARF has not been proven.
- Various other agents like growth factors, etc. have been tried. Though animal experiments are encouraging, clinical studies have been disappointing.
- Erythropoietin (EPO), commonly used for treatment of anaemia associated with chronic renal failure, has been shown to be cytoprotective in experimen-tal ARF. It acts by binding to EPO receptor and is believed to be anti-apoptotic. Translating this beneficial effect into clinical practice has not yet been accomplished.

There are no pharmacological "magic bullets" to prevent ARF. Aggressive fluid resuscitation and improving perfusion are the mainstays of preventing renal dys-function. Of the myriad agents studied, none have so far proven of any depend-able clinical usefulness.

ARF in the critically ill: a special disease?

- ARF in the critically ill, especially those with SAARF is distinct from ARF encountered on the nephrology/medical wards ("medical ARF").
- Medical ARF (including those requiring RRT) has a low mortality of about 8% where as ARF in the critically ill (especially SAARF) has a mortality of about 50–80%.
- ARF in the critically ill is usually multifactorial (e.g., sepsis, hypovolaemia, nephrotoxins) whereas medical ARF is caused by distinct causes (e.g., glomerulo-nephrites, vasculites, etc.).
- Pathologically, ARF in critically ill shows less tubular cell damage than patients who develop ARF as a single organ disease ("medical ARF").
- Critically ill patients with ARF usually require simultaneous management of other system dysfunction (e.g., respiratory, cardiovascular or gut failure).

- Management of ARF in the critically ill demands different approaches especially where fluid or nutrition management are concerned. This can be very challenging.
- Whereas many patients with "medical ARF" progress to chronic renal failure, ARF in the critically ill is reversible in most.
- Thus ARF in the critically ill should be thought of as a different or distinct disease from ARF as a single organ disease ("medical ARF").

Summary

- ARF in the critically ill has complex aetiology.
- It arises as part of multiple organ failure.
- Our knowledge of this condition is not complete given the sparsely studied pathological material in humans.
- It is not well defined, thus it is difficult to interpret various studies. It also makes it difficult to estimate its prevalence.
- ARF increases mortality in the critically ill.
- Although hypoperfusion plays an important part in its development, sepsis-associated mechanisms are important and are major factors in causing ARF in the critically ill.
- There are, as yet, no pharmacological therapies that prevent ARF.
- Finally, ARF in the critically ill patients in ICU should be looked upon as a different disease entity from that seen on the nephrology wards.

REFERENCES AND FURTHER READING

1. Lote CJ, Harper L, Savage COS. Mechanisms of acute renal failure. *Br J Anaesth* 1996; 77: 82–9.
2. Bersten AD, Holt AW. Prevention of acute renal failure in the critically ill patient. In Bellomo R, Ronco C (Eds), *Acute Renal Failure in the Critically Ill*. Berlin, Springer 1995; pp. 122–46.
3. Wan L, Bellomo R, Giantomasso DD et al. The pathogenesis of septic acute renal failure. *Cur Opin Crit Care* 2003; 9: 496–502.
4. Cunningham PN, Dyanov HM, Park P et al. Acute real failure in endotoxaemia is caused by TNF acting directly on TNF receptor-1 in kidney. *J Immunol* 2002; 168: 5817–23.
5. Lameire NH, Vriese ASD, Vanholder R. Prevention and nondialytic treatment of acute renal failure. *Cur Opin Crit Care* 2003; 9: 481–90.

6. Vriese ASD, Bourgeois M. Pharmacological treatment of acute renal failure in sepsis. *Cur Opin Crit Care* 2003; 9: 474–80.

7. Bellomo R, Kellum J, Ronco C. Acute renal failure: time for consensus. *Intens Care Med* 2001; 27: 1685–8.

8. Kishen R. Managing acute renal failure in the critically ill: where are we today? *Care Crit Ill* 2002; 18: 170–2.

9. Heyman SK, Rosenberger C. Erythropoietin: a potential remedy for renal tubular injury? *Kidney Int* 2004; 65: 737–8.

10. Ronco C, Bellomo R. The rising era of critical care nephrology. *Cur Opin Crit Care* 1997; 3: 405–7.

24

Acute lung injury and ARDS

J. Naisbitt and C. Clarke

Definition of acute respiratory distress syndrome

- The syndrome formerly known as adult respiratory distress syndrome (ARDS) was first described in 1967.
- Consensus on diagnostic criteria was finally reached in 1994 with the publication of American European Consensus Criteria (AECC) allowing simple application to clinical trials [1]. Controversy persists due to a lack of correlation with outcome.
- Many groups feel that the term ARDS should be reserved for patients at the most severe end of a spectrum of acute lung injury (ALI).

Diagnosis

The most widely used diagnostic criteria (Table 24.1) in literature differentiate ALI from ARDS by the PaO_2/FiO_2 or shunt fraction.

This definition is limited by its disregard of the level of positive end expiratory pressure (PEEP). Increased PEEP improves recruitment and oxygenation and therefore the shunt fraction considerably. It has however led to uniformity in clinical trials enabling meaningful comparisons between ventilation strategies.

An alternate diagnostic score is the Murray Lung Injury Score (LIS) [2]. The LIS is widely used in the literature and importantly is used in the current UK "CESAR" trial. There are four components to the LIS, however not all need to be assessed. A score between 1 and 4 is assigned for:

- degree of hypoxia,
- lung infiltrates,

Table 24.1. AECC criteria

Criteria	Oxygenation	Chest radiograph	Pulmonary artery wedge pressure
ALI	PaO_2/FiO_2 <300 mmHg (regardless of PEEP level)	Bilateral infiltrates	<18 mmHg when measured (or no clinical evidence of left atrial hypertension)
ARDS	PaO_2/FiO_2 <200 mmHg (regardless of PEEP level)	Bilateral infiltrates	<18 mmHg when measured (or no clinical evidence of left atrial hypertension)

- level of PEEP,
- pulmonary compliance.

The total score is divided by the number of components assessed to give the LIS. A LIS >2.5 denotes ALI/ARDS, and a score ⩾3 is one of the CESAR inclusion criteria.

Predispositions to ARDS

Simply seen as a diffuse and overwhelming inflammatory reaction of the pulmonary parenchyma, almost any cause of shock or neutrophil activation can trigger the syndrome:

- The initial insult can be directly injurious to the pulmonary epithelium (e.g. aspiration or pneumonia).
- Alternatively the injury can result as part of an extra-pulmonary systemic inflammatory process (e.g. sepsis).

Although there is undoubtedly overlap, the distinction is a focus of interest and there may be implications for ventilation strategies. Gattinoni has proposed that ARDS may be divided into "pulmonary" ($ARDS_p$) and extra-pulmonary ($ARDS_{exp}$) lung injury [3]. Patients with $ARDS_p$, typically complicating pneumonia have stiff lungs and exhibit minimal recruitment with PEEP. $ARDS_{exp}$ patients have much greater chest wall stiffness which correlates with the increased intra-abdominal pressure. $ARDS_{exp}$ patients exhibit significant recruitment with PEEP. Although

Table 24.2. Direct and indirect predispositions to ARDS

Direct lung injury	Indirect lung injury
Gastric aspiration	Sepsis
Severe pneumonia/pulmonary infection	Pancreatitis
	Hypovolaemic shock
Smoke inhalation	Trauma
Pulmonary contusion	Fat embolism syndrome
Near-drowning	Burns
	Massive transfusion
	Transfusion-associated lung injury (TRALI)
	Post cardiopulmonary bypass

these concepts are exciting studies looking at "medical" and "surgical" ARDS do not confirm Gattinoni's findings.

Predispositions do affect outcome:

- The prognosis of ARDS following aspiration or trauma is better than that of ARDS complicating sepsis.
- Multiple or combined pulmonary and extra-pulmonary insults confer drastically increased mortality.
- Genetic polymorphisms in cytokines and angiotensinogen converting enzyme have been shown to predict the development of ARDS.

Predispositions to ARDS split into pulmonary and extra-pulmonary causes (Table 24.2).

Incidence

The precise incidence of ARDS is not clear, as uniformity on diagnostic criteria has only recently been reached:

- Using AECC definitions the incidence is around 13.5 per 100,000 [4, 5].
- The incidence of ALI is higher than previously thought.
- Certain pre morbid factors (history of chronic alcohol abuse) and higher APACHE II scores confer a significantly higher incidence of ARDS.

Pathophysiology

ARDS has classically been described by three phases after the initial injury [6]:

(1) Exudative phase.
(2) Proliferative phase.
(3) Fibrotic phase.

These phases are not distinct and the sequence of events is not fully understood. An early rise in interleukin-8 has been used as a marker for high-risk patients progressing to ARDS:

- The initial injury to the alveolar epithelium can be direct or endothelially mediated.
- Rapid sequestration and activation of neutrophils as part of an inflammatory cascade involving numerous cytokines, chemokines, complement activation, arachidonic acid metabolites and activation of the coagulation cascade leads to interstitial and alveolar oedema.
- There is intra-alveolar release of super oxide radicals, proteases and other oxidants.
- Normal alveolar physiology is disrupted with the inhibition of surfactant production, destruction of type I alveolar cells and proliferation of type II cells. This results in alveolar collapse and derecruitment and increased vascular permeability. These changes are not uniform throughout West's gravitational zones and there may be areas of consolidation and alveolar collapse with near normal lung adjacent to each other. This has been confirmed on computerized tomographical (CT) scan with the posterior dependant regions more extensively affected [7].
- Functionally the patient may have a very limited area available for effective gas exchange, an important element of Gattinoni's "baby lung" hypothesis.
- Later stages of ARDS are characterized by the migration of myofibroblasts to the alveolar side of the basement membrane and disorganized deposition of collagens. There is subsequent organization of the exudates and abnormal lung repair of the pulmonary capillary membrane with fibrosis.
- Resolution of ARDS is slow. The alveolar oedema is cleared and pulmonary membranes are remodelled. The regulation of this process is thought to be humoral.

Clinical features

- After an initial latent period of up to 72 h ARDS is a progressive disease.
- A predisposing factor followed by severe hypoxia refractory to oxygen therapy, increasing respiratory distress and reducing pulmonary compliance.
- Chest radiographs may show the classical whiteout picture of diffuse alveolar oedema, pleural effusion and atelectasis of dependent zones. The radiological appearance often lags behind the clinical picture and degree of hypoxia. The fibroproliferative stages of ARDS may disrupt the pulmonary capillary bed increasing resistance leading to pulmonary hypertension and progressive right ventricular dysfunction.

Management

- The management of the syndrome remains supportive and the importance of treating the predisposing condition cannot be overemphasized.
- The mainstay of management is currently centred on ventilation strategies, which reduce ventilator-induced lung injury possibly reducing the severity of ARDS [8] (discussed below).
- Pneumothoraces, ventilator-associated pneumonia [9] and fibroproliferation can be difficult to differentiate between. Acute deterioration in a patient with ARDS should prompt thorough investigation.
- Regular microbiological review, bronchoalveolar lavage and computed tomography of the chest [10] play an important role.
- Many novel therapies have been tried but little evidence supports their routine use.

Ventilation strategies

ARDS is characterized by abnormal lung mechanics. Abnormal lung mechanics are classically demonstrated using static pressure–volume (PV) loops. It must be emphasized that obtaining these curves is a specialized procedure and these loops are not equivalent to the dynamic PV loops displayed by modern ventilators. Although PV loops have contributed much to our understanding of ARDS unfortunately the values of the inflection points on the curve may vary depending on the technique used to obtain the curve [11].

Collapsed, flooded, open diseased and near normal alveoli coexists throughout the lung. Each alveolus will have its own recruitment pressure and level of ventilation/perfusion mismatch related to the extent of disruption to its normal physiology and architecture and that of its neighbours (interdependence). The two key components of current ventilation strategies are limitation of tidal volume (and airway pressure) and alveolar recruitment.

Traditional ventilation strategies employing low levels of PEEP and large tidal volumes (10–12 ml/kg predicted body weight) may be seen to over-distend compliant areas whilst possibly not fully recruiting collapsed or flooded alveoli. "Shear stress" may exist between alveoli with differing recruitment pressures. Due to alveolar interdependence, shear stress can be dramatically increased where near normal alveoli abut upon diseased alveoli [12].

- PV loops also demonstrate an upper inflection point (flattening of the PV curve). At this point there is near maximal recruitment and increasing over distention of alveoli. Maximal inspiratory pressure should therefore be limited to just below this level. The AECC recommended limitation of trans-alveolar pressure to $<35\,cmH_2O$.
- Hickling, in retrospective and later prospective papers in the early 1990s demonstrated a significant decrease in mortality when tidal volume (and airway pressure) was limited [13]. Limitation of tidal volume and "permissive hypercapnia" was a landmark advance in our management of ARDS. During the 1990s the emphasis shifted from a concept of "barotrauma" to one of "volutrauma". Both these terms are now obsolete and have been replaced by a wider concept of ventilator-induced lung injury (VILI).
- Limiting inspiratory pressure below the upper inflection point (UIP) and setting PEEP above the lower inflection point (LIP) is an attractive theory often referred to as open lung ventilation. The recent ALVEOLI study undertaken by the ARDSNetwork attempted to investigate the importance of recruitment by PEEP in a low tidal volume strategy but was terminated early due to lack of efficacy at its first interim analysis [14].
- Assisted spontaneous ventilation and non-invasive positive-pressure ventilation are often sufficient to manage mild forms of ALI and resolving ARDS.
- Reversed I:E ratio ventilation can be utilized and frequently results in intrinsic or auto-PEEP allowing alveolar recruitment. Prolonged inspiration may allow recruitment of alveoli with long time constants.

Table 24.3. ARDSNet ventilatory strategy [12]

Variable	Setting	Comment
Ventilator mode	Volume-assist control	Relatively uncommon in UK Pressure-controlled modes are in widespread use
Tidal volume (ml/kg)	6	Reduced if necessary to keep plateau pressure $<30\,cmH_2O$
Plateau pressure	$<30\,cmH_2O$	
Rate	6–35	High rates may have generated auto-PEEP
I:E ratio	1:1 to 1:3	
Oxygenation target		
PaO_2 (kPa)	7.3–10.7	
SpO_2 (%)	88–95	
PEEP and FiO_2	Set according to a predetermined table	Range 5–24 cmH_2O

The gold standard ventilation strategy was established by the ARDSNetwork study [8]:

- 861 patients with ARDS were randomized to two groups: one receiving traditional tidal volumes of 12 ml/kg; the second low tidal volumes 6 ml/kg (lowered to 4 ml/kg where necessary to achieve target airway pressure). Mortality in the traditional group was 39.8% at 28 days in comparison to 31% in the low-volume ventilation group.
- Three other trials showed no improvement in outcome with protective strategies [15, 16, 17].
- Amato et al also showed a relative risk reduction in mortality with low tidal volume ventilation but the mortality in the traditional group was very high (71%) limiting data interpretation [18].
- Comparison of the five trials shows that the two trials that showed benefit had greater differences in tidal volume and airway pressure between the groups than the three negative trials. Amato's study is of particular interest in the titration of PEEP to a level above LIP (Table 24.3).

The implication from these studies was that in the pursuit of a normal blood gases clinicians had inadvertently caused more VILI and increased the mortality of ARDS:

- Ventilation with low tidal volumes presents problems related to an inability to clear carbon dioxide. This is particularly problematic in patients with cranial injury.
- A degree of respiratory acidosis is tolerated, the so-called permissive hypercapnia. Intriguingly acidosis is protective to the lung in animal models. No consensus exists on the level of hypercapnia that is acceptable and it is of note that the protocol of the ARDSNet trial corrected the acidosis by infusing sodium bicarbonate.
- Infusion of bicarbonate has its own problems and should be slow to prevent worsening of intracellular acidosis and excretion of carbon dioxide.
- An exciting area is the demonstration that low tidal volume strategies may beneficially alter the pattern of inflammatory mediator release in the lung [19]. We have known for 20 years that ARDS patients die not of hypoxia, but of multiple organ failure. The concept that a traditional ventilatory strategy cause further release of inflammatory mediators with ongoing inflammation has been termed "biotrauma".

Recruitment manoeuvres

Despite recent advances in lung protective ventilation strategies, critical oxygenation is commonplace in severe ARDS:

- Recruitment manoeuvres involving the application of high continuous positive airway pressures for 30 s, intermittent sighs or large tidal volumes may improve oxygenation and lung mechanics, and can be useful following ventilator disconnection. It is unknown whether regular recruitment manoeuvres influence outcome [14, 20, 21].
- The respiratory rate in the ARDSNet trial was high. It has been demonstrated that the ARDSNet strategy may cause significant intrinsic PEEP and "gas trapping". ARDSNet patients may have benefited from a degree of recruitment consequent to the high respiratory rates.
- Recruitment is an inspiratory manoeuvre. PEEP is applied in expiration. Response to a recruitment manoeuvre could indicate the need to apply more PEEP.

Adjuvant therapy

Fluid restriction

The balance of opinion is probably shifting towards keeping the injured lung dry with the important proviso that cardiac function and end organ perfusion must be maintained. Certainly administration of excessive fluid will be detrimental [22].

Prone positioning

Ventilation in the prone position may improve oxygenation in some patients allowing the reduction of inspired oxygen and PEEP. The exact mechanism is unclear but:

- the prone position may increase functional residual capacity (FRC),
- it may increase recruitment of previously "protected" lung zones,
- there is redistribution of alveolar oedema,
- there is a decrease in the physiological shunt.

Pilot studies have reported beneficial effects in oxygenation but no large trial has demonstrated an improvement in outcome [23]:

- Proning is not without logistical and clinical pitfalls (pressure sores, facial oedema, tube and line displacement, and decompensation on return to the supine position).
- Prone positioning is not routine practice but may be of use in rescue oxygenation in the most severe cases of ARDS.

High-frequency oscillatory ventilation

- High-frequency oscillatory ventilation (HFOV) can be regarded as an extreme form of lung protective ventilation.
- HFOV oscillates the lung around a constant mean airway pressure, usually higher than that applied in conventional ventilation. The pressure swings are attenuated before reaching the alveoli and HFOV may prevent VILI, reduce "biotrauma" and may be useful in the presence of air leak. Tidal volume is usually in the range of 1–3 ml/kg [24].
- A recent randomized-controlled trial involving 148 patients showed HFOV to be safe and effective in ARDS. Although the study was not powered to assess mortality high-frequency oscillation (HFO) patients had a non-significant trend towards reduced mortality at 30 days and 6 months [25].

- HFOV tends to improve oxygenation in early ARDS and there is evidence that it is most effective when applied early. HFOV may be an effective "rescue" therapy for patients with critical oxygenation.

Inhaled nitric oxide

Theoretically the administration of inhaled nitric oxide (iNO) to the ARDS patient is an attractive one:

- There is selective vasodilatation in ventilated lung areas redistributing blood to ventilated regions and improving the shunt fraction.
- The subsequent reduction in pulmonary arterial hypertension may allow improvements in right ventricular dysfunction.

Four prospective randomized-controlled studies demonstrated that iNO significantly increased oxygenation for up to 24 h but no differences in outcome were detectable between the iNO and control groups. One study reported that patients treated with iNO had a greater requirement for renal replacement therapy. A recent large study of almost 400 patients concluded that iNO was associated with short-term oxygenation improvements but had no substantial impact on the duration of ventilatory support or mortality [26]. In conclusion:

- Not all patients are responders but iNO may have a role in life-threatening hypoxia or severe associated pulmonary hypertension.
- It appears that iNO consistently improves oxygenation in 60–80% of this population but the effect may not be sustained and does not affect outcome.

Extra-corporeal membrane oxygenation

The mortalities in the two randomized-controlled trials of extra-corporeal oxygenation, published in 1979 [27] and 1994 [28] were 10% and 33%, respectively. New technology and the development of extra-corporeal removal of carbon dioxide have improved the mortality of extra-corporeal techniques but failed to show benefit over conventional therapy. Small series of selected patients, for example those with varicella pneumonia have been encouraging.

The current UK CESAR study has recruited over 100 patients. Recruitment is due to end in November 2005. Inclusion criteria are adult patients with severe but reversible respiratory failure (LIS >3). Exclusion criteria include prolonged high-pressure and high-inspired oxygen ventilation, intracranial bleed or other contraindications to limited heparinization. Extra-corporeal membrane oxygenation (ECMO) cannot be justified outside the setting of the ongoing trial.

Other novel ventilatory strategies

Partial liquid ventilation and independent lung ventilation have been trialled but failed to effect outcome. There is no role for these therapies in current best practice.

Drug therapy

Many drugs have been subject to randomized-controlled trial in ARDS. These include prostaglandin, N-acetylcysteine, surfactant and early high-dose corticosteroids. All are ineffective. Small trials have demonstrated a limited effect of pentoxyfylline in a group of patients with ARDS complicating metastatic disease and corticosteroids in late phase ARDS. A recent systematic review has concluded that the options for effective pharmacotherapy in ARDS remain extremely limited [29]. The ARDSNet group have examined the use of ketaconazole and lisophylline. In practice the only drug treatment in widespread use is corticosteroids in late phase ARDS:

- The use of low-dose methylprednisolone (2 mg/kg) during the fibroproliferative phase of ARDS, significantly improved lung injury, organ dysfunction and survival rate in 24 patients with ARDS (88% versus 38%) [30]. The results of larger randomized studies without crossover are awaited to confirm this result.
- Activated protein C (Xigris) has improved outcome in septic patients and caused interest in the role of the coagulation cascade in ARDS but trials have yet to improve outcome.

Outcome

- The in-hospital mortality for ARDS (using AECC definitions) was 61% in the UK in 2002.
- Most studies report ARDS related mortality to be in the 50–60% range.
- Lung-protective ventilation strategies as previously described are the mainstay of ARDS management.
- There is a role for late low-dose steroids.
- Combinations of adjuvant therapies may decrease mortality in the future.

FURTHER READING

Artigas A, Bernard GR, Carlet J et al. The American–European Consensus Conference on ARDS, part 2: ventilatory, pharmacologic, supportive therapy, study design strategies, and issues related to recovery and remodeling. Acute respiratory distress syndrome. *Am J Respir Crit Care Med* 1998; 157: 1332–47.

Bernard GR, Artigas A, Brigham KL et al. The American–European Consensus Conference on ARDS: definitions, mechanisms, relevant outcomes and clinical trial co-ordination. *Am J Respir Crit Care Med* 1994; 149: 818–24.

Frutos-Vivar F, Nin N, Esteban A. Epidemiology of acute lung injury and acute respiratory distress syndrome. *Curr Opin Crit Care* 2004; 10: 1–6.

Moloney ED, Griffiths MJD. Protective ventilation of patients with acute respiratory distress syndrome. *Br J Anaesth* 2004; 92: 261–70.

Sevransky JE, Levy MM, Marini JJ. Mechanical ventilation in sepsis-induced acute lung injury/acute respiratory distress syndrome: an evidence-based review. *Crit Care Med* 2004; 32: S548–53.

REFERENCES

1. Bernard GR, Artigas A, Brigham KL et al. The American–European Consensus Conference on ARDS: definitions, mechanisms, relevant outcomes and clinical trial co-ordination. *Am J Respir Crit Care Med* 1994; 149: 818–24.

2. Murray JF, Matthay MA, Luce JM et al. An expanded definition of the adult respiratory distress syndrome. *Am Rev Respir Dis* 1998; 138: 720–3.

3. Gattinoni L, Pelosi P, Suter PM et al. Acute respiratory distress syndrome caused by pulmonary and extrapulmonary disease. Different syndromes? *Am J Respir Crit Care Med* 1998; 158: 3–11.

4. Hudson L, Steinberg K. Epidemiology of ARDS. Incidence and outcome: a changing picture. In Marini J, Evans T (Eds), *Acute Lung Injury*. Springer Verlag, Berlin, 1998, pp. 3–41.

5. Luhr OR, Antonsen K, Karlson M et al. Incidence and mortality after acute respiratory failure and acute respiratory distress syndrome in Sweden, Denmark and Iceland. *Am J Respir Crit Care Med* 1999; 159: 1849–61.

6. Wright JL. The pathology of ARDS. In Russell JA, Walley RW (Eds), *Acute Respiratory Distress Syndrome*. Cambridge University Press, 1999; Cambridge.

7. Gattinoni L, Pelosi P. Pathophysiologic insights into acute respiratory failure. *Curr Opin Crit Care* 1996; 2: 8–12.

8. Brower RG, Matthay MA, Morris A et al. Ventilation with lower tidal volumes as compared with traditional tidal volumes for acute lung injury and the acute respiratory distress syndrome. *New Eng J Med* 2000; 342: 1301–8.

9. Markowicz P, Wolff M, Djedaini et al. Multicenter prospective study of ventilator asso-ciated pneumonia during acute respiratory distress syndrome. *Am J Respir Crit Care Med* 2000; 161: 1942–8.

10. Presenti A, Tagliabue P, Patroniti N et al. Computerised tomography scan imaging in acute respiratory distress syndrome. *Int Care Med* 2001; 27: 631–9.

11. Dreyfuss D, Saumon G. Pressure–volume curves. Searching for the grail or laying patients with ARDS on proscustes bed? *Am J Respir Crit Care Med* 2001; 163: 2–3.

12. Moloney ED, Griffiths MJD. Protective ventilation of patients with acute respiratory distress syndrome. *Br J Anaesth* 2004; 92: 261–70.

13. Hickling KG, Walsh J, Henderson S et al. Low mortality rate in adult respiratory distress syndrome using low volume pressure limited ventilation with permissive hypercapnia; a prospective study. *Crit Care Med* 1994; 22: 1568–78.

14. The ARDS Clinical Trials Network; National Heart, Lung and Blood Institute; National Institutes of Health. Effects of recruitment manoeuvres in patients with acute lung injury and the acute respiratory distress syndrome ventilated with high positive end-expiratory pressure. *Crit Care Med* 2003; 31: 2592–7.

15. Stewart TE, Meade MO, Cook DJ et al. Evaluation of a ventilation strategy to prevent barotraumas in patients at high risk for acute respiratory distress syndrome. *New Eng J Med* 1998; 338: 355–61.

16. Brower RG, Shanholtz CB, Fessler HE et al. Prospective, randomized, controlled clinical trial comparing traditional versus reduced tidal volume ventilation in acute respiratory distress syndrome patients. *Crit Care Med* 1999; 27: 1492–8.

17. Brochard L, Roudot-Thoraval F, Roupie E et al. Tidal volume reduction for prevention of ventilator-induced lung injury in acute respiratory distress syndrome. *Am J Respir Crit Care Med* 1998; 158: 1831–8.

18. Amato M, Barbas C, Medeiros D et al. Effect of a protective ventilation strategy on mortality in the acute respiratory distress syndrome. *New Eng J Med* 1998; 338: 347–54.

19. Ranieri VM, Suter PM, Tortorella C et al. Effect of Mechanical ventilation on inflamma-tory mediators in patients with acute respiratory distress syndrome: a randomised controlled trial. *J Am Med Assoc* 1999; 282: 54–61.

20. Villagra A, Ochagavia A, Vatua S et al. Recruitment manoeuvres during lung protective ventilation in acute respiratory distress syndrome. *Am J Respir Crit Care Med* 2002; 165: 165–70.

21. Grasso S Mascia L, Del Turco M et al. Effects of recruitment manoeuvres in patients with acute respiratory distress syndrome ventilated with protective ventilation strat-egy. *Anaesthesiology* 2002; 96: 795–802.

22. Cranshaw J, Griffiths M, Evans T. The pulmonary physician in critical care: non ventila-tory strategies in ARDS. *Thorax* 2002; 57: 823–9.

23. Gattinoni L, Tognoni G, Presenti A et al. Effect of prone positioning on the survival of patients with acute respiratory failure. *New Eng J Med* 2001; 345: 568–73.

24. Derdak S, Mehta S, Stewart TE et al. High frequency oscillatory ventilation for acute respiratory distress syndrome in adults. *Am J Respir Crit Care Med* 2002; 166: 801–8.

25. Mehta S, Lapinsky S, Hallett D et al. Prospective trial of high frequency oscillation in adults with acute respiratory distress syndrome. *Crit Care Med* 2001; 29: 1360–9.

26. Taylor RW, Zimmerman JL, Dellinger RP et al. Low-dose inhaled nitric oxide in patients with acute lung injury: a randomized controlled trial. *J Am Med Assoc* 2004; 291: 1629–31.

27. Zapol WM, Snider MT, Hill JD et al. Extracorporeal membrane oxygenation in severe acute respiratory failure. A randomised prospective study. *J Am Med Assoc* 1979; 242: 2193–6.

28. Morris AH, Wallace C, Menlove RL et al. Randomised clinical trial of pressure controlled inverse ratio ventilation and extracorporeal carbon dioxide removal for adult respiratory distress syndrome. *Am J Respir Crit Care Med* 1994; 149: 295–305.

29. Adhikari N, Burns K, Meade M. Pharmacologic therapies for adults with acute lung injury and acute respiratory distress syndrome. *Cochrane Database System Review* 2004.

30. Meduri G, Headley A, Golden E et al. Effect of prolonged methylprednisolone therapy in unresolving acute respiratory distress syndrome: a randomised controlled trial. *J Am Med Assoc* 1998; 280: 159–65.

25

The patient with gastrointestinal problems

V. Godbole

Gastrointestinal (GI) disease may be the primary reason for admission to the intensive care unit (ICU).

The GI system may also become involved in multiple organ failure, whether as source or victim is still a matter of debate.

The gut as the propagator of systemic inflammatory response syndrome

- During critical illness GI perfusion may become compromised resulting in tissue hypoxia. This in turn leads to mucosal damage and disruption of the mucosal barrier allowing pathogens and/or toxins to access the circulation.
- The liver normally removes these substances from the portal circulation but this leads to an inflammatory response with the production of cytokines and initiation of systemic inflammatory response syndrome (SIRS).
- The gut is particularly sensitive to reperfusion injury, which results in the production of oxygen-derived free radicals.

The opposing view is that the gut is an innocent bystander in shock. GI dysfunction may simply reflect the development of organ failure rather than precede it.

The gut as a source of infection

The GI tract forms a portal to the external environment. Within it is over 400 species of microbial organisms. Ordinarily they cause no problems; indeed they are an essential component of normal host defences:

- In the critically ill patient, however, they may become the source for nosocomial infections and sepsis.
- Colonisation of the upper GI tract and oropharynx occurs with the same species isolated in nosocomial infections, particularly ventilator-associated pneumonia.

Bacterial translocation

- Systemic absorption of live organisms from the GI tract.
- Well demonstrated in animal studies.
- Enteric organisms have been identified in sterile human tissue.
- Exact role played by bacterial translocation in sepsis remains unclear.

Monitoring GI perfusion

- Early detection of intestinal ischaemia may allow directed therapy to improve outcome in critically ill patients.
- Tonometry relies on measurement of GI mucosal PCO_2 to assess gut perfusion. Gastric monitors are most frequently used.
- Mucosal pH (pHi) may be calculated from PCO_2 (usually gastric, $PgCO_2$) using the Henderson–Hasselbach equation. Studies using pHi to direct therapy suggest a value of less than 7.25 is predictive of a poor outcome [1].
- pHi is a composite variable and may not adequately reflect gut perfusion. More recent studies have examined the $PgCO_2/PaCO_2$ difference as an indicator of ischaemia. However, the use of this gradient is also flawed, as $PgCO_2$ may not be representative of the rest of the GI tract.
- The benefits of using pHi and $PgCO_2$ as therapeutical indices are still being evaluated.

Selective decontamination of the GI tract

Selective digestive decontamination (SDD) was first described in 1984.

It was hoped that the incidence of nosocomial infections arising from enteric organisms would be reduced by using specific antimicrobial agents for the gut – in effect sterilising the GI tract.

The classic SDD technique consists of four aspects:

(1) A parenteral antibiotic (e.g. cefotaxime) administered for 3 days.
(2) Application of antibiotics topically within the oro-pharyngeal cavity and administration of these antibiotics enterally via nasogastric tube (e.g. polymixin B, tobramycin).
(3) Optimal hygiene to prevent cross-contamination.
(4) Monitoring effectiveness of the regime by checking regular throat-swabs and faeces.

Whilst early work demonstrated a reduction in the incidence of nosocomial pneumonia there was little evidence to suggest the use of SDD reduced ICU mortality.

Furthermore there were concerns that the use of SDD would encourage the emergence of antibiotic-resistant pathogens.

A 30-year meta-analysis by Nathens and Marshall demonstrated that mortality was significantly reduced in critically ill surgical patients, but not in medical patients [2]. The greatest effect was seen in studies where both the topical and systemic components of the regimen were used.

The incidence of pneumonia was reduced in both surgical and medical patients, whilst a reduction in bacteraemia was seen only in surgical patients.

Antibiotic resistance

A recent study from France observed an increase in methicillin resistance of *Staphylococcus epidermidis* but not *Staphylococcus aureus* [3]. Resistance amongst *Enterobacter*, *Pseudomonas* and *Acinetobacter* species remained unchanged.

Use of SDD in a Belgian ICU demonstrated significantly more Gram-positive bacteraemias and increased antimicrobial resistance, including that of methicillin resistant *S. aureus* (MRSA) [4].

In areas with a low prevalence of MRSA SDD may be a useful adjunct to treatment but many centres remain unconvinced of its overall usefulness in the general ICU and fear the long-term consequences in terms of encouraging resistant organisms.

Stress ulceration

Gastric erosion or ulceration is common in the ICU. Nearly 100% of patients will have lesions identifiable by endoscopy. Clinically significant bleeding is rare and the incidence of fatal haemorrhage lower still. However, there should be a high index of suspicion of a GI bleed in patients who have an unexpected fall in their haemoglobin (Hb) levels.

However, the mortality from overt GI bleeding remains high.

Patients most at risk include:

- head injuries,
- burns,
- multiple trauma,
- sepsis,
- prolonged intermittent positive pressure ventilation (IPPV).

It is debatable whether other ICU patients require routine stress ulcer prophylaxis.

As the underlying problem lies with gastric mucosal ischaemia, initial measures should include correction of hypoxaemia and ensuring an adequate circulating volume.

The commonest agents used in stress ulcer prophylaxis are ranitidine and sucralfate.

Ranitidine

- Histamine 2 receptor antagonist.
- Inhibits gastric acid secretion resulting in decreased volume and increased pH.

Sucralfate

- Complex of aluminium hydroxide and sulphated sucrose
- Protects gastric mucosa by:
  - adsorbing pepsin and bile salts,
  - increases prostaglandin secretion,
  - increases gastric blood flow,
  - promoting epithelial healing.

Sucralfate reduces the incidence of gastric ulcer formation when compared to placebo [5].

Which agent to use?

A major concern is the risk of developing nosocomial pneumonia, particularly with ranitidine. By reducing gastric acidity one of the body's main defences against infection is removed. This allows bacterial colonisation of the upper GI tract and oropharynx, with eventual colonisation of the trachea.

It has been observed that Gram-negative bacteria, for example, *Pseudomonas* will grow in the stomach at a pH >5 [6]. These organisms are most often implicated in ventilator-associated pneumonia.

Cook et al recruited 1200 patients for a large multi-centre study [7]. They were randomised to receive either ranitidine 50 mg 8 hourly or sucralfate 1 g 6 hourly. The incidence of clinically important bleeding was significantly less in the ranitidine group (1.7% versus 3.8%).

There was no significant difference in the rates of ventilator-associated pneumonia, length of ICU stay or mortality. The difference in the protection from bleeding led many ICUs to use ranitidine as their main prophylactic agent.

A recent meta-analysis looked at the effectiveness of each agent versus placebo. Both the incidences of bleeding and pneumonia were examined. The authors concluded "there are insufficient data on effectiveness to be able to conclude anything one way or the other" [8].

Clearly further work needs to be done in this area!

The best protection for the gastric mucosa is probably enteral feeding, and this should be established as early as possible.

Motility problems

Gastric stasis

Gastroparesis is not uncommon in the critically ill patient and may lead to failure in establishing enteral feeding.

Gastric emptying may be delayed due to:

- sepsis,
- opiates,
- abdominal surgery,
- hyperglycaemia,
- hypokalaemia.

Initial management involves the use of prokinetic agents – metoclopramide and erythromycin. Cisapride is no longer available due to its proarrhythmic activity.

Metoclopramide

- Dopamine 2 receptor antagonist.
- Promotes gastric emptying.

- Increases gut motility.
- Anti-emetic.

Erythromycin

- Macrolide antibiotic.
- Agonist at motilin receptors gives increased gut motility.

The ideal dose of erythromycin remains unclear. A recent study that demonstrated improved gastric emptying used 250 mg 6 hourly [9].

If gastric stasis persists then enteral feeding may be achieved by placement of a postpyloric tube. This is most effectively performed with endoscopic control. Blind placement of a nasojejunal tube is facilitated by erythromycin, whilst metoclopramide is ineffective [10–12].

Constipation

Constipation may be defined as a frequency of bowel movement less than three times a week. It is often overlooked in the critically ill patient, who may go for days without passing a bowel motion. The most serious consequences of constipation are GI obstruction and perforation.

Mostafa et al demonstrated an incidence of 83% in a UK ICU [13]. Constipated patients were less likely to be successful at weaning from mechanical ventilation.

The most common cause of a patient becoming constipated is the use of opiates. Other causes include immobility and total parenteral nutrition (TPN).

There are several laxatives available for the treatment of constipation. The commonest in use are osmotic laxatives (e.g. lactulose) and stimulants (e.g. senna).

Diarrhoea

Diarrhoea is an important cause of morbidity in the ICU patient. In its severest form it can lead to profound fluid loss and electrolyte disturbances. With the need for frequent bedding changes there is an increased risk of dislodging lines or even accidental tracheal extubation.

The definition of diarrhoea is even harder then that of constipation. Most practitioners accept it as being frequent, loose or watery stools:

- Diarrhoea is often attributed to enteral feed. A small study of 62 patients failed to demonstrate an increase in the incidence of diarrhoea in patients who were enterally fed [14].

- The use of antibiotics may also predispose to diarrhoea, which is a common side effect of many antibiotics.
- Infective causes for diarrhoea amongst the critically ill are rare, with the majority being due to *Clostridium difficile*. This spore-forming bacillus resides in the colon. Diarrhoea results from expression of toxins, most commonly following antibiotic therapy. Treatment is with oral metronidazole, or in severe cases the intravenous form.

Acute pancreatitis

Acute pancreatitis is a common cause of admission to the ICU.

The severity of the disease ranges from mild, which is usually managed on the surgical ward, to the severe, necrotising form that carries a mortality of up to 45%.

Aetiology

The majority of cases (70%) can be attributed to gallstones or alcohol abuse.
Other causes include:

- post-endoscopic retrograde cholangiopancreatography (post-ERCP),
- abdominal trauma,
- drug-induced (e.g. steroids, diuretics),
- metabolic (e.g. hypercalcaemia, hypertriglyceridaemia),
- infection (e.g. cytomagalovirus (CMV), mumps).

Twenty per cent are idiopathic but often associated with biliary sludge.

Prognosis

Ranson's criteria have been used for the last 20 years to predict outcome. There are 11 prognostic indicators.

- On admission:
  (1) age,
  (2) white cell count,
  (3) blood glucose,
  (4) lactate dehydrogenase,
  (5) aspartate aminotransferase (AST).

- After 48 h:
  - (6) calcium,
  - (7) PaO$_2$,
  - (8) base deficit,
  - (9) fluid deficit,
  - (10) decrease in haematocrit,
  - (11) increase in blood urea nitrogen.

Points are awarded for each factor, a higher score is associated with a worse prognosis:

- With the advent of readily available computed tomography (CT) scanning newer scoring systems based on degree of necrosis have been developed.
- In a retrospective study Company et al noted the factors that significantly related to mortality were age, upper GI bleeding, acute renal failure, respiratory failure and shock [15].
- Werner et al postulate that C-reactive protein (CRP) is "the gold standard" in predicting the severity of acute pancreatitis [16]. However, CRP is an acute phase protein not specific to pancreatitis and an increase may reflect other processes, for example development of ventilator-associated pneumonia.

Pathophysiology

- Primary insult leads to increase in free radical activity within the acinar cell.
- Normal regulation of secretory pathways is disrupted.
- Reversal of these pathways results in exocytosis and release of enzymes into the interstitium.
- This in turn initiates a local inflammatory response.
- The production of cytokines and other inflammatory mediators leads to a systemic reaction.

Management

Largely supportive:

- analgesia,
- fluids and nutrition,
- organ support as required.

Current controversies in management

Feeding

- Parenteral feeding was the traditional method of delivering nutrition in order to "rest the gut". With the publication of studies demonstrating reduced morbidity with enteral feeding the practice of feeding the gut was established [17].
- Indeed, a recent Cochrane review has suggested that whilst there is a trend towards fewer complications in patients receiving enteral nutrition (EN) this is not statistically significant [18]. (It should be remembered in medicine that the clinical significance of an intervention is usually more relevant than the statistical significance.)
- A recent meta-analysis recommends that EN is to be preferred over TPN in patients with pancreatitis [19]. EN is best administered jejunally, that is, distal to the pancreatic duct.

Antibiotics

- Infection of necrotic pancreas develops 2–3 weeks after the onset of symptoms. It is commoner in patients with a biliary aetiology. Subsequent sepsis is associated with a high mortality.
- Bacterial translocation is believed to play a part in the development of infection, as Gram-negative organisms are isolated in 75% of cases.
- Retroperitoneal air (as identified by CT scan) should alert to the presence of anaerobic bacteria.
- Antibiotics should be considered in all patients with pancreatic necrosis. Two recent meta-analyses have demonstrated reduced mortality in patients with severe pancreatitis who received prophylactic antibiotics [20, 21].
- There is evidence to show carbapenems have good penetration into infected tissue and are currently the agent of choice.

Anti-oxidants

- Oxidative stress is believed to play a part in the development of complications in severe acute pancreatitis.
- Plasma levels of ascorbic acid, carotenoids and vitamins A and E, which have anti-oxidant properties, are significantly lower in patients with acute pancreatitis [22, 23].

- The role of anti-oxidants in the treatment of severe pancreatitis is still being evaluated but a recent study has failed to identify any definite benefits from a comprehensive anti-oxidant regime in acute pancreatitis [24].

The role of surgery

Surgery is reserved for those patients with infective complications.

Recent guidelines by the International Association of Pancreatology (IAP) [25] proposed:

- Fine needle aspiration be used to confirm the presence of infection.
- Patients with sterile necrosis be treated conservatively.
- Early surgery (within 14 days) is not recommended in patients with necrotising pancreatitis unless there are specific indications.
- Interventional management should favour an organ-preserving approach.

Acute hepatic failure

The incidence of de novo liver failure is rare with the majority of the cases in the UK being due to paracetamol overdose. Even in this population the incidence is low – fulminant liver failure developing in less than 1% of UK hospital episodes. Worldwide the commonest cause is viral hepatitis.

O'Grady et al divided acute hepatic failure into three subgroups [26]:

(1) *Hyperacute*: encephalopathy developing within 7 days of the onset of jaundice.
(2) *Acute*: encephalopathy developing 8–28 days after the onset of jaundice.
(3) *Subacute*: encephalopathy that develops 5–26 weeks after the onset of jaundice.

In paracetamol-induced acute liver failure (ALF) the indicators of a poor prognosis are:

- prothrombin time (PT) >100 s,
- arterial pH <7.3,
- serum creatinine $>300\,\mu$mol/l.

More recently an elevated serum lactate (>3.0) following resuscitation was shown to correlate with a poor outcome [27].

In patients with viral or drug-induced hepatitis the poor prognostic indicators are:

- aetiology (non-A and non-B hepatitis, and drug-induced reactions),
- age <11 or >40,

- jaundice present for >7 days prior to the development of encephalopathy,
- serum bilirubin >300 μmol/l,
- PT >50 s.

Hepatic encephalopathy

Encephalopathy is due to the failure of the liver to metabolise and excrete toxins. Raised plasma ammonia levels have been implicated but other chemicals may also be involved, for example, fatty acids, aromatic chain amino acids, γ-aminobutyric acid (GABA).

It is graded as follows:

- I: Mild drowsiness
- II: Increasing drowsiness, confusion
- III: Stupor
- IV: Coma.

Patients with grade III/IV encephalopathy are at major risk of developing cerebral oedema and raised intracranial pressure (ICP):

- Treatment involves the use of mannitol and mechanical ventilation to achieve normocarbia.
- Controlled hypothermia may also have a role to play.

Lateralising signs are uncommon and should prompt a search for other causes.

Treatment

Orthoptic liver transplant is the only definitive treatment associated with improved outcome. The King's College Hospital criteria for liver transplantation are based on the prognostic indicators above [26].

Transplantation is not appropriate for all patients with ALF so prompt referral to a specialised liver unit will allow identification of potential recipients.

Management on the general ICU

Supportive ICU measures should be initiated:

- invasive cardiovascular monitoring,
- correction of hypoglycaemia,

- renal support with veno-venous haemofiltration if required,
- correction of coagulopathy should be avoided, as PT is an important prognostic indicator,
- ICP monitoring for grade III/IV encephalopathy,
- *N*-acetylcysteine for paracetamol-induced hepatic failure.

Artificial liver support:

- hybrid systems with biological tissue now emerging,
- studies with small number of patients have been encouraging,
- awaiting larger trials to evaluate benefit.

Chronic liver failure

Acute decompensation of chronic liver failure is the more common presentation of hepatic failure to the ICU. In the UK this usually occurs in patients with a history of alcohol abuse. Decompensation may result from:

- sepsis,
- GI bleeding,
- dehydration,
- large protein load.

Although the outlook for these patients is poor, ICU management may be considered if there is a reversible cause.

Management is supportive with treatment of the underlying cause.

Ascites

- Respiration may be compromised by the presence of marked ascites.
- Drainage of ascites should be controlled as sudden changes can have profound consequences on haemodynamic stability.
- Patients with ascites are at risk of developing spontaneous bacterial peritonitis.

Spontaneous bacterial peritonitis

- 30% mortality.
- Symptoms non-specific: abdominal pain, fever.
- 25% asymptomatic.

- Diagnosis: positive culture from ascitic tap with associated high ascitic neutrophil count ($>$250 cells/mm^3) and no evident intra-abdominal source of
  infection.
- Treatment: antibiotics.

Hepatic dysfunction in ICU

Two main syndromes of hepatic dysfunction occur in ICU patients [28]. Both are
relatively common and the occurrence and degree of dysfunction have adverse
prognostic significance.

- *Ischaemic hepatitis.* Due to reduced hepatic perfusion during shock. Causes
  necrosis with, often massive, elevations of AST within 24 h. Coagulopathy,
  hypoglycaemia and increased lactate (partly due to reduced hepatic clearance)
  are often seen. May predispose to the commoner.
- *ICU Jaundice.* More gradual onset (liver has considerable reserve). Associated with
  sepsis (should prompt search for occult sepsis), trauma and massive blood transfusion and is the liver component of multiple organ failure. Intrahepatic cholesta-
  sis produces marked hyperbilirubinaemia with only mild elevation of enzymes.

In both situations, Kupffer's cell (hepatic macrophage) dysfunction may predispose to bacterial or endotoxin translocation from the gut, exacerbating the hepatic
dysfunction and promoting further general organ dysfunction.

Therapeutical principles include maintaining overall cardiac output, actively
increasing liver blood flow with, for example, dopexamine, eradication of sepsis
and early enteral feeding.

Upper GI bleeding

GI bleeding is a common cause of admission to hospital but the majority
of patients do not require ICU. Most respond well to prompt and aggressive
resuscitation.

Although the incidence of upper GI bleeding has decreased the risk of
rebleeding (20%) and death (14%) remain unchanged [29].

Reasons for admission to ICU include:

- Aspiration of blood.
- Massive blood transfusion.

- Persistent shock.
- Prolonged surgery.

Causes of bleeding:

- Peptic ulcer ~50%.
- Gastric erosions ~25%.
- Varices ~10%.
- Others ~15%.

Management:

- Fluid resuscitation – Transfusion of blood and coagulation factors as required.
- Early liaison with multidisciplinary teams.
- Early diagnostic endoscopy.
- Specific treatment may be surgical or endoscopic.

Endoscopic treatment has revolutionised the management of upper GI bleeding:

- Techniques involve injecting ulcers (usually with adrenaline) and thermocoagulation.
- Routine re-look endoscopy is not recommended.
- High dose proton pump inhibitors should be used as an adjunct to treatment.

Variceal bleeds

- Patients presenting with bleeding varices have a worse prognosis due to the associated hepatic dysfunction and portal hypertension.
- After an initial bleed the risk of rebleeding is 30–40% over the subsequent 6 weeks. This carries with it an increased mortality.
- Endoscopic treatment involves sclerotherapy or banding of varices.
- A sengstaken tube may be used to tamponade the bleeding.
- Vasopressin and its derivative terlipressin, reduce blood flow through the portal system.

After successful management of an initial variceal bleed patients require definitive treatment to prevent rebleeding. This may involve:

- β-blockade,
- variceal band ligation,
- portosystemic shunt (TIPS) formation,
- liver transplantation.

Lower GI bleeding

Accounts for ~20% of GI bleeds.

  Due to:

- diverticular disease,
- colitis,
- colonic carcinoma,
- angiodysplaia.

Treatment involves resuscitation and prompt referral. Most cases will require surgical intervention.

FURTHER READING

Galley HF (Ed.) *Critical Care Focus. Vol. 9: The Gut*. BMJ Books/Intensive Care Society, London, 2002.

Kolkman JJ, Otte JA, Groeneveld BJ. Gastrointestinal luminal PCO_2 tonometry: an update on physiology, methodology and clinical applications. *Br J Anaesth* 2000; 84(1): 74–86.

Rahman T, Hodgson H. Clinical management of acute hepatic failure. *Int Care Med* 2001; 27(3): 467–76.

REFERENCES

1. Lebuffe G, Robin E, Vallet B. Gastric tonometry. *Int Care Med* 2001; 27(1): 317–9.

2. Nathens AB, Marshall JC. Selective decontamination of the digestive tract in surgical patients: a systematic review of the evidence. *Arch Surg* 1999; 134(2): 170–6.

3. Leone M, Albanese J, Antonini F, Nguyen-Michel A, Martin C. Long term (6-year) effect of selective digestive decontamination on antimicrobial resistance in intensive care, multiple-trauma patients. *Crit Care Med* 2003; 31(8): 2090–5.

4. Verwaest C, Verhaegen J, Ferdinande P, Schetz M, Van den Berghe G, Verbist L, Lauwers P. Randomized, controlled trial of selective digestive decontamination in 600 mechanically ventilated patients in a multidisciplinary intensive care unit. *Crit Care Med* 1997; 25(1): 63–71.

5. Eddleston JM, Pearson RC, Holland J, Tooth JA, Vohra A, Doran BH. Prospective endoscopic study of stress erosions and ulcers in critically ill adult patients treated with either sucralfate or placebo. *Crit Care Med* 1994; 22(12): 1949–54.

6. Marshall JC, Christou NV, Meakins JL. The gastrointestinal tract. The "undrained abscess" of multiple organ failure. *Ann Surg* 1993; 218(2): 111–9.

7. Cook D, Guyatt G, Marshall J et al. A comparison of sucralfate and ranitidine for the prevention of upper GI bleeding in patients requiring mechanical ventilation. *New Engl J Med* 1998; 338(12): 791–7.

8. Messori A, Trippoli S, Vaiani M, Gorini M, Corrado A. Bleeding and pneumonia in intensive care patients given ranitidine and sucralfate for the prevention of stress ulcer: meta-analysis of randomised controlled trials. *Br Med J* 2000; 321(7269): 1103–6.

9. Reigier J, Bensaid S, Perrin-Gachadoat D, Burdin M, Boiteau R, Tenaillon A. Erythromycin and early enteral nutrition in mechanically ventilated patients. *Crit Care Med* 2002; 30(6): 1237–41.

10. Kalliafas S, Choban PS, Ziegler D, Drago S, Flancbaum L. Erythromycin facilitates postpyloric placement of nasoduodenal feeding tubes in intensive care unit patients: randomised, double-blind, placebo-controlled trial. *J Parenter Enter Nutr* 1996; 20(6): 385–8.

11. Griffith DP, McNally AT, Battey CH et al. Intravenous erythromycin facilitates bedside placement of postpyloric feeding tubes in critically ill adults: a double-blind, randomised, placebo-controlled study. *Crit Care Med* 2003; 31(1): 39–44.

12. Silva CCR, Saconato H, Atallah AN. Metoclopramide for migration of naso-enteral tube. In: *Cochrane Review*, The Cochrane Library, Issue 4, 2003. John Wiley & Sons, Chichester, UK.

13. Mostafa SM, Bhandari S, Ritchie G, Gratton N, Wenstone R. Constipation and its implications in the critically ill patient. *Br J Anaesth* 2003; 91(6): 815–9.

14. Levinson M, Bryce A. Enteral feeding, gastric colonisation and diarrhoea in the critically ill patient: is there a relationship? *Anaesth Intens Care* 1993; 21(1): 85–8.

15. Company L, Saez J, Martinez J, Aparicio JR, Laveda R, Grino P, Perez-Mateo M. Factors predicting mortality in severe acute pancreatitis. *Pancreatology* 2003; 3(2): 144–8.

16. Werner J, Hartwig W, Uhl W, Muller C, Buchler MW. Useful markers for predicting severity and monitoring progression of acute pancreatitis. *Pancreatology* 2003; 3(2): 115–27.

17. Kalfarentos F, Kehagias J, Mead N, Kokkinis K, Gogos CA. Enteral nutrition is superior to parenteral nutrition in severe acute pancreatitis results of a randomised prospective trial. *Br J Surg* 1997; 84(12): 1665–9.

18. Al-Omran M, Groof A, Wilke D. Enteral versus parenteral nutrition for acute pancreatitis. In: *Cochrane Review*, The Cochrane Library, Issue 4, 2003. John Wiley & Sons, Chichester, UK.

19. Marik PE, Zaloga GP. Meta-analysis of parenteral nutrition versus enteral nutrition in patients with acute pancreatitis. *Br Med J* 2004; 328: 1407.

20. Golub R, Siddiqi F, Pohl D. Role of antibiotics in pancreatitis: a meta-analysis. *J Gastrointest Surg* 1998; 2(6): 496–503.

21. Sharma VK, Howden CW. Prophylactic antibiotic administration reduces sepsis and mortality in acute necrotising pancreatitis: a meta-analysis. *Pancreas* 2001; 22(1): 28–31.

22. Bonham MJ, Abu-Zidan FM, Simovic MO, Sluis KB, Wilkinson A, Winterbourn CC, Windsor JA. Early ascorbic acid depletion is related to the severity of acute pancreatitis. *Br J Surg* 1999; 86(10): 1296–301.

23. Curran FJ, Sattar N, Talwar D, Baxter JN, Imrie CW. Relationship of carotenoid and vitamins A and E with the acute inflammatory response in acute pancreatitis. *Br J Surg* 2000; 87(3): 301–5.

24. Virlos IT, Mason J, Schofield D, McCloy RF et al. Intravenous n-acetylcysteine, ascorbic acid and selenium-based anti-oxidant therapy in severe acute pancreatitis. *Scand J Gastroenterol* 2003; 38: 1262–7.

25. Uhl W, Warshaw A, Imrie C et al. IAP Guidelines for the surgical management of acute pancreatitis. *Pancreatology* 2002; 2(6): 565–73.

26. O'Grady JG, Alexander GJ, Hayllar KM, Williams R. Early indicators of prognosis in fulminant hepatic failure. *Gastroenterology* 1989; 97(2): 439–45.

27. Bernal W, Williamson N, Wyncoll D, Wendon J. Blood lactate as an early predictor of outcome in paracetamol-induced acute liver failure: a cohort study. *Lancet* 2002; 359(9306): 558–63.

28. Hawker F. Liver dysfunction in critical illness. *Anaesth Intens Care* 1991; 19(2): 165–81.

29. van Leerdam ME, Vreeburg EM, Rauws EA, Geraedts AA, Tijssen JG, Reitsman JB, Tytgat GN. Acute upper GI bleeding: did anything change? Time trend analysis of incidence and outcome of acute upper GI bleeding between 1993, 1994 and 2000. *Am J Gastroenterol* 2003; 98(7): 1494–9.

26

The comatose patient

S. Wiggans

This chapter will concentrate on the commonest causes of coma in the intensive care unit (ICU), head injury, and "stroke" (cerebral infarction and haemorrhage).

The general principles of management of these patients are applicable for other conditions that lead to coma in the ICU.

Other causes of coma and an account of other neurological conditions in the ICU can be found in "Neurological complications in critically ill patients", in the section on Further reading.

General points

- The hallmark of diffuse brain injury is loss of consciousness. Coma is unconsciousness where patients do not open eyes, obey commands or utter recognisable words.
- The depth or duration of coma may gauge the severity of the patient's condition.
- Duration of coma can only be judged in retrospect so therefore the depth of coma as quantified by the glasgow coma scale (GCS) is widely used as an index of the severity of injury. GCS:

Eye opening		Verbal response		Motor response	
Spontaneous	4	Oriented	5	Obeys commands	6
To voice	3	Confused speech	4	Localises pain	5
To pain	2	Inappropriate words	3	Withdraws	4
None	1	Incomprehensible	2	Abnormal flexion	3
		sounds		Extension	2
		None	1	None	1

Score 3–15: mild head injuries, 14 or 15; moderate, 9–13; severe, 8 or less.

General care of the comatose patient

- Skilled nursing care, especially with regard to pressure area care and protection of joints.
- *Physiotherapy* – both respiratory care and prevention of contractures in immobile limbs.
- *Nutrition and hydration* must be maintained.
- *Stress ulcer prophylaxis* – head injuries are at particular risk (Cushing's ulcer).

Aims of intensive care

- Detect and treat complications of primary injury that may cause delayed damage.
- Prevent delayed hypoxic/ischaemic damage – largely through control of intracranial pressure (ICP).
- Provide optimal conditions for recovery of brain function – natural recovery only at present, perhaps therapy aided neurological recovery in the future.

Principles of neuroprotection

- Factors causing increases in ICP should be avoided.
- Encourage venous drainage and therefore minimise ICP by:
  - neck maintained in neutral position;
  - minimise the use of positive end expiratory pressure (PEEP) where possible;
  - nurse with head up by 10°.
- Indications, complications and management of ICP monitoring will be discussed in the section on Head injury in this chapter.
- Avoid hypotension. There is a loss of normal blood pressure (BP)/cerebral blood flow (CBF) autoregulation. Normal relationship:

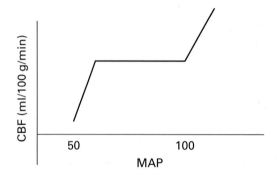

Normally CBF is constant between mean arterial pressure (MAP) of 50–100, auto-regulation. This relationship may be lost in, for example, head injury. Therefore the head injury patient is predisposed to ischaemic brain damage at levels of MAP normally considered satisfactory:

- Hyperventilation to reduce ICP. Controversial. See below.
- Mannitol to reduce ICP. Mannitol 0.5–1.0 g/kg if above ineffective. Continue until osmolarity reaches 320 mosm/l. Furosemide is often used as either an adjunct or an alternative.
- Normoglycaemia. Animal studies and studies on stroke patients clearly show increased neuronal damage after global brain ischaemia in the presence of hyperglycaemia [1]. Increasing evidence exists that maintaining normoglycaemia is important in all critical care patients [2].
- Fever is thought to be harmful – by increasing cerebral metabolic oxygen requirements. Despite early studies suggesting that controlled hypothermia improved outcome [3], a recent multi-centre study claimed no benefit [4]. Improved outcome *may* be possible if the side effects of cooling (abnormalities of fluid balance, electrolytes, coagulation and haemodynamic parameters) are treated aggressively [5].
- Steroids have no proven role in the management of head injury or stroke [6]. A large multi-centred randomised trial examining the effects of corticosteroid (methylprednisolone) infusion for 48 h after head injury (the MRC CRASH trial) has shown a higher risk of death in the group given steroids [7].
- Indomethacin infusion (a cerebral vasoconstrictor) reduces ICP but there may be a rebound if stopped suddenly.
- Experimental strategies. Interest is focusing on neuroprotective drugs (animal studies so far) for example, free radical scavengers, inhibitors of lipid peroxidation, glutamate antagonists and calcium channel blockers.
- Calcium channel blockers prevent Ca influx in an ischaemic area and decrease cell damage. Their smooth muscle relaxing properties also reduce vasospasm.
- On theoretical grounds, the combination of barbiturates (to reduce cerebral oxygen demand) and positive inotropic drugs (to maintain cardiac output and MAP) is attractive but remains experimental.

The problem of hyperventilation

- CBF and therefore ICP is directly related to PCO_2 with a fall in PCO_2 of 1 mmHg being normally associated with a fall in ICP of approximately 1.3 mmHg. This effect may be short lived due to brain and cerebrospinal fluid (CSF) pH compensation.

- In controlled studies *prophylactic* hyperventilation (i.e. in the absence of raised ICP) resulted in a slightly worse outcome compared to the control group [8]. The danger of hyperventilation is that it may produce excessive cerebral vasoconstriction and ischaemia.
- It seems illogical somehow to treat brain ischaemia by a measure that reduces CBF. No other organ in the body is treated in this way.
- Hyperventilation will shift the haemoglobin (Hb) oxygen dissociation curve to the left impairing tissue oxygenation, regardless of any contested effect on CBF.
- An interesting study on head injury patients compared different therapies to lower ICP – 25 g intravenous (IV) mannitol, 3 min of CSF drainage via ventriculostomy and increase in respiratory rate of 4/min [9]. For similar decrease of ICP, hyperventilation caused decreases in jugular venous saturation (SJO_2), implying worsening cerebral oxygenation by reducing CBF, while mannitol increased SJO_2. CSF drainage was in between but not nearly as bad as hyperventilation:
- Thus, mannitol improved CBF while decreasing ICP and this study supports many centres avoidance of "routine" hyperventilation.
- Although the routine use of hyperventilation is debatable there is no doubt that hypercapnia is harmful and should be avoided.
- The majority of centres still practice *therapeutical* hyperventilation for short-term control of raised ICP. Many use SJO_2 measurements as a guide. Jugular saturations less than 55–60% may indicate that hyperventilation is harmful.

ICP monitoring

- Although the origin of raised ICP after head injury is still debated, rational management of the injured brain depends on knowledge of cerebral perfusion pressure (CPP) that is, MAP – ICP.
- Changes in ICP are difficult to identify clinically.
- ICP monitoring has been widespread since the 1970s after several reports indicated a reduced mortality in severe head injuries (GCS <9) subsequent to its use. However, it is impossible to separate the contribution of ICP monitoring to this improved survival from other advances, for example, routine computed tomography (CT) scanning.

- Nevertheless, there is a definite association between raised ICP and poor outcome although cause and effect have never been proven. Certainly, uncontrollable increases in ICP represent overwhelming brain damage.
- Several large, non-randomised trials have shown a beneficial effect on head injury mortality from the use of ICP monitoring [10, 11].
- ICP measurement is more useful when combined with measurement of SJO_2. With this information, a therapy such as hyperventilation (which can lower CBF) can be more accurately judged.
- Less than 50% of severe head injuries in Europe receive ICP monitoring [12].

Indications

- GCS <9.
- Evidence of raised ICP on CT scan.
- Any CT abnormality.
- Post craniotomy for mass lesion.
- Space occupying mass lesion.
- Traumatic coma as part of multiple trauma requiring intermittent positive pressure ventilation (IPPV).

Contraindications

- Frank coagulopathy.
- Obvious infection at insertion site.
- Paediatric head injury, unless in specialised centres.

Complications of ICP monitoring

- Haemorrhage requiring neurosurgical intervention – perhaps 5% in some studies.
- Infection.
- Occlusion of fluid filled monitoring systems.

Complications are low compared to other ICU interventions:

- One study [13] from Italy of ICP monitors inserted by ICU staff as opposed to neurosurgeons found the incidence of morbidity (3.3%) to be comparable to that of central venous pressure (CVP) monitoring. There were no intracranial haematomas attributed to the monitor in their 5 years study.

- Another study found that ICP monitors are safe with the main problem being accidental removal. ICP monitoring led to therapeutical changes in 81% of patients [14].
- Older studies suggest a 10% incidence of infection. It is believed that the incidence with modern solid state or fibreoptic systems (i.e. not fluid based system) will be considerably less (3% in Ref. [8]). Of course, the disadvantage of the modern systems is that CSF drainage for therapeutical reduction of ICP is not possible.

Control of raised ICP

The skull contains brain, blood and CSF within a rigid closed container. An increase in volume of one must be accompanied by a decrease in another or pressure will rise (Monro-Kellie Doctrine). Initially the volume increase, whether it be due to haematoma or increased CBF (hyperaemia), is compensated by displacement of CSF followed by later *large* increases in ICP for a *small* further increase in volume. This may lead to:

- acute hydrocephalus due to obstruction of CSF flow,
- reduced CBF,
- brainstem herniation at the foramen magnum ("coning").

Although the normal ICP is <10 mmHg there is general agreement that treatment is indicated when ICP is ≥20 mmHg. The mainstays of treatment are diuretics (mannitol and/or furosemide) and therapeutical hyperventilation as discussed previously. Transient elevations occur during turning, physiotherapy, etc. and do not usually require treatment. A bolus of sedation in the ventilated patient may be all that is required to prevent these transient elevations in the patients most at risk, for example, already elevated ICP. Care should be taken, however, to maintain CPP. In all cases of persistent elevation of ICP, a cause should be sought (e.g. obstructed venous drainage of the head). "Fighting" the ventilator should be excluded. When no cause is apparent repeat CT may be indicated. Thiopentone is often used as a second or third line agent.

Head injury

Approximately 100,000 patients with head injuries are admitted to hospital each year in the UK of which approximately 10,000 are severe. Most studies show a preponderance of males to females of between 2:1 and 4:1. The peak ages are in the second and third decades. Common causes are:

- road traffic accident (RTA),
- falls,
- assault,
- gunshot (especially in USA).

Younger cases are commonly a result of RTA – lower incidence of mass lesions on CT scanning. Older cases are commonly a result of falls – higher incidence of mass lesions. Depending on aetiology, 10–50% are intoxicated on admission. Fifty per cent of multiple injury patients include a central nervous system (CNS) component and brain injury is present in 75% of deaths from RTA.

Pathophysiology

Primary brain injury

- Occurs within milliseconds.
- Prevention is the only effective treatment.

The fact that some patients who subsequently die are conscious at the scene of an accident, implies that there are secondary or delayed injuries which may be preventable or reversible.

Secondary brain injury

In most cases later secondary damage is focal (i.e. related to contusions and/or haematomas) but may also be due to metabolic changes, raised ICP *and* extracranial events such as hypoxaemia, hypotension and hypercarbia.

CT scanning

- CT remains the scanning method of choice in head injuries and can evaluate skull fractures, major contusions, haematomas and the cervical spine.
- CT can only provide information about ICP *at the time of scanning.*
- Effacement of basal cisterns is usually present when ICP >20.
- In general, scanning should be delayed until oxygenation and systemic BP are satisfactory.

- Despite early studies suggesting that only a small proportion of patients with a normal CT scan develop raised ICP, recent studies suggest that severely injured patients with a normal scan are at substantial risk of developing intracranial hypertension [15].
- The prognosis in severe head injury is best when haematomas are diagnosed by CT and evacuated prior to the patient's deterioration from subsequent rises in ICP or local mass effect. With increasing use of CT scanning, smaller mass lesions or "smear" haematomas may be found.
- For patients at risk of delayed haemorrhage or oedema, repeat CT scanning may be necessary (e.g. at 24 h, 72 h and 7 days). Unexpected deterioration (clinically or persistent rises in ICP) should prompt a repeat scan to exclude the development of secondary hydrocephalus or intracranial bleeding.

Indications for urgent CT scanning

NICE guidelines for the management of head injury state the following are indications for *immediate* request of CT. Imaging should be performed (imaging carried out and results analysed) within 1 h of the request having been received by the radiology department (see Further reading in this chapter).

- GCS <13 at any point since the injury.
- GCS 13 or 14 at 2 h after the injury.
- Suspected open or depressed skull fracture.
- Any sign of basal skull fracture.
- Post-traumatic seizure.
- Focal neurological deficit.
- More than one episode of vomiting.
- Coagulopathy (clotting disorder, warfarin, etc.) if amnesia experienced since the injury.
- Age 65 years or over if amnesia experienced since the injury.

In addition, the following are indications for CT within 8 h of the *injury*.

- Amnesia for greater than 30 min of events before impact.
- Dangerous mechanism of injury.

Management

As for all trauma patients, *ABC* and *VIP* principles are crucial. If these are not maintained appropriately the neurological outcome is likely to be poor because of secondary ischaemic/hypoxic brain damage, even if the patient "survives".

General management

Airway must be maintained. Neck should be immobilised in cervical collar due to association of head injury with cervical spine injury until cervical spine shown to be intact.

Breathing. Indications for intubation include:

- loss of protective laryngeal reflexes,
- GCS <9,
- severe facial and/or multiple injuries,
- hypercapnia, hypoxaemia or marked tachypnoea,
- preparation for transfer,
- seizures.

Circulation. Head injury in the absence of other injuries is almost never associated with hypotension. Normal MAP should be maintained or even supranormal MAP if ICP is raised (see below).

Ventilation. Twenty per cent may be hypoxic without chest injury as a result of:

- neurogenic pulmonary oedema,
- aspiration,
- ventilation and perfusion (V/Q) mismatch,
- pulmonary emboli (includes fat emboli after long bone fractures),
- nosocomial pneumonia (high incidence).

Appropriate respiratory care will maintain appropriate oxygenation. PEEP should be avoided or at least minimised where possible as it can restrict cerebral venous drainage and therefore contribute to raised ICP.

Duration of ventilatory support is controversial in head injured patients:

- If ICP monitoring is employed, IPPV is continued until ICP is stable and has settled to near normal. Increasing ICP during weaning leads to re-sedation.
- If no ICP monitoring, many now suggest a minimum period of sedation and ventilation of 3 days to allow the oedema to settle. Some centres repeat the CT scan prior to allowing the patient to awaken.

Infusion. Appropriate fluids should be administered. The presence of other injuries will necessitate appropriate volume resuscitation. Fluid infusion will not necessarily increase ICP [16]. Volume infusion is therefore "safe". Dextrose containing and hypotonic fluids should be avoided.

Perfusion. CPP must be maintained especially in the presence of raised ICP (CPP = MAP − ICP). Increasing emphasis in the literature is being placed on maintaining CPP at >70. It would also seem as if maintaining CPP by increasing MAP is almost to be preferred to maintaining CPP by lowering ICP, especially if ICP is resistant to therapy [17].

Additional measures

- Attention to the principle of neuroprotection (see above).
- Nasogastric tube for gastric decompression (gastric atony common).
- Early enteral nutrition – patients with head injury can be markedly catabolic.
- Stress ulcer prophylaxis.
- Physiotherapy.
- Antibiotics prophylactically if ICP monitored. Prophylactic antibiotics are not indicated otherwise in head injury [18].
- Some authorities recommend routine anticonvulsants (e.g. phenytoin).
- Nimodipine if traumatic subarachnoid injury present, to reduce associated vasospasm.

Outcome and quality control

The mortality from severe head injuries is 30–50% in most series. Factors suggesting a poor outcome include:

- low GCS,
- increase age,
- significant haemorrhage,
- significant systemic injuries.

Fifty per cent who die do so from uncontrolled increases in ICP (often early).

A small number of patients will be left in a persistent vegetative state or alert but totally dependent. The numbers of these are *not* increased in studies involving aggressive management strategies shown to reduce mortality. Recovery may continue for up to 24 months but most improvement occurs in first 6 months.

In a study of 41 US trauma centres [19] the outcomes varied from 43% below expected to 52% above expected. 70% of this variation in outcome was found in patients with *moderate* head injuries rather than severe. The outcomes varied enormously between different centres. The implication is that the quality of pre-hospital and ICU care can be expected to have a profound effect on the outcome after head injury.

Stroke

Subarachnoid haemorrhage

- Studies vary but approximately 10 per 100,000 per year.
- Ten per cent of all cerebrovascular accidents (CVA).
- Aneurysms identified in 75–80% but no discrete bleeding source found in 15–20%.
- Hypertension is a significant risk factor for the development and for rupture of aneurysms.
- Peak age is 55–60 years.
- Females more than males.

Pathophysiology of rupture

The resulting increase in ICP reduces CBF and is responsible for the decrease in conscious level in all but the mildest cases. This increase in ICP may help stop the bleeding by a "tamponade" effect. Patients admitted in a deep, persistent coma develop persistent increases in ICP, secondary vasospasm and cerebral oedema.

There is a surge in catecholamine levels, which can cause:

- myocardial ischaemia,
- arrhythmias,
- tachycardias,
- prolonged QT interval on the electrocardiograph (ECG, itself associated with ventricular arrhythmias,
- decreases in serum K (due to the action of adrenaline on the β-2 receptor),
- neurogenic pulmonary oedema.

Clinical presentation

- Headache in 85–95%.
- Nausea and vomiting.
- Decreased conscious level.
- Photophobia.
- Variety of neurological deficits.

Diagnosis

- CT scanning. Mainstay of diagnosis and gives information on location of bleed and likely origin. May also indicate the likelihood of development of vasospasm, for example, in the presence of significant amounts of blood in the basal cisterns.

- Magnetic resonance imaging (MRI) scanning. Although not the initial investigation of choice may show even very small aneurysms.
- Lumbar puncture (LP). Very sensitive especially the presence of xanthochromia (yellow discoloration of the CSF due to the presence of altered blood). A CT scan should be done first to detect increased ICP as performing an LP in a patient with increased ICP can cause brain herniation.
- Angiography. Needed to define the source of bleeding and the presence of other aneurysms.

Non-operative management

- Non-operative management is associated with a high mortality.
- Attention to the principles of neuroprotection (see above).
- Surgical referral is indicated in all patients apart from those in persistent coma.
- Re-bleeding occurs in 16–25% of patients in the first 2 weeks with a peak incidence at 4–9 days [20].
- If surgery is not feasible measures should be taken to lessen the risk of re-bleeding (e.g. control hypertension) and to prevent vasospasm. Simple measures such as prescribing laxatives to prevent constipation and subsequent straining may be helpful. The use of antifibrinolytics to reduce re-bleeding increases mortality [21].
- Interventional neuroradiology (see below).

Prevention and treatment of vasospasm

The two mainstays of treatment to prevent vasospasm are:

- *Nimodipine.* Given IV as soon as possible at a rate of 1–2 mg/h (less if BP unstable) and continued for 5–14 days. This is followed by oral nimodipine, 60 mg 4 hourly, to complete 21 days of treatment. This therapy has been clearly shown to improve outcome [22].
- *"Triple H" therapy* (hypervolaemia, haemodilution and hypertension). Generous fluid therapy (±vasopressors), to maintain a high BP and lower viscosity, will reduce the incidence of vasospasm [23]. This must *only* be practised following aneurysm clipping.
- *Before or after surgery,* hypotension and hypovolaemia should be avoided.

Surgical intervention

The timing of surgical intervention has always been controversial. In the 1960s surgery was delayed and outcome was often poor. In the 1970s and 1980s early surgery was claimed to offer better results. It seems that there are similar results for surgery at 0–3 days and at 11–14 days. The worst outcome seems to be for surgery between days 7–10 due to the development of vasospasm. In other words, early or late surgery but *not* in between [24]. IV nimodipine should be continued for 5 days postoperatively.

Interventional neuroradiology

An endovascular route may be used to treat aneurysms. "Coiling" of aneurysms was originally developed as an alternative technique for patients not suitable for standard surgical intervention (e.g. medically unfit or surgically difficult). However, a multi-centred randomised trial comparing radiological and surgical management has suggested "coiling" is superior to "clipping", if both treatment options are appropriate [25].

Prognosis

One-third will die before reaching medical attention. Of the remaining about one third will die or remain severely disabled. An international co-operative study found that 58% returned to their premorbid state [26].

Cerebral infarction

Ischaemic stroke is a common cause of coma in patients admitted to many ICUs. However, the role of ICU is controversial.

On the one hand, prognosis is undoubtedly poor following a major cerebral ischaemic event:

- Realistically, IPPV in the absence of definitive therapy able to restore brain function cannot be expected to improve survival.
- A retrospective review of almost 1000 patients concluded that IPPV only delays an inevitable fatal outcome in patients with respiratory failure following ischaemic stroke [27].
- Another study suggests discontinuing IPPV for patients who remain comatose for more than 72 h following stroke [28].

On the other hand, some centres dispute this nihilistic attitude:

- "Stroke units" for "brain attack" (analogous to coronary care units for heart attack) result in reduced mortality and complications for stroke patients compared to medical wards [29]. However, this may be due, in part, to better rehabilitation rather than better acute care.
- Despite some increased incidence of intracranial haemorrhage, treatment with recombinant tissue plasminogen activator within 3 h of the onset of an ischaemic stroke improves outcome [30].
- The challenge (beyond the reach of most units) is to diagnose infarction (i.e. rule out haemorrhage) within 3 h by CT scanning to identify those who are candidates for thrombolysis.
- Surgical decompression to reduce ICP is being investigated for patients with massive hemispheric infarction with initial encouraging results [31].

Management

- Attention to the principle of neuroprotection (see above).
- Treat severe hypertension but take care not to produce ischaemia from hypotension.
- ICP monitoring is of limited value in massive stroke.
- Look for sources of emboli, for example, echocardiogram to look for valve lesions or intracardiac thrombi, auscultate carotid arteries for bruits. Consider antiplatelet drugs or anticoagulants if emboli likely.
- Nimodipine orally may have slight protective effect when given within 12 h but the results are not as impressive as for subarachnoid haemorrhage. IV nimodipine causes too much hypotension and should not be given.

FURTHER READING

Diringer MN. Intracerebral hemorrhage: pathophysiology and management. *Crit Care Med* 1993; 21: 1591–603.

Gentleman D, Dearden M, Midgley S, Maclean D. Guidelines for resuscitation and transfer of patients with serious head injury *Br Med J* 1993; 307: 547–52.

Hacke W, Stingele R, Steiner T, Schuchardt V, Schwab S. Critical care of acute ischemic stroke. *Intens Care Med* 1996; 21: 856–62.

NICE Guidelines. Head Injury: Triage, assessment and early management of head injury in infants, children and adults. June 2003.

Wijdicks EF. Neurologic complications in critically ill patients. *Anesth Analg* 1996; 83: 411–19.

REFERENCES

1. Weir CJ, Murray GD, Dyker AG, Lees KR. Is hyperglycaemia an independent predictor of poor outcome after acute stroke? Results of a long term follow up study. *Br Med J* 1997; 314: 1303–6.

2. Van den Berghe G, Wouters P, Weekers F et al. Intensive insulin therapy in critically ill patients. *New Engl J Med* 2001; 345: 1359–67.

3. Marion DW, Obrist WD, Carlier PM, Penrod LE, Darby JM. The use of moderate therapeutic hypothermia for patients with severe head injuries: a preliminary report. *J Neurosurg* 1993; 79: 354–62.

4. Clifton GL, Miller ER, Choi SC et al. Lack of effect of induction of hypothermia after acute brain injury. *N Engl J Med* 2001; 344: 556–63.

5. Polderman KH, Tjong Tjin Joe R, Peerdeman SM, Vandertop WP, Girbes ARJ. Effects of therapeutic hypothermia on intracranial pressure and outcome in patients with severe head injury. *Intens Care Med* 2002; 28: 1563–73.

6. Alderson P, Roberts I. Corticosteroids in acute traumatic brain injury: a systematic review of randomised controlled trials. *Br Med J* 1997; 314: 1855–9.

7. Roberts I, Yates D, Sandercock P, Farrell B et al. Effect of intravenous corticosteroids on death within 14 days in 10008 adults with clinically significant head injury (MRC CRASH trial): randomised placebo-controlled trial. *Lancet* 2004; 364: 1321–8.

8. Muizelaar JP, Marmarou A, Ward JD, Kontos HA, Choi SC et al. Adverse effects of prolonged hyperventilation in patients with severe head injury: a randomized clinical trial. *J Neurosurg* 1991; 75: 731–9.

9. Fortune JB, Feustel PJ, Graca L, Hasselbarth J, Kuehler DH. Effect of hyperventilation, mannitol and ventriculostomy drainage on cerebral blood flow after head injury. *J Trauma* 1995; 39: 1091–9.

10. Miller JD, Becker DP, Ward JD. Significance of intracranial hypertension in severe head injury. *J Neurosurg* 1977; 47: 503–16.

11. Marshall LF, Smith RW, Shapiro HM. The outcome with aggressive treatment in severe head injury. Part 1: The significance of intracranial pressure monitoring. *J Neurosurg* 1979; 50: 20–5.

12. Stocchetti N, Penny KI, Dearden M et al. Intensive care management of head injured patients in Europe: a survey from the European Brain Injury Consortium. *Intens Care Med* 2001; 27: 400–6.

13. Bochicchio M, Latronico N, Zappa S, Beindorf A, Candiani A. Bedside burr hole for intracranial pressure monitoring by intensive care physicians. A 5-year experience. *Intens Care Med* 1996; 22: 1070–4.

14. Eddy VA, Vitsky JL, Rutherford EJ, Morris Jr JA. Aggressive use of ICP monitoring is safe and alters patient care. *Am Surg* 1995; 61: 24–9.

15. O'Sullivan MG, Statham PF, Jones PA, Miller JD, Dearden NM et al. Role of intracranial pressure monitoring in severely head-injured patients without signs of intracranial hypertension on initial computerized tomography. *J Neurosurg* 1994; 80: 46–50.

16. Schmoker JD, Shackford SR, Wald SL, Pietropaoli JA. An analysis of the relationship between fluid and sodium administration and intracranial pressure after head injury. *J Trauma* 1992; 33: 476–81.

17. Andrews PJD. What is the optimal perfusion pressure after brain injury – a review of the evidence with an emphasis on arterial pressure. *Acta Anaesthe Scand* 1995; 39(Suppl 105): 112–4.

18. Antimicrobial prophylaxis in neurosurgery and after head injury. Infection in neurosurgery working party of the British Society for Antimicrobial Chemotherapy. *Lancet* 1994; 344: 1547–51.

19. Klauber MR, Marshall LF, Luerssen JG. Determinants of head injury mortality: importance of the low risk patient. *Neurosurgery* 1984; 24: 3.

20. Rosenorn J, Eskesen V, Schmidt K, Ronde F. The risk of rebleeding from ruptured intracranial aneurysms. *J Neurosurg* 1987; 67: 329–32.

21. Fodstad H, Forsell A, Liliequist B. Antifibrinolysis with tranexamic acid in aneurysmal subarachnoid haemorrhage: a consecutive controlled trial. *Neurosurgery* 1981; 28: 21–3.

22. Allen GS, Ahn HS, Preziosi TJ. Cerebral artery spasm – a controlled trial of nimodipine in patients with subarachnoid haemorrhage. *New Eng J Med* 1983; 308: 619–24.

23. Kassell NF, Peerless SJ, Durward QJ, Beck DW, Drake CG et al. Treatment of ischemic deficits from vasospasm with intravascular volume expansion and induced arterial hypertension. *Neurosurgery* 1982; 11: 337–41.

24. Guy J, McGrath BJ, Borel CO, Friedman AH, Warner DS. Perioperative management of aneurysmal subarachnoid hemorrhage. Part 1: Operative management. *Anaesth Analg* 1995; 81: 1060–72.

25. Molyneux A, Kerr R, Stratton I et al. International Subarachnoid Aneurysm Trial (ISAT) of neurosurgical clipping in 2143 patients with ruptured intracranial aneurysm: randomized trial. *Lancet* 2002; 360(9342): 1267–74.

26. Kassell NF, Torner JC, Haley C. The international cooperative study on the timing of aneurysmal surgery. Part 1: Overall management results. *J Neurosurg* 1990; 73: 18–32.

27. El-Ad, B, Bornstein N, Fuchs P, Korczyn AD. Mechanical ventilation in stroke patients: is it worthwhile? *Neurology* 1996; 47: 657–9.

28. Grota J, Pasteur W, Khwaja G, Hamel T, Fisher M et al. Elective intubation for neurological deterioration after stroke. *Neurology* 1995; 45: 640–4.

29. Langhorne P, Williams BO, Gilchrist W, Howie K. Do stroke units save lives? *Lancet* 1993; 342: 395–8.

30. The National Institute of Neurological Disorders and Stroke rt-PA Stroke Study Group. Tissue plasminogen activator for acute ischemic stroke. *New Engl J Med* 1995; 333: 1581–7.

31. Rieke K, Schwab S, Krieger D, von Kummer R, Aschoff A et al. Decompressive surgery in space-occupying hemispheric infarction: results of an open, prospective trial. *Crit Care Med* 1995; 23: 1576–87.

27

The critically ill asthmatic

J. Barker and G. Brear

The chapter highlights two main features:
- Acute severe asthma should be considered the unstable angina of respiratory medicine.
- Asthma kills.

Incidence

In many countries, in the 30–40 years up to 2000, there was a steep rise in hospital admissions for asthma, accounting for ≈100,000 per year in England and Wales, half of which were <15 years of age. In children, males have a higher admission rate than females, the opposite being true for adults. In the UK there had been a similar but less marked increase in asthma deaths, which latterly seems to be falling slowly probably because of better long-term prophylactic treatment.

Over the period 1995–2001, acute severe asthma accounted for 1.7% of admissions to adult general critical care units across England, Wales and Northern Ireland. Of these, 57% were mechanically ventilated within the first 24 h. Unit mortality was 7.1% and hospital mortality 9.8%[1].

Causes

Asthma is an inflammatory disease of the lower airways that may be associated with specific identifiable allergy (atopic or extrinsic asthma) or not (non-atopic or intrinsic asthma). The latter starts more commonly in mid- and late adult life.

It is a disease of exacerbation with either full remission or persistence of symptoms (chronic severe asthma). Exacerbation may be due to:

- specific allergen exposure – environmental, food or occupational,
- air pollution – gaseous or particulate,
- treatment non-compliance,
- infection – viral or bacterial,
- thunderstorms.

Many exacerbations have no identifiable cause.

Differential diagnosis

The diagnosis may be obvious, but in adults, especially in the absence of a previous history of asthma or failure to respond to appropriate treatment, the following alternatives should be considered:

- chronic obstructive airways disease,
- left ventricular failure,
- upper airways obstruction,
- pulmonary embolus.

Medical management

Much of the following broadly follows the British Thoracic Society Guidelines [2] on asthma management.

Prevention of exacerbation

Avoiding severe exacerbation is preferable and is helped by:

- avoidance of allergens,
- monitoring of peak flows and a written asthma action plan,
- avoid reliance just on short acting bronchodilators,
- prophylactic anti-inflammatory treatment (inhaled steroids, etc.),
- longer acting β-agonists (e.g. Salmeterol),
- prompt treatment of worsening symptoms (e.g. oral steroids, hospitalization),
- prompt treatment of bacterial infections when appropriate.

Presentation and signs of severity

Asthmatics may die before admission to hospital or intensive care unit (ICU) because of one or more of the following identifiable and preventable factors [3, 4]:

- Doctors failing to assess severity by objective measurement.
- Patients and their relatives underestimating the severity of attacks.
- Under treatment of attacks (e.g. under use of oral corticosteroids).
- Very rapid progression from uncontrolled to life-threatening asthma.

The majority appears to have significant psychosocial factors contributing to their deaths and most occur in patients with chronic severe asthma.

Note: Hypoxia suppresses symptom perception in asthma.

Many clinical signs of acute severe and life-threatening asthma are unreliable. The following are the most reliable.

Acute severe asthma

- Peak expiratory flow rate (PEFR) is 33–50% of best previous recorded or predicted.
- Inability to complete a sentence in one breath.
- Tachycardia >110 beats/min.
- Respiratory rate >25 breaths/min.

Life-threatening asthma

- Peak flow rate <33% of best previous recorded or predicted.
- Exhaustion, confusion, depressed level of consciousness or coma.
- Shock or dysrhythmia.
- Silent chest, cyanosis or feeble respiratory effort.

Not all patients with acute severe or life-threatening asthma display all features. Extreme caution should be exercised in the presence of *any* of them.

The importance of blood gas estimation

Physical signs can be unreliable. A PEFR >33% predicted is rarely associated with CO_2 retention. All patients with oxygen saturation <92% or who have

life-threatening features should have arterial blood gases measured. The following indicate a very severe attack:

- acidosis–respiratory or metabolic,
- severe hypoxia (PaO_2 <8 kPa, 60 mmHg),
- normal or raised $PaCO_2$.

Initial treatment

The following measures should be taken immediately:

- Oxygen in high concentration. Clinically important CO_2 retention is not aggra-
  vated by high-concentration oxygen in asthmatics.
- High-dose nebulized (oxygen driven) β_2-agonists.
- Intravenous (i.v.) hydrocortisone 200 mg.

The patient should receive no sedatives and should have a chest X-ray to exclude
pneumothorax. Response to treatment must be monitored with PEFR and repeat
blood gas estimation. If life-threatening features are present include:

- Nebulized ipratropium 0.5 mg in addition to the β_2-agonist.
- Aminophylline 250 mg i.v. over 20 min – not to be given if already on oral theophylline. Alternatively 250 μg salbutamol or terbutaline i.v.

If the patient improves with the above:

- continue a high-concentration oxygen,
- give oral prednisolone 40–50 mg daily or hydrocortisone 100 mg 6 hourly,
- regular nebulized β_2-agonists,
- monitor the patient's saturations, blood gases and PEFR closely.

If the patient does not improve in 15–30 min:

- continue oxygen and steroids as above;
- give β_2-agonists more frequently (up to 15–30 min or even continuously);
- add ipratropium 0.5 mg 6 hourly;
- consider aminophylline infusion 750–1500 mg/24 h – dose depending on size;
- consider salbutamol or terbutaline infusion as an alternative to aminophylline.

Response to treatment must be monitored with PEFR, "clinical" assessment of the
patient and blood gas estimations if life-threatening features persist or oximetry
is <92%.

Indications for admission to ICU

Intensive care admission is indicated if:

- the PEFR deteriorates despite treatment,
- hypoxia persists or worsens,
- hypercapnea or acidosis persists or worsens,
- the patient has impaired consciousness or exhaustion,
- respiratory effort deteriorates clinically,
- the patient is comatose or has a respiratory arrest.

Staff able to intubate reliably must be immediately available.

Indications for intubation

Absolute indications for intubation and mechanical ventilation include:

- coma,
- respiratory arrest or ineffectual respirations,
- exhaustion.

Other considerations for early intubation include:

- progressive hypoxaemia despite increasing inspired oxygen,
- progressive hypercapnea (note that a normal $PaCO_2$ may denote a rising level passing through the normal range),
- progressive acidosis particularly if metabolic,
- ineffectual cough/retained secretions.

These non-mandatory indications should be used in conjunction with the general state and appearance of the patient.

The most experienced intubator available must carry out intubation. A standard, rapid sequence method with pre-oxygenation should be used and gastric aspiration prevented using cricoid pressure. The standard fibreoptic bronchoscopes in ICU general use will usually only fit down an endotracheal (ET) tube >7.5 mm.

Mechanical ventilation of the asthmatic patient

Two broad overlapping groups of patients requiring mechanical ventilation are recognized.

Acute asphyxic asthma [5]

It is characterized by:

- often short onset of action from relatively normal respiratory function baseline,
- extremely severe airflow obstruction overwhelming relatively normal respiratory muscles,
- response to treatment may be rapid (but often not).

These patients are very difficult to ventilate using standard parameters [6] – which often causes:

- cardiovascular instability,
- high airway pressures,
- severe air trapping with intrinsic positive end-expiratory pressure (PEEP),
- high risk of barotrauma,
- mortality from obstructive shock, tissue hypoxia or pneumothorax.

Acute severe asthma

It is characterized by:

- lengthier onset of attack – may be days,
- often not from normal respiratory function baseline,
- more secretions and airway oedema problems,
- moderate or severe airway obstruction but respiratory muscle fatigue may be a significant problem,
- response of airway disease to treatment may be very slow – steroids can take many days to work,
- at one end of spectrum, may be relatively easy to ventilate with standard settings,
- if respiratory muscle fatigue is the major problem then rapid recovery occurs.

Cardiovascular instability and barotrauma can be avoided by limiting peak and mean airway pressures, extending expiratory time, minimizing intrinsic PEEP, maintaining oxygen saturations >92% and supporting cardiac output [7].
    This can be achieved by:

- low respiratory rates (down to 1–2/min, if necessary by manual ventilation, in extreme cases),
- low tidal volumes and low inspiratory flow rates to keep peak airway pressures <50 mmHg,

- long I:E ratios to allow adequate expiration to occur,
- high-concentration oxygen to maintain adequate saturations.

This strategy will result in high concentrations of $PaCO_2$, but patients are more at risk from hypoxia, low cardiac output and barotrauma than from hypercapnea.

Pressure-controlled ventilation can be used but tidal volumes have to be monitored very closely since the fluctuating changes of airway resistance typical of asthma affects tidal volume greatly.

Anecdotal therapies

There are reports of benefit for the following treatments in the resistant asthmatic. Most are controversial or anecdotal reports only. They should be considered after the above management fails.

i.v. magnesium sulphate

- Used in both adults and children.
- Reports of improvement and even avoidance of intubation and mechanical ventilation.
- Optimal dose is unclear but as a guide, 8–16 mmol over 30–60 min followed by 64 mmol over 24 h is a regimen suggested for arrhythmias.

Volatile anaesthetic agents

- Halothane, isoflurane and sevoflurane are the most commonly used.
- Patients are usually already intubated and ventilated.
- They are bronchodilators but may be associated with cardiovascular side effects, and halothane may cause hepatotoxicity with repeated use.

Ketamine

- An i.v. anaesthetic agent that has bronchodilating properties.
- Anecdotal reports of ketamine used as an adjunct to standard bronchodilators, substituting as sedative of choice.
- Side effects include hallucinations, psychosis and increase in blood pressure.
- Less likely to be respiratory depressant and the airway better maintained than with many other anaesthetic agents.

Helium–oxygen mixture

- Use of helium–oxygen mixture in asthma is controversial.
- Available in various oxygen concentrations.
- Less dense than air and offers less resistance to gas flow. Encourages laminar rather than turbulent flow in medium and larger airways.
- Work of breathing may be reduced and the onset of respiratory muscle fatigue delayed in awake patients.
- Has been shown to reduce dyspnoea and pulsus paradoxus and improve PEFR in children with status asthmaticus.
- It has been suggested that may help in the first hour of use [8].

Bronchoscopy and bronchial lavage

- Bronchoscopy can be helpful in removing the mucous (particularly in the upper lobes) plugs that may cause bronchial occlusion and worsen gas exchange.
- Tenacious secretion can be difficult to aspirate through the small channel of a fibreoptic bronchoscope – saline (not water) instillation can help and the procedure may need repeating.
- Single, whole-lung saline lavage has been used although it may be associated with an increase incidence of pneumonia.

Extracorporeal membrane oxygenation (ECMO)

- ECMO has been used in some patients with success, although it has many practical and other problems.
- Indications have included hypoxaemia and shock unresponsive to treatment, excessively high $PaCO_2$ and excessively low pH.
- It is associated with a high incidence of a serious side effect (e.g. bleeding).
- It is only available in specialist centres.
- It is only considered as last resort in centres where the technique is available.

Leukotriene receptor antagonists

- Sporadic early reports with i.v. preparation suggest possible benefit.
- Seems to work rapidly when as adjunct to other therapy.
- Relatively few side effects.
- Not yet widely available.

Cardiorespiratory arrest in asthmatics

Very little has been written of the management of cardiorespiratory arrest in the asthmatic patient. The following applies:

- Resuscitation is often unsuccessful or associated with residual cerebral anoxic damage.
- Standard resuscitation guidelines do not address the specific problem of cardiorespiratory arrest due to acute severe asthma.
- Inappropriate application of standard guidelines may turn a respiratory arrest into a cardiorespiratory arrest and death.
- Cardiac arrest may be secondary to hypoxia, electrolyte disturbance or obstructive shock.
- The cardiac arrest is often due to electromechanical dissociation (EMD) or asystole.

The general recommendation during resuscitation of 12 breaths/min with 3–4 s for exhalation is inappropriate in intubated asthmatics following respiratory arrest, whose passive exhalation time may be measured in minutes. The following problems arise:

- High levels of intrinsic PEEP.
- Marked air trapping and increases in residual capacity.
- High intrathoracic pressures.
- Obstructive shock with progressive reduction in cardiac output leading to cardiac arrest and cerebral hypoxic damage.
- Ineffectual external cardiac massage.
- High risk of tension pneumothorax and other barotrauma.

The following measures should be considered in these extreme circumstances:

- Low respiratory rates of 1–4 slow manual breaths/min.
- Apnoeic oxygenation with intratracheal oxygen insufflation (as performed during brain stem testing [9].
- Manual extrathoracic compression to mimic active exhalation and reduce intrathoracic volume.
- High suspicion of tension pneumothorax – if in doubt insert bilateral chest drains.
- If external cardiac massage ineffective in producing output – early recourse to internal cardiac massage.

Asthmatics can survive cardiorespiratory arrest but the longer the above methods are inappropriately delayed, the more likely cerebral anoxic damage will result. Patients die of a lack of cardiac output and tissue hypoxia, not of hypercapnea from hypoventilation.

Prognosis and causes of mortality

- In England and Wales there are ≈2000 deaths per year in adults from asthma.
- From the ICNARC database increasing age and cardiopulmonary resuscitation (CPR) or neurological insult before ICU admission are associated with mortality
- Over a quarter of deaths occurred after discharge from ICU.
- Despite fears of deaths related to *over* treatment, most asthmatic deaths are associated with *under* treatment.
- Many deaths may be preventable with early recognition of exacerbation and prompt treatment particularly with systemic steroids.
- Mortality rates vary greatly in a reported series of mechanically ventilated asthmatics – from 28% to 0 – is it explained by different types/severity and the threshold for intubation between units?
- The commonest causes of death are asphyxia, cardiovascular insufficiency, cerebral hypoxia, pneumothorax and overwhelming infection.
- Many deaths occur in patients who are known to be bad asthmatics and/or who have recently been seen by a doctor for asthma.

FURTHER READING

Cockcroft DW. Management of acute severe asthma. *Ann Aller Asthma Imm* 1995; 75: 83–9.
Levy BD, Kitch B, Fanta CH. Medical and ventilatory management of status asthmaticus. *Intens Care Med* 1998; 24: 105–17.
McFadden ER. Acute severe asthma. *Am J Respir Crit Care Med* 2003; 168: 740–59.

REFERENCES

1. Gupta D, Keogh B, Chung KF, Ayres JG et al. Characteristics and outcome for admissions to adult, general critical care units with acute severe asthma: a secondary analysis of the ICNARC Case Mix Programme Database. *Crit Care* 2004; 8: R112–21.
2. British Guideline on the Management of Asthma. *Thorax* 2003; 58(Suppl 1): 1–94.

3. Cochrane GM, Clark T. A survey of asthma mortality in patients between ages 35 and 64 in Greater London hospitals in 1971. *Thorax* 1975; 30: 300–5.

4. A confidential enquiry into deaths caused by asthma in an English health region: implications for general practice. *Br J Gen Pract* 1996 Sep; 46(410): 529–32.

5. Wasserfallen JB, Schaller MD, Feih LF, Perret CH. Sudden asphyxic asthma: a distinct entity? *Am Rev Respir Dis* 1990; 142: 108–11.

6. Tuxen DV. Detrimental effects of positive end-expiratory pressure during controlled mechanical ventilation of patients with severe airflow obstruction. *Am Rev Respir Dis* 1989; 140: 5–9.

7. Darioli A, Perret C. Mechanical controlled hypoventilation in status asthmaticus. *Am Rev Respir Dis* 1984; 129: 385–7.

8. Ho AMH, Lee A, Karmakar MK, Dion PW, Chung DC, Contardi LH. Heliox vs air–oxygen mixtures for the treatment of patients with acute asthma: a systematic overview. *Chest* 2003; 123(3): 882–90.

9. Frumin MJ, Cohen G. Apnoeic oxygenation in man. *Anaesthesiology* 1959; 20: 789–98.

28

The critically ill diabetic

I. McConachie

Diabetes is a common medical condition: almost 5% of the population, although a much smaller proportion, are insulin-dependent diabetics. Consideration of diabetes in this text is worthwhile not least due to the important points regarding fluid therapy in diabetic hyperglycaemic coma.

Diabetic coma, the commonest endocrine emergency, falls into three categories:

- *Hypoglycaemic coma*: easy to understand and treat once recognised. Therefore not discussed here.
- *Diabetic ketoacidosis* (DKA).
- *Hyperosmolar non-ketotic coma.*

DKA

DKA is relatively common:

- approximately 5% of insulin-dependent diabetic patients per year,
- mainly under the age of 40 years but can also affect elderly patients,
- said to affect women more than men.

Precipitated by infection in 30%, management errors in 15% but no obvious cause in 40%. Previously undiagnosed diabetes is the cause in 10% of DKA.

The hallmarks of DKA are:

- *Hyperglycaemia*: Lack of insulin causes the increase in blood sugar by decreasing cellular glucose uptake, increasing protein breakdown (thus promoting gluco-neogenesis) and glycogenolysis.
- Dehydration (5–10l of water) lost by osmotic diuresis, hyperventilation and vomiting.

- Loss of electrolytes, approximately 500 mmol in total of both Na and K.
- Acidosis (ketosis and, in later stages, lactic acidosis from tissue hypoperfusion).

Much of the fluid lost, comes from the intracellular space and therefore is relatively hypotonic. Therefore, although distinction is made between DKA and hyperosmolar non-ketotic coma (HNC) this is slightly arbitrary as DKA patients are always significantly hyperosmolar. Ketosis progresses to ketoacidosis when fluid loss exceeds intake due to:

- osmotic diuresis,
- vomiting,
- renal compensation overwhelmed by decreasing renal function.

Presentation

The average time of onset of condition to presentation is approximately 3 days.
   Commonly present with combinations of the following:

anorexia	vomiting	thirst
weakness	polyuria	weight loss
reduced conscious level	blurred vision	abdominal pain
gastrointestinal bleed	hyperventilation	tachycardia
ketones on breath	hypotension	hypothermia (rarely fever)

It is dangerous to assume that the abdominal pain is due to DKA. Conversely, it would be inappropriate to take a patient with DKA for laparotomy!
   Laboratory signs are:

- Increased blood sugar, haematocrit, urea, white blood corpuscles (WBC), triglycerides.
- Decreased pH, bicarbonate, serum K, Mg and phosphate.

The raised WBC is not necessarily an indicator of associated infection.
   The interpretation of serum Na is more complex. It is well demonstrated but underappreciated that an elevated serum glucose "dilutes" the plasma Na resulting in an inappropriately low measured Na [1]. The plasma Na decreases by approximately 1 mmol/l for each 3 mmol/l rise in blood sugar.
   In addition, if the Na is measured by a flame emission spectrophotometer technique an elevated hyperlipidaemia (as in DKA) will cause a "pseudohyponatraemia" due to the increase of the "solids" component of plasma. Thus a low

Na may be "normal" in DKA, a normal Na may be "high" and a high Na signifies marked hyperosmolarity.

Indications for admission to ICU

Most DKA patients do not need to go to ICU. Indications include:

- *airway compromise,*
- *severe acidosis,* unless rapidly responsive to fluid therapy,
- *hypotension,* unless rapidly responsive to fluid therapy,
- *hypoxia,*
- severe coexisting *medical conditions,*
- *lower threshold* in the elderly patient.

In one large American study, DKA was the admitting diagnosis in 7.6% of patients [2]. This is probably an overestimate for UK practice.

Management

General

- The airway must be protected; by tracheal intubation if necessary.
- A nasogastric tube is essential due to the gastric atony.
- Urinary catheter, risk of renal shutdown outweighs the risk of infection.
- Close observation, regular electrolyte and blood sugar measurements.
- Infection screen but no routine antibiotics unless clinical evidence of infection.
- Subcutaneous heparin prophylaxis due to risk of thrombosis.
- CVP monitoring if hypotensive despite initial rapid fluid therapy.
- Elderly patients, severely acidotic patients, patients who do not respond to colloid infusion or patients developing adult respiratory distress syndrome (ARDS) (see below) warrant a pulmonary artery flotation catheter (PAFC).

Fluid and electrolyte therapy

Fluid replacement is the first priority taking precedence over the administration of insulin. Delay may lead to a poor outcome. Fluid therapy alone will:

- reduce the blood sugar by dilution (by up to 20%),
- restore cardiac output, organ blood flow, cardiac output and blood pressure and correct acidosis,

- restore renal function which will aid the correction of acidosis,
- deliver insulin to its tissue receptors.

The choice of fluid is controversial between 0.9% saline, 0.45% saline and colloids. Arguments in favour of 0.9% saline being the main fluid:

- Restores plasma volume and interstitial fluid.
- Na content being higher than plasma may prevent too rapid decreases in osmolarity.
- Clinically found to be sufficient and effective for many DKA.

Arguments against large volumes of 0.9% saline:

- Danger of late hyperchloraemic acidosis [3].
- Danger of late hypernatraemia.
- May over expand the interstitial space while not replenishing the intracellular space.
- Patients have lost more water than Na.

Arguments in favour of 0.45% saline:

- Closer in composition to that of fluid deficit.
- Replenishes all fluid spaces equally.
- Avoids hypernatraemia.

Arguments against 0.45% saline:

- Slow to expand plasma and interstitial spaces.
- Potentially more rapid fall in plasma osmolarity (see below re cerebral oedema).

Arguments in favour of colloid:

- Initial rapid correction of plasma volume and shock.

Arguments against colloid:

- Not necessary for less severe cases that is those not admitted to ICU.

A suggested approach is:

(1) Initial 1000 ml N saline rapidly if hypotensive.
(2) 2000 ml of colloid rapidly if hypotension or acidosis are severe or no response in BP to above.

(3) Continue with 0.45% saline at approximately 500 ml/h for 4 h then approximately 250 ml/h so as to aim for 4–6 l of fluid in 24 h. Be prepared to adjust according to responses.

(4) No 0.9% saline or colloid if Cl >110 or Na >150.

(5) When blood sugar <20 mmol/l switch fluids to dextrose 5% or dextrose/saline.

(6) Give K early in form of KCl at 20 mmol/h unless K is very high (due to the acidosis) or there is no urine output. Rate may have to be increased if K is very low. If K is very low Mg should also be checked. Consider giving some of the K as K phosphate if Cl high or serum phosphate very low, but at lower rates of infusion.

Insulin

Soluble insulin should be given at a rate of 5–10 U/h. Previously recommended higher doses are rarely necessary [4]. The aim is to bring the blood sugar down relatively slowly over 24 h to avoid precipitate falls in osmolarity.

Adsorption of insulin to plastic syringes is irrelevant as the infusion rate and dose are titrated to the clinical effect. Occasionally higher rates of insulin infusion are required.

Bicarbonate

Bicarbonate administration is usually unnecessary and potentially dangerous:

- rapid falls in K as acidosis corrected,
- shifts Hb dissociation curve to the left inhibiting tissue oxygenation,
- 8.4% Bicarbonate is extremely hyperosmolar,
- Danger of "overshoot".

There may be no difference in outcome with bicarbonate therapy [5] and it is recommended that bicarbonate be reserved for those patients with pH <7.0 or electrocardiogram (ECG) signs of hyperkalaemia; 8.4% Na bicarbonate should be avoided or diluted in 0.45% saline. The same degree of acidosis in DKA is better tolerated than in lactic acidosis due to the lesser degree of tissue hypoxia. Interestingly the degree of acidosis does not correlate with the degree of hyperglycaemia [6].

Phosphate

Often low. In theory replacement should replenish the low levels of 2,3 diphos-phoglycerate (2,3DPG) in red blood corpuscles (RBC) and aid oxygen release from Hb [7]. However, the harmful effects of a low 2,3DPG on Hb oxygen affinity are mitigated by the presence of acidosis and routine phosphate administration, with its dangers of hypocalcaemia is not recommended.

Complications of DKA

Common complications of severe DKA and, therefore, complications seen in DKA patients admitted to ICU are as follows:

Cerebral oedema

It may occur from too rapid lowering of osmolarity either by overhydration or rapid lowering of blood sugar. It is commoner in children than adults and is associated with an increased mortality. Unnecessary administration of bicarbonate may cause a paradoxical cerebro spinal fluid (CSF) acidosis and cerebral oedema as carbon dioxide crosses the blood–brain barrier but bicarbonate cannot. Animal studies strongly support the rapid reduction and fall in osmolarity rather than the degree of acidosis as the main mechanism [8].

In a small study [9], patients with DKA underwent CT brain scans before and after rehydration with fluids of differing Na content and osmolarity. The brains of patients with DKA were denser than control patients without DKA (thought to represent dehydration). There were no differences in brain density after 24 h of fluid therapy with either of the intravenous fluid choices suggesting that fluid osmolarity and Na content are not major factors in the development of cerebral oedema. Reasons why some patients, but not others, develop cerebral oedema, even following expert management, are unclear.

ARDS

ARDS can lead to a requirement for intermittent positive pressure ventilation (IPPV) in severe DKA. The cause is the thought to be related to severe acidosis and its effects on membrane permeability. Physiological shunt may increase despite no increase in lung water [10]. Curiously, even when adjusted for other variables, it seems as if septic diabetic patients develop ARDS less frequently than other septic non-diabetic patients [11]. The reasons for and significance of this is unclear.

Miscellaneous

- Hypoglycaemia is a common complication of therapy of DKA [12].
- A recent study found that 14% of patients admitted to the ICU with DKA suffer significant upper GI haemorrhage [13].

Prognosis

Reported mortality from DKA varies in the literature but in the ICU is probably about 5%. There were no deaths in patients admitted with DKA in a recent study [2] but the authors admit that the patients had a lower severity of illness score than other patient groups in the study. Many deaths are due to preventable metabolic complications. Increasing age and coexisting disease significantly increase mortality [14]. The mortality is probably better correlated with the osmolarity rather than the degree of acidosis. Development of either ARDS or cerebral oedema is a poor prognostic sign.

Length of stay in the ICU is related to the underlying cause of the DKA [2].

HNC

In HNC the abnormalities of lipid metabolism seen in DKA do not occur and therefore ketosis and acidosis is not a feature. The reason for this difference is not known for certain but one theory is that residual insulin levels may be sufficient to prevent this. Hyperglycaemia is severe, water loss is often greater (up to 25% total body water) and hyperosmolarity is marked. Most patients are over the age of 50 and infection is a common precipitating cause. Mortality may approach 50%.

Hyperosmolarity *is* a feature of DKA and therefore overall presentation and management *are* similar with several important differences:

- onset is slower: over 5–10 days,
- aggressive fluid loading may lower osmolarity too rapidly; therefore slower rehydration may be appropriate. 0.45% saline recommended,
- often more sensitive to insulin, therefore uncommon to require >5 U/h,

- empirical antibiotics are indicated due to the high incidence of associated infection,
- Thromboembolic complications are common, including hemiplegia, therefore full anticoagulation is indicated.

FURTHER READING

Boord JB, Graber AL, Christman JW, Powers AC. Practical management of diabetes in critically ill patients. *Am J Resp Crit Care Med* 2001; 164: 1763–7.

Delaney MF, Zisman A, Kettyle WM. Diabetic ketoacidosis and hyperosmolar nonketotic syndrome. *Endocrinol Metab Clin North Am* 2000; 29: 683–705.

Krentz AJ, Nattrass M. Acute metabolic complications of diabetes mellitus: diabetic ketoacidosis, hyperosmolar nonketoic syndromes and lactic acidosis. In Pickup J, Williams G. (Eds), *Textbook of Diabetes Volume 1*. Blackwell, 1997; Oxford.

REFERENCES

1. Worthley LIG. Handbook of emergency laboratory tests. Churchill Livingstone, New York, 1996, pp. 14–5.
2. Freire AX, Umpierrez GE, Afessa B, Latif KA et al. Predictors of intensive care unit and hospital length of stay in diabetic ketoacidosis. *J Crit Care* 2002; 17: 207–11.
3. Oh MS, Banerji MA, Carrol HJ. The mechanism of hyperchloraemic acidosis during the recovery phase of diabetic ketoacidosis. *Diabetes* 1981; 30: 310–3.
4. Kitabachi AE. Low dose insulin therapy in diabetic ketoacidosis. Fact or fiction? *Diabet Metabol Rev* 1989; 5: 337–41.
5. Viallon A, Zeni F, Lafond P, Venet C et al. Does bicarbonate therapy improve the management of severe diabetic ketoacidosis? *Crit Car Med* 1999; 27: 2690–3.
6. Brandt KR, Miles JM. Relationship between severity of hyperglycaemia and metabolic acidosis in diabetic ketoacidosis. *Mayo Clin Proc* 1988; 63: 1071–4.
7. Clerbaux T, Reynart M, Willems E, Frans A. Effect of phosphate on oxygen–haemoglobin affinity, diphosphoglycerate and blood gases during recovery from diabetic ketoacidosis. *Inten Care Med* 1989; 1: 495–8.
8. Silver SM, Clark EC, Schroeder BM, Sterns RH. Pathogenesis of cerebral oedema after treatment of diabetic ketoacidosis. *Kidney Int* 1997; 51: 1237–44.
9. Azzopardi J, Gatt A, Zammit A, Alberti G. Lack of evidence of cerebral oedema in adults treated for diabetic ketoacidosis with fluids of different tonicity. *Diabetes Res Clin Pract* 2002; 57: 87–92.

10. Laggner AN, Lenz K, Kleinberger G, Sommer G, Drumi W, Schneeweiss B. Influence of fluid replacement on extravascular lung water (EVLW) in patients with diabetic ketoacidosis. *Intens Care Med* 1988; 14: 201–5.

11. Moss M, Guidot DM, Steinberg KP, Duhon GF et al. Diabetic patients have a decreased incidence of acute respiratory distress syndrome. *Crit Care Med* 2000; 28: 187–92.

12. Malone ML, Klos SE, Gennism VM, Goodwin JS. Frequent hypoglycaemic episodes in the treatment of patients with diabetic ketoacidosis. *Archiv Int Med* 1992; 152: 2472–7.

13. Faigel DO, Metz DC. Prevalence, etiology and prognostic significance of upper gastrointestinal haemorrhage in diabetic ketoacidosis. *Dig Dis Sci* 1996; 41: 1–8.

14. Connell FA, Louden JM. Diabetes mortality in persons under 45 years of age. *Am J Public Health* 1983; 73: 1174–9.

29

The cardiac surgical patient in the ICU

J. Dunning and C. Harle

Approximately 30,000 cardiac surgical operations are performed annually in the UK. Almost all of these patients are admitted to either a general or a cardiac intensive care unit (ICU) for initial postoperative management. These patients often have clinical issues peculiar to cardiac surgery. This makes a sound understanding of the preoperative and postoperative decision making process together with an understanding of the operative techniques used, essential for intensivists involved in the care of these patients.

Preoperative

History and examination

These patients will frequently have undergone comprehensive investigation before their operation, particularly in regard to their primary cardiac pathology. Nonetheless a thorough examination and full review of the notes is needed, as these patients frequently have other pathology including carotid arterial disease, femoral arterial disease, abdominal aneurysmal disease, respiratory and renal disease which may not have been recognised or have progressed since their last examination.

Risk assessment

Since the advent of national publication of centre-specific and surgeon-specific mortality data for all cardiac operations, cardiac surgical patients are rigorously assessed in order to estimate their perioperative mortality risk. The Parsonett score has been superseded by the Euroscore and most patients have their mortality risk assessed by this score. The score estimates the patient's percentage risk of mortality and thus a patient with a Euroscore of 5 has a 5% risk of death. This score is illustrated in Table 29.1 [1, 2].

Preoperative pharmacological considerations

- Ideally, clopidogrel should be stopped at least a week before surgery in order to reduce the risk of postoperative bleeding. Patients on warfarin for atrial fibrillation (AF) should also have this discontinued preoperatively. In low risk patients undergoing coronary artery bypass grafting (CABG), aspirin should probably be stopped about 5 days before surgery.
- Beta-blockers should be continued through to the morning of surgery. They protect against intra-operative ischaemia and reduce the incidence of post-operative dysrhythmias.
- Angiotensin-conversion enzyme (ACE) inhibitors should be stopped 2 days preoperatively as ACE inhibition contributes to vasodilatation and a resistance to vasoconstrictors such as noradrenaline.
- Patients on high doses of nitrates should have these continued and a nitroglycerin (GTN) infusion may be commenced with anaesthesia.
- Diabetes should be meticulously managed, to avoid hyper or hypo glycaemia in the perioperative period.
- Other antihypertensive medication may be continued until the time of operation.
- It is important that ACE inhibitors, beta-blockers, aspirin, statins and antihypertensive agents are recommended postoperatively along with the patient's non-cardiac medication and mechanisms to ensure that this is not omitted should be in place.

Preoperative investigations

- Pre-operative full blood count (FBC), and clotting screen are important, as pre-operative anaemia and postoperative transfusion is associated with significant morbidity. Leukocytosis may indicate systemic infection or inflammation, which may be greatly exacerbated by cardiopulmonary bypass (CPB). A new low platelet count may indicate heparin-induced thrombocytopenia, which is not uncommon in patients who have been receiving unfractionated heparin (UH) or low-molecular weight heparin (LMWH).
- Urea and electrolytes: preoperative hypokalaemia is often associated with diuretic use and predisposes to perioperative dysrhythmias. Hypokalaemia is an independent predictor of increased postoperative mortality.

Table 29.1. The Euroscore

Risk factors	Definition	Weights (score)
Patient-related factors		
Age	Per 5 years or part thereof over 60 years	1
Sex	Female	1
Chronic pulmonary disease	Long-term use of bronchodilators or steroids for lung disease	1
Extracardiac arteriopathy	Any one or more of the following: claudication, carotid occlusion or >50% stenosis, previous or planned intervention on the abdominal aorta, limb arteries or carotids	2
Neurological dysfunction	Disease severely affecting ambulation or day-to-day functioning	2
Previous cardiac surgery	Requiring opening of the pericardium	3
Serum creatinine	>200 mol/l preoperatively	2
Active endocarditis	Patient still on antibiotic treatment for endocarditis at the time of surgery	3
Critical preoperative state	Any one or more of the following: VT or VF or aborted sudden death, preoperative cardiac massage, positive pressure ventilation before anaesthesia, preoperative inotropic support, intra-aortic balloon counter pulsation or preoperative acute renal failure. (Anuria or oliguria <10 ml/h)	3
Cardiac-related factors		
Unstable angina	Rest angina requiring i.v., nitrates before induction of anaesthesia	2
LV dysfunction	Moderate (LVEF 30–50%) or	1
	Poor (LVEF <30%)	3
Recent MI	<90 days	2
Pulmonary hypertension	Systolic PA pressure >60 mmHg	2
Operation-related factors		
Emergency	Carried out on referral before the next working day	2
Other than isolated CABG	Major cardiac procedure other than or in addition to CABG	2
Surgery on thoracic aorta	For disorder of ascending aorta	3

i.v.: intravenous; VT or VF: ventricular tachycardia or fibrillation; LV: left ventricle; LVEF: left ventricular ejection fraction; MI: myocardial infraction.

- Renal impairment as evidenced by elevated serum Creatinine ($>$120 μmol/l) is associated with an increased mortality and where possible, surgery should be delayed while this is further investigated.
- Methicillin-resistant *Staphylococcus aureus* (MRSA) colonisation should be identified, and eradication therapy and antibiotics directed towards these multi-resistant organisms should be given.
- Chest radiography can identify lung pathology in patients with a history of smoking and cardiac disease such as lung malignancy, cardiac failure or chronic obstructive pulmonary disease (COPD). Calcification of the ascending aorta should be identified, as this will significantly increase the risk of stroke perioperatively.
- Electrocardiography (ECG) is an essential test, both as a baseline reference and to identify dysrhythmias, heart block, ischaemia or recent myocardial infarction (MI).
- Echocardiography is useful to assess the ventricular function, valvular pathology, structural anomalies, volume resuscitation and success of valve repair or replacement surgery. It is also useful to identify aortic pathology.
- Cardiac catheterisation will have been performed in virtually all patients; this provides detailed imaging of coronary anatomy, data on ejection fraction, chamber pressures and aortic root anatomy.

Operations

CABG

About 80% of CABG operations in the UK are performed using CPB, with systemic anticoagulation. 20% of operations are performed off pump, using a system of stabilisers to allow the operation to proceed without arresting the heart. Putative benefits may include reduced mortality and neurological morbidity in specific patient subgroups, although this remains controversial [3].

Conduit usually includes the left internal thoracic (also called the left internal mammary artery or LIMA artery which is usually anastomosed to the left anterior descending branch of the left main coronary artery), and saphenous vein grafts to other vessels. Occasionally a radial artery may also be used as conduit.

Valve surgery

Aortic and mitral valves may be replaced with either mechanical or biological valves. Mitral valve repair is an increasingly successful surgical intervention for regurgitant mitral valve disease, preserving the native mitral valve cusps and subvalvular apparatus, reducing the need for lifelong anticoagulation. The tricuspid valve is infrequently replaced, and occasionally repaired with annuloplasty. The pulmonary valve is also infrequently replaced.

Aortic arch surgery

This is performed for either dissection or aneurysm. These are high-risk operations, and occasionally deep hypothermic circulatory arrest (DHCA) with systemic cooling of the patient to 15–22°C is required. Coagulopathy and bleeding frequently occur following complicated aortic surgery.

Postoperative care

Postoperative cardiac surgical patients differ from other postoperative patients in many respects. CBP initiates a range of inflammatory cascades causing a systemic inflammatory response, the severity of which is unpredictable. The period of low, non-pulsatile flow during CPB may contribute to cerebral and mesenteric ischaemia, which may be exacerbate subclinical vascular disease.

The CPB circuit contains about 2 litres of priming solution, which may contribute to extravascular oedema. The patient may have also undergone a period of induced hypothermia, and they are frequently mildly hypothermic and usually intubated and ventilated on return to the ICU.

Anticipation of common postoperative complications along with an understanding of monitoring strategies employed is vital for effective postoperative care. Postoperative care will generally be assisted by significant input from the surgical team as well as from the resident intensivists.

Monitoring

ECG

Continuous ECG monitoring identifies dysrhythmias, and early ST segment changes, which may herald early graft occlusion and ischaemia.

Pulse oximetry

Continuous pulse oximetry supplements intermittent arterial blood gas analysis and may identify hypoxaemia.

Invasive monitoring

Along with ECG and oximetry, invasive arterial blood pressure monitoring, central venous pressure (CVP) monitoring and hourly urine output are minimum, mandatory monitoring standards. Pulmonary artery flotation catheters (PAFC) and other means of monitoring cardiac output may guide volume replacement and the use of inotropic and vasopressor drugs.

Mediastinal drainage

Continuous mediastinal drainage measurement is routinely employed, with documentation initially at ¼ to ½ hourly intervals:

- Drainage of 100 ml/h is regarded as moderate drainage.
- 200 ml/h is regarded as high.
- 400 ml/h is severe, and is invariably a trigger for re-operation.
- The absence of measurable drainage from the drains may be misleading as bleeding can occur into the chest cavity, and not be reflected in the drainage.

Urine output

Oliguria is an ominous finding in these patients, and may reflect hypovolaemia, hypotension and/or poor splanchnic perfusion. Oliguria frequently precedes acute renal failure. Urine output should be recorded hourly, and hourly urine outputs of less than 0.5 ml/kg is a cause for concern.

Chest radiography

A postoperative chest X-ray (CXR) will identify the correct placement of central lines, Swan-Ganz catheters and mediastinal drains. It may also identify pneumo-thorax or occult bleeding into the left or right hemi-thorax, especially when the pleura have been opened.

Blood gas monitoring

Blood gas analysis should be performed at regular intervals to guide ventilatory strategy, as well as to monitor metabolism and to identify anaemia and electrolyte abnormalities.

Haematology

A FBC should be requested early in order to quantify thrombocytopaenia, or anaemia, and if there is a suspicion of bleeding, a coagulation screen can help guide treatment. The activated clotting time (ACT) is routinely checked, as high ACTs are associated with increased bleeding.

Postoperative complications

Bleeding

Excessive postoperative bleeding is common, and between 1% and 5% of patients may require re-operation for bleeding. Bleeding and transfusion of blood and blood products is associated with increased morbidity and mortality. Early identification, and distinction between surgical bleeding and coagulopathy is essential. Quantification of, and rational intervention for coagulopathy and/or surgical bleeding may reduce morbidity associated with inappropriate blood transfusion. Bleeding may be "surgical", or related to coagulopathy, or both.

Investigation of coagulopathy

In addition to the ACT, and the clotting screen (International Normalised Ratio (INR), prothrombin time (PT), activated partial thromboplastin time (APTT)), specific tests exist that are in common usage in cardiac ICU. The Hepcon™ machine uses protamine titration to estimate heparin levels, and gives an accurate indication of residual heparin that may require supplemental protamine.

The Thrombelastogram® (TEG) is a point of care test which can graphically illustrate reduced clotting factors, platelet dysfunction or inadequate heparin reversal.

Surgical bleeding

- Perioperative changes in blood pressure, cardiac output and regional blood flow occur frequently in these patients, and bleeding from the operative field may not manifest during the operative time.
- Sudden bleeding after haemodynamic changes, bleeding from specific drain sites, as well as sustained or high-volume blood loss raise the suspicion of ongoing surgical bleeding. Early surgical exploration and intervention to stop bleeding is indicated in cases of surgical bleeding.

Coagulopathy

Coagulopathy is often multi-factorial, and may be associated with the following.

Thrombocytopenia/platelet dysfunction

Modest reductions in platelet numbers will increase bleeding in patients on antiplatelet medications at the time of surgery are more so than in controls who have not taken antiplatelet drugs. Platelet transfusion is associated with increased risk of serious adverse outcome, and the decision to transfuse platelets has to be balanced against potential risks.

Depletion of clotting factors

A prolonged PT associated with continued bleeding suggests coagulation factor deficiency, and treatment with fresh frozen plasma (FFP) may be indicated. In the context of markedly abnormal coagulation with a low fibrinogen count, particularly after administration of large FFP, blood and platelet transfusion, consideration should be given to administration of cryoprecipitate.

Inadequate heparin reversal

The ACT is a crude measure of heparinisation. A prolonged ACT does not necessarily imply residual heparin. Heparin rebound is the reappearance of anticoagulant activity, despite apparently adequate neutralisation with protamine. This may be due to delayed release of heparin from binding sites on plasma proteins after elimination of protamine. The clinical contribution of measured heparin rebound to ongoing bleeding has not been shown to be significant in many studies. Protamine has serious side effects, and before it is given to postoperative patients, consideration must be given to the pharmacokinetics of heparin, and the doses of both heparin and protamine already given in the operating theatre. Ideally it should only be given when there is clear evidence for circulating heparin. The Hepcon™ device, and the Thrombelastograph® can demonstrate quantitative and qualitative heparin recirculation, respectively, and where they are available; they should be used to guide supplemental administration of protamine. Protamine to heparin dose ratios of 2.6:1 have been shown to actually increase the ACT. It is easy to exceed this dose of protamine if it is given empirically based on total doses of heparin given, without considering the elimination and excretion of heparin during the surgery. If protamine is given, the ACT *must* be rechecked, as excessive protamine can make bleeding worse, and a rise in ACT following supplemental protamine suggests this to be the case. Routine and repeated administration of protamine in response to prolonged ACTs in the postoperative period is neither rational nor safe. Protamine should not be given in dose ranges in excess of 2.6:1 of circulating heparin levels [4, 5].

Prothrombotic drugs

In bleeding patients, aprotinin and tranexamic acid have been shown to reduce postoperative bleeding and should be considered [6]. There is growing interest in the use of recombinant factor VIIa in the management of severe life-threatening haemorrhage.

Miscellaneous

Judicious use of positive end-expiratory pressure (PEEP), and elevation of the back of the bed can reduce bleeding.

Hypothermia and shivering can exacerbate coagulopathy and bleeding, and active warming should be employed in hypothermic patients who are bleeding.

Tamponade

Mediastinal drains cannot be relied on to drain all blood loss from the pericardium. Accumulated blood in the pericardium can block the mediastinal drains. Hypotension with high CVP and oliguria suggest tamponade and it should be specifically excluded by echocardiography, radiography or re-operation. Tamponade may occur more slowly and manifest with increased inotrope requirement, metabolic acidosis and oliguria. Low cardiac index should alert physicians to this possibility.

The risk of tamponade decreases considerably after 6–12 h. However late tamponade may occur, particularly after removal of epicardial pacing wires up to 4 or more days postoperatively.

Hypotension

This should be approached systematically in order to avoid a cascade of complications due to end-organ hypoperfusion and also to identify treatable causes:

• *Preload*: This should be addressed first. Hypovolaemia is a common reason for hypotension post-cardiac surgery. CPB is associated with haemodilution,

capillary leakage and postoperative vasodilatation, all of which cause intravascular hypotension. Fall in CVP, urine output, and pulmonary arterial wedge pressure,
and increasing arterial pulse pressure variability suggest hypovolaemia and fluid
replacement should be initiated (Table 29.2).

- *Afterload*: If intravascular volume is deemed adequate, but hypotension persists, this may be due to vasodilatation. The inflammatory response to CPB,
and patient warming contribute to this. Clinical examination should reveal
warm peripheries and low dose noradrenaline is commonly needed. If increasing doses are required a Swan-Ganz catheter should be considered, to guide
management.
- *Contractility*: Persistent hypotension with appropriate pre- and afterload conditions suggest "pump failure". Remediable causes of low cardiac output
including dysrhythmia, ischaemia, tamponade and other mechanical causes
must be sought and addressed. Inotropic drugs (see Table 29.3) should be commenced, and consideration given to the placement of an intra-aortic balloon
pump (IABP).

Table 29.2. Fluid replacement therapy

Crystalloid 1 ml/kg/h (dextrose/saline)	Maintenance therapy
Colloid (gelatine, hetastarch), 10–20 ml/kg	Boluses as required to treat hypovolaemia
Blood	To give if Hb <7.5–8 g/dl
Platelets, FFP	Guided by coagulation studies

Table 29.3. Vasoactive drugs in common usage

Drug with dose (μg/kg/min)	HR	SVR	CI	PAWP	MAP
Dopamine (3–10)	++	+	+	+	−/+
Adrenaline (0.01–0.6)	++	−/+	+++	−+	+
Noradrenaline (0.01–0.3)	+	+++	+	++	++
Milrinone (0.35–0.75)	+	−	++	−	+
Isoprenaline (0.01–0.1)	+++	−	+++	−	−/+
Dopexamine (0.5–6.0)	++	−	++	−	+
Dobutamine (5–20)	++	−	++	−	+

HR: heart rate; CI: cardiac index; SVR: systemic vascular resistance; PAWP: pulmonary arterial
wedge pressure; MAP: mean arterial pressure.

Pneumothorax

Pneumothorax is a common complication due to either intentional or uninten-
tional opening of either pleura, particularly when positive pressure ventilation is
employed. Surgeons may or may not have placed a drain into the pleura and
the presence of a drain does not exclude the possibility of pneumothorax.
Pneumothorax may present with increasing ventilatory requirements in ventilated patients, hypoxaemia, and hypotension with or without a high CVP.
Pneumothorax should be excluded by clinical examination, followed only by
CXR if the patient is stable.

Tension pneumothorax should be considered early in the management of
patients with acute circulatory collapse, and immediate drainage is necessary.

Graft occlusion/perioperative MI

Repeated studies suggest that the incidence of postoperative graft occlusion is in
the order of 5% [7]. Graft occlusion correlates poorly with conventional signs
of MI. Graft occlusion may occur because of technical failure or thrombosis. MI
may occur in the absence of graft occlusion due to distal embolisation of air or
debris during the operation.

ST elevation in the territory of one of the grafted vessels should alert physicians
to this possibility, as should dysrhythmias, in particular ventricular tachycardia or
fibrillation (VT or VF). Widespread myocardial depression may indicate subendo-
cardial infarction due to inadequate myocardial protection intra-operatively and
Troponin T or I may help retrospective diagnosis of perioperative MI [8]. If blood
pressure is adequate, intravenous nitrates may be indicated, but if blood pressure
is low, an IABP and possibly re-operation with revision of the anastomoses should
be considered.

Ischaemic bowel

This is a feared complication, which is difficult to diagnose and treat and is often
fatal. It occurs in around 2–3% of patients, but when it occurs, mortality may be
as high as 60% [9, 10]. It may be caused by perioperative rupture of atheroma in
the mesenteric arteries, emboli or ischaemia induced by perioperative hypoperfusion. Intubated patients may not complain of abdominal pain and the first
signs are often metabolic acidosis with falling systemic vascular resistance and
increasing requirement for vasoconstrictors. Absent bowel sounds, abdominal

distension and abdominal pain (in extubated patients), and a high index of suspicion, should generate urgent abdominal surgical referral. Prompt surgical intervention is imperative in this situation.

Renal failure

Oliguria (<0.5 ml/kg/h) is a common postoperative complication and may be caused by renal insult secondary to hypotension or a low cardiac output state combined with the effects of CPB. Prompt treatment is required to prevent acute tubular necrosis. Primary intervention should be directed at optimising renal blood flow paying attention to volume replacement, cardiac output and renal perfusion pressure. The role of diuretics and of dopamine agonists remains controversial; however, diuresis is desirable while awaiting renal recovery, and their use is often associated with natriuresis and diuresis. Severe hyperkalaemia, acidosis, uraemia and marked fluid overload may require haemofiltration.

Prevention and identification of stroke

The incidence of stroke varies from under 1% in patients under 65 years to over 10% in elderly patients with ascending aortic atheromatous disease. Symptomatic carotid arterial disease should be treated with preoperative or intra-operative carotid endarterectomy. Minimisation of aortic manipulation in patients with aortic atheroma may also reduce the risk of stroke, but patients with focal neurology or abnormal behaviour on attempted extubation may have suffered a stroke. Computerised tomography (CT) scanning when the patient is stable for transfer to the radiology department will confirm the diagnosis.

Dysrhythmia

Twenty percent of cardiac surgical patients will develop AF postoperatively. This is often transient and related to endogenous or exogenous catecholamines. Serum electrolytes, oxygenation and hydration should all be optimised, and potassium should be kept above 4.5 mmol/l. Antidysrythmics or rate controlling drugs may be used and occasionally synchronised DC cardioversion may be required if AF causes significant hypotension. Overdrive pacing is also occasionally attempted using atrial epicardial pacing wires.

Ventricular dysrhythmias may also occur and electrolyte correction, intravenous lignocaine, amiodarone and defibrillation may be required to correct this.

Epicardial pacing

Epicardial pacing wires are commonly placed onto the right atrium and/or the right ventricle. Patients undergoing valve surgery and especially mitral valve surgery are particularly susceptible to damage of conduction pathways intraoperatively. Atrial pacing is indicated for sinus bradycardia or slow junctional rhythms, atrioventricular pacing is useful in complete heart block or second-degree heart block, and ventricular pacing is effective in slow AF with a slow ventricular rate.

The IABP

An IABP has two major beneficial effects. On inflation, it provides increased diastolic blood pressure, which improves coronary blood flow. Deflation occurs just prior to systole, reducing afterload, and decreasing the work of the heart.

The IABP is usually inserted via the right femoral artery, and the balloon lies in the descending thoracic aorta, 1–2 cm distal to the left subclavian artery. After insertion, the left radial pulse should be checked to ensure that the tip has not entered or occluded the left subclavian artery and a CXR should be performed to confirm correct placement.

Heparin infusion should be considered to prevent thrombosis around the IABP and the balloon should never be left in situ without active counterpulsation for more than a few minutes.

Inflation should occur just after the aortic valve closes (the dicrotic notch on the arterial trace or the peak of the T-wave) and deflation should occur prior to systole (or the R-wave) in order to ensure that the end-diastolic pressure is as low as possible. Inflation and deflation may be adjusted manually in order to optimise it, although the most modern IABPs have an automatic setting to optimise this (Figure 29.1).

The complication rate is around 2–5% [11] and an IABP is contraindicated in severe aortic regurgitation or severe aorto-iliac atheromatous disease. The complications are listed in Table 29.4.

Mechanical cardiac support is increasingly being used electively as a bridge to cardiac transplantation, or as salvage in critically ill cardiac patients. Left

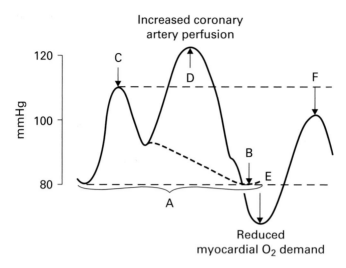

Figure 29.1 An arterial trace augmented by an IABP. A, one complete cardiac cycle; B, unassisted aortic end-diastolic pressure; C, unassisted systolic pressure; D, diastolic augmentation; E, assisted aortic end-diastolic pressure; F, reduced systolic pressure.

Table 29.4. Complications of IABP

Complication	Prevention/treatment
Limb ischaemia	Regular assessment of peripheral pulses by Doppler ultrasound
Thromboembolism/ insertion site bleeding	Regular monitoring of ACT and titration of i.v. heparin
Balloon rupture/leak	Blood down the drive line heralds this uncommon complication but the IABP must be immediately removed to prevent thrombus forming in the semi-inflated balloon, preventing subsequent removal
Aortic dissection	Haemodynamic instability may herald this life-threatening complication
Renal failure/GI ischaemia	Misplacement of the IABP with the lower portion of the balloon placed intra-abdominally

GI: gastrointestinal; i.v.: intravenous.

and right ventricular assist devices (LVADs, RVADs), and biventricular assist devices (BIVADs) as well as mechanical pump devices (Impella device) and extracorporeal membrane oxygenation (ECMO) are used with varying degrees of success in different centres, for a variety of clinical reasons. Familiarity with the application and restrictions of these technologies are essential for their successful use.

FURTHER READING

Gothard J, Kelleher A, Haxby E. *Anaesthesia in a Nutshell Series: Cardiovascular and Thoracic Anaesthesia.* Butterworth Heinmann, 2003.

Treasure T, Hunt I, Keogh B, Pagano D. *The Evidence for Cardiothoracic Surgery.* TFM, 2004.

REFERENCES

1. Parsonnet V, Dean D, Bernstein AD. A method of uniform stratification of risk for evaluating the results of surgery in acquired adult heart disease. *Circulation* 1989; 79(6: Pt 2): 1–12.

2. Roques F, Nashef SA, Michel P, Gauducheau E et al. Risk factors and outcome in European cardiac surgery: analysis of the EuroSCORE multinational database of 19030 patients. *Eur J Cardio-Thorac Surg* 1999; 15(6): 816–2.

3. Van Der Heijden GJMG, Nathoe HM, Jansen EWL, Grobbee DE. Meta-analysis on the effect of off-pump coronary bypass surgery. *Eur J Cardio-Thorac Surg* 2004; 26: 81–4.

4. Mclaughlin KE, Dunning J. In patients post cardiac surgery do high doses of protamine cause increased bleeding? *J Interact Cardiovasc Thorac Surg* 2003; 2: 424–6.

5. Butterworth J, Yonggu AL, Prielipp RC, Bennett J et al. Rapid disappearance of protamine in adults undergoing cardiac operation with cardiopulmonary bypass. *Ann Thorac Surg* 2002; 74: 1589–95.

6. Wong BI, McLean RF, Deemar KA, Harrington EM et al. Aprotinin and tranexamic acid for high transfusion risk cardiac surgery. *Ann Thorac Surg* 2000; 69:808–16.

7. Canos DA, Mintz GS, Berzingi CO, Apple S et al. Clinical, angiographic, and intravascular ultrasound characteristics of early saphenous vein graft failure. *J Am Coll Cardiol* 2004; 44: 53–6.

8. Botha P, Nagarajan DV, Lewis PS, Dunning J. Can cardiac troponins be used to diagnose a perioperative myocardial infarction post cardiac surgery? *Interact J Cardiovasc Thorac Surg* 2004 (in press).

9. Allen KB, Salam AA, Lumsden AB. Acute mesenteric ischaemia after cardiopulmonary bypass. *J Vasc Surg* 1992; 16: 391–5.

10. Christenson JT, Schmuziger M, Maurice J, Simonet F et al. Gastrointestinal complications after coronary artery bypass grafting. *J Thorac Cardiovasc Surg* 1994; 108: 899–906.

11. Ferguson JJ, Cohen M, Freedman RJ, Stone GW et al. The current practice of intra-aortic balloon counterpulsation: results from the Benchmark Registry. *J Am Coll Cardiol* 2001; 38: 1456–62.

30

Cardiac arrest

I. McConachie

Cardiac arrest is cessation of effective circulation due to asystole, ventricular fibrillation (VF) or pulseless electrical activity (PEA, previously known as electromechanical dissociation EMD).

- Brain damage will occur within 4–6 min (unless protected by hypothermia). Therefore this is the ultimate cardiac emergency.
- One of the truly landmark papers in the 20th century was that on closed chest cardiac resuscitation in 1960 by Kouwenhoven.
- This was the start of the modern concept of cardiopulmonary resuscitation (CPR).

This chapter will briefly review current guidelines for basic life support (BLS) and advanced life support (ALS) and discuss some of the controversies in resuscitation research. The practical aspects of BLS and ALS are not covered in detail as these are best learnt at formal resuscitation courses.

All hospital doctors should be proficient at CPR and should receive regular training/practice at BLS and ALS.

Causes

- Asystole is the first diagnosed rhythm in approximately 30% of cardiac arrest victims. In some, especially out-of-hospital arrests this will be due to untreated VF (especially if bystander CPR has not been initiated). In hospital, asystole may be due to severe coronary artery disease and myocardial infarction (MI). Occasionally hypoxia and other acute, severe medical conditions may result in asystolic arrest. Rarely asystole may be due to excess vagal stimulation or carotid sinus hypersensitivity.

- "Sudden death" outside hospital is a major form of cardiac death. The majority of these are VF or pulseless ventricular tachycardia (VT) and are due to ischaemic heart disease. If untreated, all VF will degenerate into asystole. One study of over 1700 patients found that if the paramedics arrived within 4 min 53% were found to have VF/VT. With time the incidence of VF/VT decreased to 27% at 20 min [1]. Bystander CPR maintained VF.

- PEA usually has a potentially reversible cause, for example,

Hypovolaemia	Tension pneumothorax
Hypoxia	Tamponade
Hyperkalaemia	Drug Toxicity
Hypokalaemia	Thromboembolism
Hypothermia	

Survival

Overall, results are, to say the least, disappointing. Survival depends, in part, on the institution of bystander CPR and the time from arrest to defibrillation. Survival of up to 25% in out-of-hospital arrests is possible with rapid bystander CPR: survival is often higher for arrests in public than arrests at home.

One might expect survival from arrests in hospital to be better due to rapid availability of trained personnel and equipment but overall results are equally poor. This is due to the presence of other pathology than ischaemic heart disease in many of these patients. The exception is cardiac arrest due to VF in CCU for which survival is high because of immediate defibrillation, though many of these patients will not receive formal CPR.

Factors increasing survival

- VF versus asystole.
- Rapid CPR.
- Rapid defibrillation: survival of out-of-hospital arrest 43% if BLS <4 min and defibrillation, <8 min [2].
- Short duration of CPR.
- Witnessed arrest.

- Bystander CPR if out-of-hospital.
- Defibrillation at scene if out-of-hospital.
- Effectiveness of CPR (see later).
- Skill and training of resuscitation personnel.
- Location of arrest in hospital: favourable if arrest in CCU. Although cardiac arrest under anaesthesia is rare, these have highest resuscitation success rates.

BLS protocols

Reference should be made to the latest guidelines as listed in Further reading. This brief summary assumes two rescuers. In summary:

- First establish the need for intervention by feeling carotid pulse.
- Call for expert help.
- *First rescuer*: If no sign of respirations, assess and open airway by tilting head backwards and lifting jaw. Inflate lungs using equipment provided in your institution at a ratio of 1 breath per 5 cardiac compression (2:15 if only one rescuer).
- *Second rescuer*: If no signs of circulation, provide external cardiac massage (ECM) using two interlocked hands over lower third of sternum. Aim for cardiac compression rate of approximately 100/min.
- Monitor BLS for return of pulse and breathing.
- *Remember*: Early BLS and defibrillation shown to improve outcome.

Exceptions to the above include a witnessed VF arrest in CCU where BLS need not be performed if defibrillation can be immediately performed (unless defibrillation unsuccessful!). A precordial thump may be attempted while defibrillator mobilised.

Mechanisms of ECM

- *Original theory*: Heart squeezed between sternum and vertebral column with blood expelled with each compression. Relaxation "sucks" blood back into the thorax. Some animal studies lend some credence to this theory.
- *Thoracic pump theory*: Coughing during cardiac arrest can generate effective systolic pressures suggesting that high intrathoracic pressures can promote cardiac output. In this theory the heart serves as a conduit and increasing thoracic

pressures during ECM expel blood out of the heart down a pressure gradient between intrathoracic and extrathoracic vasculature.

Controversies in BLS/ECM

Awareness of the thoracic pump theory of cardiac output during ECM led to refinements which could be expected lead to increased output.

Active compression/decompression

A "kitchen sink plunger" type of mechanism attached to the chest which improved ventricular filling and forward flow by "sucking" blood into the chest has been investigated. However, a large trial has found no differences in outcome [3].

Abdominal counterpulsation

Pressure on the abdominal aorta during ECM to improve filling of the heart again showed initial promise.

Pneumatic vest

Circumferential pressure on the thorax with a pneumatic system increase intrathoracic pressure and again showed initial promise.

However, the message from all these adjuncts to standard ECM is that non-supplant standard ECM at present.

Duration of compressions

Increasing the duration of compressions to about 50% of the ECM cycle is beneficial in animals and is a useful practical "side effect" of increasing the rate of compressions to approximately 100/min.

Open chest massage

Usefulness is limited to trauma and in the operating theatre especially during cardiac surgery. Such heroics do not lend themselves to routine performance by cardiac arrest teams. Similarly, placing the arrested patient onto cardiopulmonary bypass is limited mainly to cardiac surgery patients.

Infectious diseases

There is no doubt that fear of human immunodeficiency virus (HIV) transmission is limiting the application of BLS techniques by lay bystanders. This is despite education that HIV has not been reported to be transmitted by saliva contact.

Nevertheless it is prudent to take precautions (tuberculosis (TB) and viruses such as herpes can definitely be transmitted during BLS). All hospital personnel should have access to devices such as pocket masks, etc. which should negate the necessity for "mouth to mouth" resuscitation.

However, this has no impact on the fear of lay bystanders. It has, therefore, been suggested [4] that lay CPR should concentrate on ECM only (i.e., no "mouth to mouth"), particularly if there is only one rescuer. The rationale is based on animal studies showing that ventilation during CPR is not as important as ECM.

Clinical studies clearly show:

- Bystander ventilation only gives no increased survival *cf.* no resuscitation.
- Bystander ECM only gives increased survival.
- No further increased survival with both ECM and ventilation.

ALS protocols

BLS alone will rarely result in successful resuscitation. The purpose of BLS is to maintain organ blood flow until techniques can be applied to restore spontaneous circulation.

Summary of ALS principles:

- Maintain CPR/BLS.
- Precordial thump if VF witnessed followed by immediate defibrillation if necessary.
- Verify rhythm. Defibrillate with 200, 200 then 360 J. Care with paddle positions. *Note*: Eighty percent of successful defibrillations occur in first three shocks. Many modern defibrillators employ biphasic technology which is more efficient than monophasic defibrillation shocks that are used in older devices. The UK Resuscitation Council recommends following manufacturers advice regarding shock energy for biphasic devices rather than adhering to protocols developed for the older monophasic units.
- Appropriate intravenous access (see below).

- Ensure oxygenation and intubation if appropriate personnel present. Oxygenate prior to attempting intubation and avoid prolonged attempts without reoxygenation.
- In general, patients do not die of failure to intubate, they die of failure to oxygenate. However, intubation is probably worthwhile if only to protect against aspiration of stomach contents.
- Drug administration is simplified in latest guidelines (see Further reading). Basically consists of 1 mg of adrenaline every 3 min. Atropine, 3 mg, may be given *once* in asystole.
- Be aware of potentially reversible causes of EMD (see Causes).

Immediate transthoracic external pacing is recommended in some protocols for management of asystole but does not occupy a position of priority in the European guidelines (possibly due to lack of routine access to the equipment).

Drug controversies in ALS

Adrenaline

One milligram boluses of Adrenaline intravenously is currently the recommended drug of choice in almost all circumstances in cardiac arrest. However, this is despite a lack of convincing clinical evidence showing that adrenaline improves survival or neurological outcome. Certainly there are animal studies showing improved myocardial and cerebral blood flow and survival but patient studies are conflicting.

The rationale for the administration of adrenaline includes:

- α vasoconstricting effect raising coronary and cerebral perfusion pressures. This improves the chances of successful defibrillation in VF.
- The $\beta 1$ effect may coarsen fine VF or promote VF in asystole. Its positive inotropic effects are of lesser importance.
- Positive chronotropic effects may be useful if bradycardia occurs.

Because of favourable animal studies higher doses have been tried (up to 10 mg) but have not led to improved survival. In fact, disappointingly, neither "normal"- or "high"-dose adrenaline produced improved survival compared to placebo in a recent study [5].

Vasopressin

Disenchantment with clinical results from the use of adrenaline have resulted in other vasoconstrictors being investigated. For example, in a randomised controlled study the use of 40 μg of vasopressin (a non-catecholamine vaso-pressor) produced increased 24 h survival compared to 1 mg of adrenaline [6]. A larger European multicentre study comparing two injections of 40 μg of vaso-pressin with 1 mg of adrenaline found improved survival and hospital discharge in the vasopressin group. They also showed that the combination was more effec-tive than either drug alone in refractory cardiac arrest [7]. Although these results are encouraging it is still too early for widespread adoption of vasopressin in ALS.

Atropine

The rationale for the use of atropine comes from studies showing high-endogenous catecholamine levels during cardiac arrest (implying presumably a limited effect from additional exogenous catecholamines) and a relatively high-vagal tone [8]. However, atropine administration has not been shown to improve survival from cardiac arrest and its role is currently secondary to that of adrenaline.

Calcium chloride

Although calcium salts have a positive inotropic action its use has not been shown to improve survival in cardiac arrest. Now the use should be restricted to hyperkalaemia, hypocalcaemia or arrests secondary to overdosage of calcium-blocking drugs. There is also concern that high blood levels of calcium could pre-cipitate coronary spasm in patients with ischaemic heart disease and also potentially increase cerebral damage during periods of ischaemia. For similar reasons dextrose containing fluids should be avoided during cardiac arrest.

Sodium bicarbonate

No longer routinely administered due to concerns regarding the production of a hyperosmolar state, "overshoot" alkalosis (detrimental effect on oxyhaemoglo-bin dissociation curve limiting oxygen release at the tissues) and hyperna-traemia. The use of bicarbonate is best reserved for prolonged resuscitation (i.e., pH <7.1) where the myocardium may be directly compromised. Most useful in hyperkalaemic arrest or arrest following tricyclic antidepressant overdosage.

Antiarrhythmic administration

The usefulness of many antiarrhythmic drugs during cardiac arrest is limited by their negative inotropic properties.

- Lidocaine is currently widely used during prolonged VF arrests and to prevent recurrence of VF. Although controversial this use is supported by studies showing improved outcome from sustained VF arrests [9]. Interestingly, lidocaine is known to increase defibrillation threshold.
- Bretylium lowers defibrillation threshold and is beneficial in sustained VF. Convincing evidence for improved *survival*, however, is lacking.
- The cardiac depressant effect of amiodarone is relatively mild and well tolerated. An important randomised, controlled trial of out-of-hospital cardiac arrest has been presented at a major scientific meeting. The ARREST trial found that a 300 mg bolus of amiodarone improved survival to hospital compared to placebo [10]. If this is substantiated by further studies and the improved survival translates to improved survival to discharge this will have important implications.

Route of drug administration

- Initial administration of drugs is best via good peripheral venous access. Drug injections should be well flushed.
- With prolonged resuscitation central venous catheterisation may be appropriate *if* performed by experienced personnel (pneumothorax from unskilled central venous attempts is counterproductive!). Many find it difficult to catheterise a central vein during ECM – but this is not an indication to stop CPR.
- If no vascular access possible, adrenaline, lidocaine and atropine may all be given via the endotracheal tube at twice the normal dose, preferably diluted to 10 ml. Blood levels of drugs given by the endotracheal route are unpredictable.
- Intracardiac injection is no longer recommended due to the potential for trauma.

Monitoring effectiveness of CPR

Cardiac output only, at best, 10–30% of normal during CPR. Flow is especially poor to organs below the diaphragm. Presence of a carotid pulse is not a reliable *quantitative* indicator of cardiac output. Pupillary responses during CPR are not helpful, beware of the effects of adrenaline and atropine.

Indicators of effective CPR:

- Arterial pressure tracing if arterial line *in situ*, especially with diastolic >40 mmHg.
- Measured CO_2 in expired gas or end tidal CO_2. Measured with simple hand held device attachable to breathing circuit. Chemical indicators provide a semi-quantitative indicator of pCO_2. Increases with CPR indicate increasing cardiac output and pulmonary artery blood flow and a likely successful outcome.

Indicators of ineffective CPR:

- As above, lack of increasing end tidal CO_2 predicts a poor outcome.
- Worsening metabolic acidosis indicates poor tissue blood flow. Venous pH may be more useful than arterial as will better reflect the acid–base state of the tissues.

Complications of CPR

- Ineffective ECM, including situations where circulation has been reestablished but neurological outcome is poor because of relatively ineffective ECM.
- Stomach distension, potentially leading to regurgitation and pulmonary aspiration.
  - Arguably fear of this complication is one of the main reasons for endotracheal intubation of the patient.
- Rib and sternal fractures.
- Laceration of liver and other abdominal organs has been reported.
- Complications of central vascular access (e.g., pneumothorax).
- Potential proarrhythmic effects of drugs administered. Certainly, tachycardia following successful resuscitation is widespread.
- Complications of defibrillation – including burns to patient, shocks to operator (no deaths reported) and explosion of glyceryl trinitrate (GTN) patches. It is recommended that patches be removed and to keep paddles 10–15 cm away from pacemakers.

Neurological outcome

- One study found that an arrest time prior to resuscitation (or "down time") >6 min and CPR time >15 min *always* produced neurological impairment. However, down times <6 min *and* CPR times of <30 min resulted in satisfactory neurological recovery in 50% of patients [11]. One implication of this is to limit resuscitation attempts to <15 min where down time exceeds 6 min.

- Scoring systems have been developed using various clinical signs to try and predict the likelihood of neurological recovery but, unfortunately, none are sufficiently accurate to enable definite pronouncements on prognosis to be made in advance.
- Electroencephalogram (EEG) monitoring may occasionally be useful and improves our ability to predict outcome.
- Many believe that lack of corneal reflexes or pupillary light reflexes after 24 h indicates a uniformly poor outcome.
- Some points from the literature:
  - Most who recover show rapid improvement in the first 24–48 h.
  - Coma persisting more than 4 h makes neurological damage more likely.
  - Long duration of coma (especially >4 days) leads to very poor outcome.

Post resuscitation care

- Depends on underlying cause of the arrest. Specific causes may obviously need specific treatment.
- VF associated with MI – treatment largely that of MI.
- In USA, many patients undergo emergency cardiac catheterisation with aggressive reperfusion attempted in some centres.
- Control blood glucose. Hyperglycaemia is associated with a worse neurological outcome.
- Blood pressure (BP) autoregulation is impaired – avoid hypo or hypertension.
- Occasionally patients have a low-cardiac output and develop multiple organ failure. The myocardial dysfunction is suggestive of some degree of "myocardial stunning". Animal studies support the use of dobutamine.
- Drug therapy to improve neurological outcome is still experimental and has much interest, so far fruitless, in the use of Ca blockers.
- Intracranial pressure is not usually increased. Recent research confirms that, as for head injuries, routine hyperventilation in an attempt at "cerebral salvage" can *lower* cerebral blood flow.
- Many centres offer intermittent positive pressure ventilation (IPPV) and intensive care unit (ICU) care in an effort to optimise haemodynamics and oxygenation but there is no evidence that this approach improves outcome in this rather depressing clinical situation.

Hypothermia

There have been two prospective randomized trials published comparing mild hypothermia with normothermia in comatose survivors of out-of-hospital cardiac arrest [12, 13]. Although there were some adverse effects in the hypothermia group, overall survival and recovery of neurological was improved compared to normothermia. On the basis of the published evidence to date, the International Liaison Committee on Resuscitation recommends:

- Unconscious adult patients with spontaneous circulation after out-of-hospital cardiac arrest should be cooled to 32–34°C for 12–24 h when the initial rhythm was VF.
- Such cooling may also be beneficial for other rhythms or in-hospital cardiac arrest.

Family presence during CPR

Traditionally this has been seen as a distraction and has been discouraged due, in part, to fears of medicolegal consequences. However, family members being present at the resuscitation is now seen as beneficial to the grieving process and should be allowed if the family wish to be present.

Training

- In general, studies showing best survival in out-of-hospital arrests are those in which early bystander CPR is initiated. Therefore, community wide programmes of BLS modelled on Seattle and Belgian experience would seem important.
- Unfortunately poor knowledge amongst doctors is still a problem [14]. This is despite the studies clearly demonstrating that patient survival varies with knowledge of correct management as well as availability of equipment. All doctors (indeed all health care personnel) should undergo training and practice of CPR skills. The majority of hospitals now have full time Resuscitation Training Officers for this purpose. Six monthly reinstruction has been shown to maintain adequate skills.

FURTHER READING

Advanced Life Support Working Group of the European Resuscitation Council. The 1998 European Resuscitation Council guidelines for adult advanced life support. *Br Med J* 1998; 316: 1863–9.

Basic Life Support Working Group of the European Resuscitation Council. The 1998 European Resuscitation Council guidelines for adult single rescuer basic life support. *Br Med J* 1998; 316: 1870–6.

Cao L, Weil MH, Sun S, Tang W. Vasopressor agents for cardiopulmonary resuscitation. *J Cardiovasc Pharmacol Ther* 2003; 8: 115–21.

REFERENCES

1. Herlitz J, Ekstrom L, Wennerblom B, Axelsson A, Bang A, Holmberg S. Type of arrhythmia at EMS arrival on scene in out-of-hospital cardiac arrest in relation to interval from collapse and whether a bystander initiated CPR. *Am J Emerg Med* 1996; 14: 119–23.

2. Eisenberg MS, Bergner L, Hallstrom A. Cardiac resuscitation in the community: Importance of rapid provision and implications for program planning. *J Am Med Assoc* 1979; 241: 1905–9.

3. Stiell IG, Hebert PC, Wells GA, Lapacis A et al. The Ontario trial of active compression–decompression for in-hospital and prehospital cardiac arrests. *J Am Med Assoc* 1996; 275: 1417–23.

4. Berg RA, Wilcoxson D, Hilwig RW, Kern KB et al. The need for ventilatory support during bystander CPR. *Ann Emerg Med* 1995; 26: 342–50.

5. Woodhouse SP, Cox S, Boyd P, Case C, Weber M. High dose and standard dose adrenaline do not alter survival, compared with placebo. *Resuscitation* 1995; 30: 243–9.

6. Lindner KH, Dirks B, Strohmenger HU, Prengel AW et al. Randomised comparison of epinephrine and vasopressin in patients with out-of-hospital ventricular fibrillation. *Lancet* 1997; 349: 535–7.

7. Volker W, Krismer AC, Arntz HR, Sitter H. A comparison of vasopressin and epinephrine for out-of-hospital cardiopulmonary resuscitation. NEJM 2004; 350: 105–13.

8. Little RA, Frayn KN, Randall PE, Stoner HB et al. Plasma catecholamines in patients with acute myocardial infarction and in cardiac arrest. *Q J Med* 1985; 214: 133–40.

9. Herlit J, Ekstrom L, Wennerblom B, Axelsson A, Bang A et al. Lidocaine in out of hospital ventricular fibrillation. Does it improve survival? *Resuscitation* 1997; 33: 199–205.

10. Kern KB. Drug therapy in advanced cardiac life support. *Cur Opinion Crit Care* 1998; 4: 161–4.

11. Abramson NS, Safar P, Detre KM et al. Neurologic recovery after cardiac arrest: effect of duration of ischaemia. *Crit Care Med* 1985; 13: 930–1.

12. Bernard SA, Gray TW, Buist MD et al. Treatment of comatose survivors of out-of-hospital cardiac arrest with induced hypothermia. *New Engl J Med* 2002; 346: 557–63.

13. The Hypothermia after Cardiac Arrest Study Group. Mild therapeutic hypothermia to improve the neurologic outcome after cardiac arrest. *New Engl J Med* 2002; 346: 549–56.

14. Tham KY, Evans RJ, Rubython EJ, Kinnaird TD. Management of ventricular fibrillation by doctors in cardiac arrest teams. *Br Med J* 1994; 309: 1408–9.

Index